ADVANCES IN **SPORT** AND **EXERCISE** SCIENCE SERIES

Genetics and Molecular Biology
of **Muscle Adaptation**

For Churchill Livingstone

Commissioning Editor: Sarena Wolfaard, Dinah Thom
Project Manager: Andrew Palfreyman
Designer: Stewart Larking
Illustrations Manager: Bruce Hogarth
Illustrator: Richard Morris

ADVANCES IN **SPORT** AND **EXERCISE** SCIENCE SERIES

Genetics and Molecular Biology of Muscle Adaptation

Neil Spurway MA PhD

Emeritus Professor of Exercise Physiology, University of Glasgow, Glasgow, UK

Henning Wackerhage PhD

Senior Lecturer in Molecular Exercise Physiology, University of Aberdeen, Aberdeen, UK

Series Editors

Neil Spurway MA PhD

Emeritus Professor of Exercise Physiology, University of Glasgow, Glasgow, UK

Don MacLaren BSc MSc PhD CertEd

Professor of Sports Nutrition, School of Sport and Exercise Sciences, Liverpool John Moores University, Liverpool, UK

Foreword by

Stephen D. R. Harridge PhD

Professor of Human and Applied Physiology, Kings College, London, UK

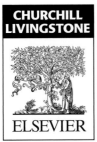

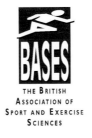

THE BRITISH
ASSOCIATION OF
SPORT AND EXERCISE
SCIENCES

EDINBURGH LONDON NEW YORK OXFORD PHILADELPHIA ST LOUIS SYDNEY TORONTO 2006

CHURCHILL
LIVINGSTONE
ELSEVIER

First published 2006

ISBN 10: 0 443 10077 2
ISBN 13: 978 0 443 10077 2

British Library Cataloguing in Publication Data
A catalogue record for this book is available from the British Library.

Library of Congress Cataloging in Publication Data
A catalog record for this book is available from the Library of Congress.

Notice
Knowledge and best practice in this field are constantly changing. As new research and experience broaden our knowledge, changes in practice, treatment and drug therapy may become necessary or appropriate. Readers are advised to check the most current information provided (i) on procedures featured or (ii) by the manufacturer of each product to be administered, to verify the recommended dose or formula, the method and duration of administration, and contraindications. It is the responsibility of the practitioner, relying on their own experience and knowledge of the patient, to make diagnoses, to determine dosages and the best treatment for each individual patient, and to take all appropriate safety precautions. To the fullest extent of the law, neither the publisher nor the editor and contributors assume any liability for any injury and/or damage to persons or property arising out or related to any use of the material contained in this book.

The Publisher

Printed in Italy

Contents

H2   오후

Foreword

It was difficult to have foreseen, even 20 years ago, that exercise science would have evolved so rapidly to now embrace such aspects of biology as genetics, cell and molecular biology. As the physiologist Joseph Barcroft noted back in the 1930s, 'exercise is not a mere variant of the condition of rest, it is the essence of the machine' (Barcroft 1934). Exercise is fundamental to our understanding of the way the body works. As we seek to understand the mechanisms underlying the responses to exercise, we have embraced new technologies which have allowed us to take a more reductionist approach, right down to the level of our genes, in the search for answers.

Our gene pool evolved when the physical demands of survival were much greater than they are today. Frank Booth (2002) has recently proposed that our bodies are likely to have been designed for significantly higher levels of physical activity than are currently being undertaken by most of the general population. He argues that characteristics such as a more hypertrophied left ventricle, as observed in many elite athletes, are our more natural phenotype, whereas the characteristics of the 'normal' heart are a result of relative disuse. This genetic inheritance also haunts our inactive 21st century lifestyle, where the abundance of affordable, highly calorific food is combined with ever greater means of avoiding physical activity. A product of this is the emergence of an obesity epidemic and the dramatic increase in the incidence of type II diabetes, even amongst the young.

The sequencing of the human genome has proved the impetus for accelerating our understanding of the role of our genes in health and disease. Our search for genes that may be key determinants of sporting ability has begun in earnest. Genetic association studies linking single gene variations to performance traits have hinted, but certainly not proven, the importance of certain genes in predicting athletic performance. Whether it be a polymorphism in the angiotensin converting enzyme (ACE) gene pointing towards superior endurance performance, or a polymorphsm in the actinin 3 gene pointing towards superior power and speed, the fact remains that it is extremely unlikely that sports performance can be predicted only on the basis of genotype.

All tissues, organs and cells are the result of the interaction of different proteins. Whether structural, motor or hormonal, all proteins result from the same fundamental processes: the transcription into mRNA of the genetic information encoded in our DNA as adenonucleotide base pairs, and its subsequent translation into functioning proteins by the building yards of the cells, the ribosomes. We need to know more about the complex regulation of gene expression and how processes such as alternative splicing of genes result in a greater number of proteins than predicted by the number of genes alone.

Whilst genetics is the study of heredity and variation, the use of molecular biological techniques, such as microchip gene arrays and quantitative PCR (polymerase chain reaction) technology, has allowed the identification and quantification of genes that are regulated by exercise. This is on a timescale of minutes and hours, as opposed to the weeks and months required for phenotypic changes to be measured. The relatively new discipline of 'proteomics', that studies variations in protein rather than gene expression, has arisen and is itself now being superseded by the study of protein – protein interactions or 'metabolomics'. One might say that we are beginning to come full circle in recognizing that all these factors combine to result in the functioning of the organism, namely, 'physiology'! Or perhaps it should now be termed 'physiomics'? Indeed, the Nobel Laureate Sir James Black once said that the future lay in a 'progressive triumph of physiology over molecular biology' (Boyd 1993). Maybe this is going too far. The combination of the two provides a powerful set of tools for helping us understand some of the fundamental ways in which the cells, tissues, organs and systems of our bodies work and are regulated.

Molecular exercise physiology has arrived and is here to stay. What Neil Spurway and Henning Wackerhage have so eloquently achieved in this book is an evaluation of the molecular and cellular processes that have a direct relevance for sport and exercise science. This book is an invaluable reference for both scientists and students with an interest in exercise science, and provides an opportunity to probe more deeply into the fundamental underlying processes of exercise physiology.

Stephen D. R. Harridge PhD

References

Barcroft J 1934 The architecture of physiological function. Cambridge University Press, New York, p 286

Booth F W, Chakravarthy M V, Spangenburg E E 2002 Exercise and gene expression: physiological regulation of the human genome through physical inactivity. Journal of Physiology 543: 399–411

Cited in Boyd C A R, Noble D (eds) 1993 The logic of life. The challenge of integrative physiology. Oxford University Press, Oxford

Preface to students

What have we here?

This book breaks new ground. Whether it does so well or badly will be for you to judge.

At the end of one chapter we cite Perusse and Bouchard, who wrote as long ago as 1994:

The greatest challenge at this time is to improve understanding of the potential of genetic and molecular medicine among the physical activity scientists, to train a new generation of these scientists to undertake these genetic studies, and to establish several competing centres of excellence where such investigations would be carried out routinely. Too few physical activity scientists and laboratories are involved in genetic and molecular biology research ... Corrective measures and coordinated efforts are needed to explore the current revolution in the biological sciences, particularly in DNA technology and the study of the human genome.

We would have written 'genetics and molecular biology' instead of 'genetic and molecular medicine' in the first sentence, but in every other respect we agree entirely.

In our eyes no textbook, in the more-than-decade since that was written, has responded adequately to its challenge. The one commendable approach to a response we have seen is itself very recent: it is Mooren & Völker's *Molecular and Cellular Exercise Physiology* (2005). Yet even these authors devote only one of their 19 chapters to genes, gene expression and the modification of that expression in exercise, and one other to the adaptive responses of skeletal muscle fibres. To us, by contrast, these are the core components of molecular exercise physiology – not to mention being more than sufficient for one course module! So they are the essential themes of this book, and the topics of its four major chapters, numbered 3–6.

In Chapter 3 we ask how people's muscles differ, tackling the question in a comparative–zoological perspective without which only a narrow-minded answer can be given; it also devotes considerable space to techniques of investigation, particularly those involving histochemistry and immuno-histochemistry. Chapter 4 is an even more emphatically 'methods and background' chapter, but this time it is preparing the ground for the final two. It considers DNA, genes, their transcription and translation into proteins, and the regulation of all these by signal transduction pathways. It puts these processes into an exercise context whenever possible, but does so in general terms. Chapter 5 looks in specific detail at endurance training. Here, we explore how this form of exercise activates signal transduction pathways which regulate the formation of motor proteins, the production of mitochondria and new blood vessels, and the growth of the heart. Chapter 6 does the same for resistance training: we consider the effect of exercise and nutrition on protein synthesis followed by an overview of the signal transduction that regulates these responses. The common aim of Chapters 5 and 6 is to try to explain the adaptation to training. A particular theme of ours is that many coaches and sports scientists use the 'supercompensation' model (Viru 2002) in trying to explain how training works. That model does describe glycogen recovery after exercise, but it fails to describe or explain most of the other adaptations we have mentioned.

All these chapters, particularly but not only Nos 3 and 4, place weight on methods of investigation, and the Appendix provides detailed lab protocols for several of them. Before these major chapters, however, No. 2 asks how studies of people – particularly twins and family groups – have been designed to get some handle on the relative influences of nature and nurture on physical performance and muscle characteristics. Chapter 2 is shorter than any of 3–6, but it is intended for study at the same level, and its references, like theirs, are predominantly to the research literature. Only Chapter 1 is different in this respect: it is a short sketch of the histories of life and of the human species, written at the 'popular science' level. We believe it is not sensible to go into detail about genes and gene expression without some perspective on how these genes, and the biochemistry they bring into being, came about. However, we do not expect many students of exercise or sport science to embark upon research into these matters; hence the different kind of treatment.

Background requirements

The more you know before starting any course, the easier you will find it. But authors of textbooks, even for senior students, have to try and make only realistic assumptions about the backgrounds of their readers. In this book we of course assume that you have good general knowledge of training methods, and the specificity of most of them. We also assume a solid grasp of muscle physiology, to the level of the interactions of myosin and actin in force generation, biochemical pathways for the supply of ATP, and the performance of whole muscle in both static and dynamic exercise of varying intensities and durations. More general aspects of exercise physiology and biochemistry are also assumed. Every one of these topics should be known to the level of the penultimate university year – 'know' not necessarily meaning that you can instantly from memory put on paper, say, the complete tri-carboxylic acid cycle, but that you remember what it is, in broad terms what it does, and where you can remind yourself of more details if you need them. The equivalent should be true of at least 90% of the complete background we have mentioned, and if it is true of 99% you will be considerably better placed throughout Chapters 3–6.

For understanding Chapter 2, some knowledge of statistics will also be necessary, though not more than is covered in the sort of course included as part of every well-designed sport or exercise science degree curriculum. If you are rusty on this, have the notes to hand as you study our chapter. The more you remember of basic genetics too, the easier you will find much of the book, but particularly again Chapter 2. However, we have tried to limit the knowledge assumed to that covered in school-level human biology; to have done more genetics than this will enable you to move with greater facility through quite a lot of our text, but it is not essential. Finally, there is molecular genetics – the interface of biochemistry with basic genetics. We do not assume *any* of this: everything necessary is explained within this text. Yet obviously, if you do know some of it already, you will find life easier.

That completes the routine duties of a Preface. The two short sections which follow touch on more philosophical questions about which you are not in the least obliged to be concerned, but we include them in case you are.

'Role' and 'function'

These words appear from time to time in most chapters of the book. A few scientists avoid them, feeling that they imply design or purpose in living systems, so that by using them one is tacitly asserting that these systems are subservient to some divine plan. This is *not* our intention! *By the 'role' or 'function' of a structure or process we simply mean its contribution to the life of the organism.*

Longer phrases, which embody all the meaning we attach to 'role' and 'function', are ones like 'contribution to survival value' or, as two words for one, 'adaptive advantage'. The single everyday words we have used are simply neater. Whatever the form of words, however, this search for role, function or survival-value is basic to the physiologist's enterprise (Spurway 2005). It does *not* have theological connotations!

Evolution

The second potential misunderstanding goes in exactly the opposite direction. It is that some potential readers, especially in the USA, may conclude from our acceptance of evolution that we are putting forward atheistic propaganda. In fact it is no more our purpose to do that than to make tacit theistic claims.

Our approach does absolutely assume the broadly Darwinian account of how human beings have come to exist. We believe it impossible to discuss anything to do with genetics in any other terms. The many millions of living species were not separately created but evolved, by natural selection acting upon mutations and other forms of variation, from a common origin at an almost unimaginably distant time. One purpose of Chapter 1 is to illustrate how mechanisms which are alike in widely different species owe their similarity to these species having shared origins. In later chapters the fact that the underlying mechanisms are this much alike will continually be found essential to both the process of research and the understanding of its findings.

Thus it is true that we cannot accept as literal fact the accounts of creation given in the scriptures of any of the world's great religions. Nor is it our purpose here to indicate whether we ourselves find them true symbolically and poetically. Science is concerned with mechanisms in the physical world – with 'how' questions – and in this book we are writing science. Questions of meaning, of purpose in the ultimate sense – 'why' questions – are not our business here. We must stress, however, that in requiring our readers to accept an evolutionary standpoint we are not *requiring* them to adopt an atheistic one. Of course, there are those who have argued trenchantly that this is the implication of the evolutionary account: Monod (1972), Dawkins (1986) and Dennett (1995) have done so with particular verve. Many others, however, see things completely the other way: Miller (1999), Haught (2000), Ruse (2001), Drees (2002) and Peters (2002) are among recent authors who have written especially well to this effect. The essential difference between the two groups is whether a process which, *at the level accessible to scientific analysis*, must be described as chance – the chance variations upon which natural selection cannot fail to act – is thereby demonstrated as purposeless at a more fundamental level. *We make no such assertion!*

Acknowledgements

NS owes a particular debt to Dr Richard Wilson for discussions, extending over several months, of Chapter 2. He is also grateful to Drs Vincent Macaulay, Harper Gilmore and Ian Montgomery for most helpful guidance on aspects of Chapters 1, 2 and 3 respectively. HW expresses warm thanks to Dr Marco Cardinale and Professors Steven Harridge, Michael Rennie and Craig Sharp for searching comments on drafts of Chapters 4–6. Finally, both authors are extremely grateful to Professor Bengt Saltin for reading the book in proof, and writing the Foreword.

References

Bouchard C, Perusse L 1994 Heredity, activity level, fitness and health. In: Bouchard C, Shephard R J, Stephens T (eds) Physical Activity, Fitness and Health. Champaign, IL, Human Kinetics: p 106–118.

Dawkins R 1986 The blind watchmaker. London, Longman (republished Penguin Books, 1988).

Dennett DC 1995 Darwin's dangerous idea: Evolution and the meanings of life. London, Allen Lane (Penguin Press).

Drees WB 2002 Creation: From nothing until now. London, Routledge.

Haught JF 2000 God after Darwin: A theology of evolution. Boulder CO, Westview Press.

Miller KB 1999 Finding Darwin's God: A scientist's search for common ground between God and evolution. New York, Harper Collins.

Monod J 1972 Chance and necessity. London, Collins.

Mooren FC, Völker K 2005 Molecular and cellular exercise physiology. Champaign, IL, Human Kinetics.

Peters K 2002 Dancing with the sacred: Evolution, ecology and God. Harrisburg, PA, Trinity Press International.

Ruse M 2001 Can a Darwinian be a Christian? The relationship between science and religion. Cambridge, University Press.

Spurway NC 2005 Can physiology be both Popperian and ethical? In: McNamee M (ed) Philosophy and the Sciences of Exercise, Health and Sport: Critical Perspectives on Research Methods. London, Routledge p 34–55.

Viru A 2002 Early contributions of Russian stress and exercise physiologists. Journal of Appied Physiology 92: 1378–1382.

Chapter 1

Origins

Neil Spurway

LEARNING OBJECTIVES:

After studying this chapter, you should be able to . . .

1. Give a general account of the development of life on earth from pre-biotic molecules to human beings.
2. Indicate the stages at which it seems likely that the biochemical pathways, and then the anatomical/physiological systems, utilized in present-day athletic performance became established.
3. Discuss the implications of our species' genetic background both for our sporting capabilities and for healthy living in the modern world.

> 'What is abundantly clear is that all life – from bacterium to elephant – shares common characteristics at the level of molecules. There is a common thread that runs through the whole of biological existence. Individual genes on the ribosomal RNA are common to all life, and these are complex structures. It is hugely improbable that such genetic similarities arose by chance. These molecules run through life in the same way as the musical theme runs through Brahms's Fourth Symphony. There is a set of variations which superficially sound very different but which are underpinned by a deeper similarity that binds the whole. The beauty of the structure depends upon the individuality of the passing music, and also upon the coherence of the construction. That vital spark from inanimate matter to animate life happened once and only once, and all living existence depends on that moment. We are one tribe with bacteria that live in hot springs, parasitic barnacles, vampire bats and cauliflowers. We all share a common ancestor.'
>
> Fortey (1997) p 39–40

THE BEGINNINGS

Earth was formed about 4550 million years (Myr) ago. By 3800 Myr life had almost certainly begun. Fortey's picture, quoted above, that there was only one start to animate life, is not the only one held by researchers: others suspect that there were many starts, triggered by the energy of intense unfiltered sunlight, but only one of them survived to evolve into the modern biosphere. However, all agree that RNA, and even more so DNA, which have been the backbones of more advanced evolution, cannot have been formed at the beginning – they are too complex, and the biochemistry required to make them is too advanced. Yet inheritable pattern there had to be, and one idea is that the original pattern ('template' may be a better word) was not carried by biological molecules at all, but on inert minerals such as clays (Cairns-Smith 1990). Some time after this, RNA would have formed and led to the synthesis of polypeptides and simple proteins. But once DNA-based inheritance arrived, in the footsteps of the RNA, its stability yet ease of replication made it totally dominant. Every serious scientific investigator agrees about this, and about Fortey's key point, that the other main components of biochemical machinery are common to all forms of life now existing. But the fact that the same genetic code – the same triplets of just four among the many possible bases leading, via RNA as intermediary, to the same 20 of the 64 possible amino acids – the fact that this same code is found in every living form from algae to elephants does lend credence to the suggestion that all modern life derived from just one primordial cell. If so, it was an Adam (or Eve) indeed!

(Incidentally, it has recently been realized that utilization of less than 1/3 of possible amino acids, each encoded by a number of different DNA triplets, has probably protected life from potentially catastrophic errors (Freeland & Hurst 2004).)

Life, as we would recognize it, was initially prokaryotic – consisting of simple cells, with neither nuclei nor organelles. Very probably the earliest of these were heat-loving ('hyperthermophilic') bacteria, living in hot springs or underwater outlets of hot materials from beneath the earth's hard crust. The atmosphere was, in chemical terms, an entirely reducing one, and all metabolism *anaerobic*. So when the muscles of a 21st Cy 800 m runner resort to anaerobic ATP production for the drive to the finish, they are utilizing the most primitive energy supply available to life on earth. The fact that there was little or no oxygen in the atmosphere at that early time is demonstrated by the observation that iron-containing minerals in the oldest rocks do not have the oxidized, red-brown colour of later ones. Oxygen, indeed, would have been toxic to the initial life forms, as it is to many of the anaerobic bacteria existing in air-free ecological niches to this day. It would also have given rise to high-altitude ozone, and so filtered out a large percentage of the ultraviolet light which had powered pre-biotic synthesis of organic molecules – a process which would cease to be necessary once biological systems existed to do the same job.

Reference to *ATP* also invites comment. Phosphates are found in the very earliest rocks, contemporary with the postulated start of life; and among the molecules formed when simulations of the early earth's surface chemistry are irradiated with ultraviolet light, or sparked with artificial lightning, are those of the so-called 'high-energy' phosphates, specifically including ATP. Though this is not the place to go into detail on the point, it should be remembered that what is being described by the term 'high energy' is not the energy of the bond as such but the energy released when it is hydrolysed – and that this is only high in living cells because the products of the hydrolysis are present at very low concentrations. A good account is given in Chapter 3 of Nicholls & Ferguson (1992). Since phosphates were available and have such appropriate properties it is considered that they must have been utilized, from very early days, in much the way they are still. Nor should it be forgotten that both RNA and DNA contain considerable amounts of phosphate. DNA, at least, probably came after aerobic metabolism, but once both were fully operating, production of ATP may well have been limited by the available phosphate supply.

Only a little later than the heat-loving and other 'archaebacteria', green and blue-green bacteria began to form (Fig. 1.1). At first they did so in the sea, but after a while these second-generation bacteria began to invade the surface of the earth, living in mats and then in multi-layered colonies ('stromatolites'). Much the same kinds of colony occur in some parts of the world to this day. The green and blue-green bacteria performed two versions of a process which also still goes on, and the later of the two versions was to have a particularly profound consequence. The process is *photosynthesis*, the vital mechanism whereby the energy of photons is captured by pigments and utilized to drive metabolism. In the simpler form of modern photosynthesis, 'cyclic photosynthesis', the result is ATP. This would have been immensely useful to primitive bacteria, and it is considered certain that it did take place, although its mechanism was not necessarily identical to the modern one in all details. However, cyclic photosynthesis would leave no incontrovertible trace. In this it contrasts markedly with *non-cyclic photosynthesis* – which is what people almost always mean when they just speak of 'photosynthesis', without a modifying adjective. This is the mechanism by which CO_2 is captured and combined with water to form carbohydrate molecules *and release oxygen into the atmosphere*. (A lucid and colourfully illustrated textbook account of photosynthesis is given by Starr & Taggart, 2003 – who also provide an excellent outline of the origin and evolution of life.)

Even if non-cyclic photosynthesis started with a rather simpler light-capturing pigment than chlorophyll, any molecule capable of transferring energy from a captured photon to drive organic syntheses had to be sophisticated, and therefore

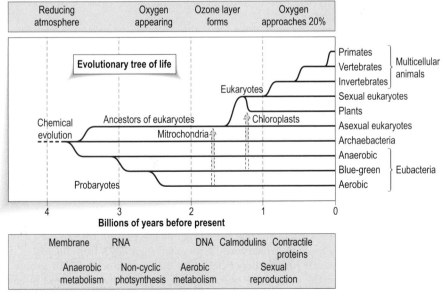

Figure 1.1   An evolutionary 'tree of life', roughly sketching time–relations of the divergences of some of its main branches. Atmospheric conditions indicated in words above the diagram, biochemical developments beneath it.

complex to manufacture. Some investigators do not believe it began until ~2500 Myr ago – almost half way from the planet's formation to the present day. Starr & Taggart accept this figure. Others note that the very first fossils, microscopic spheres and threads, looking very like modern blue-green bacteria, have been identified in rocks at very least 3000 Myr old, and conclude that the process of releasing oxygen must have begun by then. Whenever it did begin, it did not have a free hand in raising the oxygen content of the atmosphere because many minerals, including but not only those containing iron, would have absorbed this highly reactive element almost as fast as it could be made – initially, indeed, just as fast. Ultimately, however, it was produced faster than it was sequestered: iron-containing rocks became red by ~2000 Myr ago. Oxygen had come into its own, and was changing the world (Fortey 1997). From the standpoint of biochemistry the biggest change resulting would have been the development of *aerobic metabolism*, with its order of magnitude greater energy yield from carbon-based fuel molecules. Even though the oxygen content of the atmosphere was at this stage still very low – a few percent of present atmospheric level – this would have sufficed for *oxidative phosphorylation* to begin in single-celled organisms. But the limited range of diffusion ensured that the single cells could not become large, and substantially more oxygen would be necessary to support sizeable multi-cellular life forms.

EUKARYOTES

Thus, although our story has now covered more than half the age of the earth, life is still morphologically very simple. All organisms are prokaryotic and unicellular, even though they may live together in strings and mats. Reproduction is rapid, as it still is for modern bacteria, but each cell division simply consists in producing two cells identical to the one from which they came – cloning. Only when there is a mutation in the primitive DNA can change occur. Two developments are necessary to speed things up: eukaryotic cells, and sex.

The eukaryotic cell has its main DNA held within one membrane-bound structure, the *nucleus*, and key aspects of its metabolism located in cytoplasmic organelles such as *mitochondria* and *chloroplasts*, which are also membrane-bound.

The favoured view of how the organelles were formed is that of Margulis (1970). She proposed that aerobic bacteria were taken up into the cytoplasm of anaerobic ones and some, instead of being digested, survived – indeed flourished in their protected, nutrient-rich new environment – and thereafter supplied their hosts with ATP. They would thus have become the first mitochondria. Even now, mitochondria retain some of their own DNA, their inner membranes are similar to the plasma membranes of bacteria, and they divide by fission, independently of the cells in which they lie (Ch. 5). By a similar mechanism, primitive aerobic bacteria could have taken up oxygen-evolving photosynthetic bacteria, which became the first chloroplasts. Such non-destructive uptake of one cell by another, leading to mutually beneficial partnership, is termed *endosymbiosis*. There is less confidence about the development of the nucleus, but it seems likely that infoldings of the plasma membrane (which readily occur in many modern prokaryotes) segregated their DNA from the rest of the cytoplasm in ways which proved beneficial to its different function. This group of processes, resulting in the emergence of eukaryotes, is generally considered to have taken place ~1400 Myr ago.

As for sex, this is only meaningful in the context of eukaryotes, but there is evidence that it first expressed itself quite early (in geological terms) after their appearance. A large deposit of a fossil seaweed dating from 1200 Myr was found as recently as 1999, in rocks in Arctic Canada. This seaweed is almost indistinguishable from a modern red alga, and both large and more numerous small spores – primitive female and male gametes – can be clearly identified in the fossil deposit. The evolutionary significance of sexual reproduction is that the genes of two different cells are mixed in their progeny, so that a new source of variation, in addition to mutation itself, was introduced to the biosphere. The consequence would be more rapid diversification than before.

If we think again of the 800 m runner, we can say that by the time which our history has reached – with the earth about 3/4 its present age – not only the pattern of her initial and late-burst anaerobic metabolism, but that of the aerobic metabolism which contributes more economically to the middle part of the race, has now been established. Almost certainly, so has the role of calcium in regulating many bio-chemical processes, for calmodulin molecules only a little different from each other – in biochemical language, having structures which are 'highly conserved' – are found throughout the modern plant and animal kingdoms, which immediately indicates that they must have come into operation early in the development of life. Evidence from its amino-acid composition in fact places its origin no later than the earliest eukaryotes (Baba et al 1984). More recent methods pursue such questions at the level of the DNA specifying the molecule's structure. Figure 1.2, showing the degree of match between calmodulin genes over the range of vertebrate animals, is an example of how this kind of study is represented; the underlying techniques are considered in Chapter 4.

We have seen that this biochemical armoury had developed in cells whose basic structure (nucleated, with organelles) was like that of our modern runner's own cells,

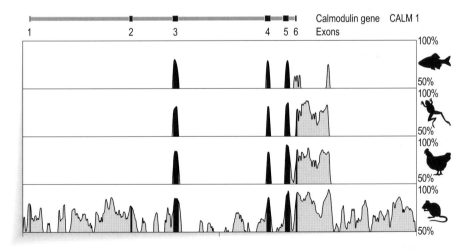

Figure 1.2 Simplified 'ECR' (evolutionarily conserved regions) plot showing the similarity between CALM1, the main gene determining the form of human calcium-sensing protein, calmodulin, and those of the genes determining the expression of homologous proteins in rat, chicken, frog and fugu (a bony fish). The six parts of the human DNA which will be transcribed into protein ('exons') are shown in red on the gene (upper line) and numbered. The plots in the rows below show the percent homologies higher than 50% between human and other sequences. The larger the percentage, the higher the conservation between humans and the species in that row. The figure shows that exons 3, 4 and 5, which are between them responsible for the great majority of the protein's structure, are strikingly similar (evolutionarily highly conserved) between all species represented. From Ovcharenko et al (2004), with permission.

and that they had arrived at the fundamental means by which she could inherit traits from both her parents equally. Nevertheless, 1000–1200 Myr ago, life was still some way from the development of complex multicellular organisms, with different organs contributing their contrasting functions to the life of the whole. By 800 Myr, it seems that this development had begun. Among the more striking indications is that the number of stromatolites began to decline dramatically: they were a concentrated food-source for tiny, soft-bodied, but multicellular animals. Also, at much this time – certainly well established by 700 Myr – tracks and burrows were left in sediments on the floors of shallow seas. These imply *muscle*: we could call this the last key requirement, at the cellular level, for our runner to have the potential of emerging from the subsequent processes of evolution. Modern invertebrates even have different types of voluntary muscle fibre, akin to those of vertebrates treated in detail in Chapter 3, so it is quite possible that their pre-Cambrian precursors did too; but this can only be speculation, because the tissues concerned were too soft to affect the fossil record and there seem to be no grounds for more confident deduction.

THE CAMBRIAN PERIOD AND AFTER

Although they prompted reflections on our own condition, the invertebrate animals we have just considered were themselves still small. More oxygen was needed for bigger ones to develop, and one suggestion is that it was the break-up of a continent which was the final trigger. Having many small land-blocks provides far more beaches than one great mass, and the sand of these beaches would bury organic remains which would otherwise have used up oxygen in their final decay. Whatever the reason, or combination of reasons, for the increased amount of oxygen, a huge change occurred about 545 Myr ago – the 'Cambrian explosion'. In this period, which was a short space of time in geological terms, marine animals enlarged and diversified at a rate previously unimaginable, and many of the fossil forms from that time are complex and beautiful – trilobites are well-known examples of the early Cambrian developments. Vertebrates as well as invertebrates also appeared, and there are clear indications of predation from before 500 Myr ago, so some of the animals were already carnivorous.

During the next 450 million years the earth's continents underwent massive movements. They moved horizontally, to the South Pole and back to straddle the Equator, producing massive swings of temperature. And they moved vertically, dipping under the sea at one stage, rising into great mountain ranges at another. The consequent changes in habitat promoted ever faster evolutionary adaptations. Variety flourished at many periods, but alternated with great extinctions. Around 400 Myr ago, in the Devonian period, a line of backboned fishes, with simple lungs and lobed fins which could evolve into legs, invaded the land, feeding on the plants which had preceded them by perhaps 40 Myr. These lobe-finned fishes adapted to produce first amphibians, then reptiles – the latter step deriving from the development of eggs which could survive terrestrially rather than having to exist in water. From the reptiles both mammals and finally birds evolved, and co-existed with the reptiles for con- siderable time. As was pointed out in a beautiful book, written 50 years ago yet still well worth reading (Berrill 1955), the fact that 'we are fish out of water' is the reason why 'we are so wet inside that we splash if we fall from a tall building onto a sidewalk', and need many litres of water a day if we are to survive in a desert. It is also the reason why our extracellular body fluids still have an electrolyte composi- tion similar to that of the sea – not the modern sea, which is much saltier, but that of 400 Myr or more ago, to which Devonian fish were equilibrated. (This fact was reflected upon almost a Cy ago in one of the great literary works of physiology – Henderson 1913 p 187–190.) But Berrill continues, 'More than this, of course, we suffer from the lack of support of water'. Until birth, 'a baby is supported comfortably by the liquid within the membranes and only the mother feels the weight of her burden. But once birth has occurred, and the buoyant water has been replaced by insubstantial air, the infant is held down, as though by a giant magnet, wherever it is put'. We may add that many of the problems modern humans have, with posture and with joints, stem from their subsequent lifelong contest against gravity.

Gravity and inertia (which impedes acceleration, braking and turning) present a further challenge, well worth considering in a book whose main theme is to be muscle. It concerns the limit to the ability of animals to supply their muscles with oxygen. There are constraints for both water-breathers (using gills) and air-breathers (using lungs), but they are different, and humans are air-breathers. It might be imagined that, once animals became air-breathing, there need be virtually no limit to their capacity to supply their muscles with oxygen via their pulmonary and cardiovascular systems: after all, the amount of oxygen which can be taken in that way in given time is so much greater than can be similarly absorbed from water, that an aerobic system which had worked in the marine environment must surely find the gaseous one rich beyond its dreams? But there are constraints – a balance of *pros* and *cons*. The more of an animal's body that is given over to breathing and blood-pumping, i.e. the larger its thoracic cage, the more the oxygen which can be got to the muscles when they are working flat out. But the more also is the burden of bones, respiratory and cardiac muscles, and lung tissues, which the animal must carry around all the rest of the time: they would not only impose high costs in terms of energy expenditure, but reduce mobility in starts, stops and turns, and hence in the ability to capture food. Because 'the rest of the time' is massively predominant – like, say, 99.9% of the total – no animal now known has evolved so massive a thoracic system that all its muscle fibres can be wholly aerobic. Instead, all have a mixture of aerobic and anaerobic muscle fibres – to a first approximation, of red type 1 and white type 2 (Ch. 3) – but use the aerobic ones whenever they can and recruit their anaerobic partners only for the highest-intensity work. We can observe that this is the situation of all current animals. However, logic indicates that it must have prevailed throughout the life of all mobile creatures on this earth. After all, the early atmospheres had less oxygen than now.

Up to this point, our account of animal development has been based almost entirely on the evidence from fossils – preserved relatively hard tissues, or occasionally the tracks left by a creature's movement. Conclusions about soft tissues, notably muscle, have only been deduced indirectly from that fossil record. Recently, however, it has become possible to draw some conclusions about soft-tissue evolution by direct studies of those tissues, and their embryological development, in modern species with contrasting evolutionary histories. An impressive example is that of Neyt et al (2000) who applied sophisticated immunohistochemical techniques (such as described in Chs 3 and 4 of this book) to compare muscle development in a teleost (bony fish) and an elasmobranch (cartilaginous fish). In the teleost, fin muscles develop from the same embryological site as do the limb muscles of all legged animals, but in the elasmobranch the site of fin-muscle origin is different. Now the bony fish diverged from the cartilaginous ones before the lobe-finned sub-group of the bony ones, the 'sarcopterygians', themselves separated from the others and subsequently invaded the land. Neyt et al are therefore able to conclude that the genetic mechanism controlling the formation of limb muscles evolved before the lobe-finned fishes. Clearly, this point is more detailed than our main account in this chapter, but we cite it to illustrate how modern methods are beginning to provide solid evidence about stages in the evolution of muscle which occurred a very long time ago.

Returning now to the fossil record and the chronological account based upon it, we saw previously that the lobe-finned fish gave rise first to amphibians and then to reptiles. This took place during the period of about 180 Myr after the lobe-fins first appeared on land and breathed air. By Triassic times, ~220 Myr ago, some of the reptiles had become dinosaurs. Initially these were quite small and lived alongside large, mammal-like, plant-eating reptiles. It was in the Jurassic, starting a little before 200 Myr ago, that the dinosaurs became huge and dominant – as Stephen Spielberg's films have made us all aware!

More important to the human story, however, are the little mammals, inhabiting the rich undergrowth at the dinosaurs' feet from about 190 Myr ago. Warm-blooded and temperature controlled, although not originally placental, these insignificant-looking creatures were to survive the cataclysmic meteor impact of 65 Myr ago, which is considered to have been what caused the sudden, almost total extinction of the dinosaurs. Preserved skulls indicate that the ground-dwelling mammals relied more on smell than sight. However, when the dinosaurs had gone, the mammals could safely come out into the open, and some of them climbed trees. The fossil record of 50 Myr ago includes a small, tree-dwelling creature, an early lemur. Its *foramen magnum*, the hole at the base of the skull where the spinal cord enters, is near the back, showing that this animal still hung its head forward and slightly downward from the body – not at all like a modern primate. Yet its eye-sockets are large, implying that there had by that time been selection against the sense of smell to favour that of vision. Furthermore, compared to earlier plant and insect-eaters, its eyes had begun to move from the side to the front of the head, giving it a degree of stereoscopic vision; and stereoscopy is immensely useful in judging distances, such as from branch to branch – invaluable for the survival of a tree-dweller. Also its thumb could, to an extent, be opposed to the hand, improving dexterity over the simple, five-digits-in-one-plane anatomy of earlier non-hoofed mammals. The distance from ourselves is still very great, but further crucial evolutionary steps had been taken. The primate line had begun.

PRIMATES

About 20 million years after the early lemurs appeared, the line that was to lead to modern monkeys broke away from that leading to apes and humans – and this latter line came down from the trees to spend some of its time on the ground. About 20 Myr ago anthropoid apes lived in Europe, Asia and Africa. One of these, *Proconsul*, was so named by Louis Leakey in 1931 to suggest that he was a precursor of a chimpanzee then famous in the London zoo, nicknamed Consul. *Proconsul's* brain is markedly larger than that of any predecessors, and his eyes look straight forward, in fully stereoscopic vision. Proconsul is now considered to be the first unequivocal ape in the fossil record.

Until the last few years it was almost universally assumed that the whole of subsequent evolution towards *Homo sapiens* took place in Africa. Darwin had thought this, and few dared challenge Darwin! But there is a blank of about 10 million years in the African fossil record, in which upholders of that theory have to contend that the flukes either of preservation or of finding have so far infuriatingly hidden a particularly intriguing part of the story of specifically human evolution. Recent thinking is, instead, that the early apes migrated out of Africa around 17 Myr ago, diversifying and flourishing in various lushly forested parts of Europe and Asia for the several million years in which the African record is blank, before being driven back towards the Equator by climate change (Begun 2003). During this period away from Africa the great apes appeared. While still mainly tree-living they almost certainly took to hanging below branches and swinging from one to another, rather than walking on all fours along the upper surfaces as monkeys do and *Proconsul*, although already tail-less, had still done. This changed posture required more flexible joint structures in both fore and hind limbs, while the forelimbs also became longer. (They would shorten again in the human line once the trees had been fully left behind.) Back in Africa, 6–8 Myr ago, there appeared the last common ancestor of humans and what are now agreed to be our closest relatives, differing from us in only about 1.6% of our DNA, namely chimpanzees – hence Jared Diamond's splendid and challenging book, describing the human being as 'The Third Chimpanzee' (Diamond 1992). This common ancestor was, in Begun's words, 'a knuckle-walking, fruit-eating, forest-living chimp-like primate that used tools, hunted animals, and lived in highly complex and dynamic social groups, as do living chimps and humans'. But this was an increasingly dry world, extensive tracts of which had few trees. So an ecological niche had developed for non-forest dwellers. The consequence was that 'one ape – the one from which humans descended – eventually invaded open territory by committing to life on the ground'.

The Appearance of Hominids

Thus it is now almost universally agreed that, despite the 10-Myr gap after *Proconsul*, recognizably human creatures, *hominids,* first appeared back in Africa. Most probably it was in the sweep of land stretching from south-western Ethiopia, through and to the east of the Great Rift Valley, and thence south to the northern part of South Africa. The predominant terrain here is savannah – extensive dry grassland, broken by occasional small clumps of trees. On it there now roam great herds of herbivores such as zebra and many different antelopes, plus small numbers of lions and lesser carnivores whose prey the grass-eaters are. (A moment's thought will explain why there must always be far fewer predators than prey!) The situation was already much like this 2–3 Myr ago. Our ancestors of those days would have felt entirely familiar with modern antelopes and lions, but they would not have recognized us as one of themselves. If we compare the skeletons, particularly the skulls, of the earliest hominids with our own, the differences are still immense. Evolution has been fast for us yet slow for the quadrupeds with whom we shared those lands. Why?

Almost certainly the explanation is that, when the African climate turned dry, the lions and zebras, the cheetahs and gazelles, were already beautifully adapted for it and under no pressure to change, so they did not. As Bronowski (1973) put it, the savannah became for them 'a trap in time as well as space; they stayed where they were, and much as they were'. By contrast, the early hominids were only marginally adapted to savannah life. They survived, but they needed to change considerably if they were to flourish. The first big change is signalled by preserved footprints as well as the bones of feet. Those from 2 Myr ago are very like our own, although little of the rest of the body is. They indicate that by then our ancestors had begun to walk upright. Knuckle-running was no longer their mode of progression.

Another indication of upright posture is at the other end of the skeleton in the *foramen magnum*. In the forebears of human kind, the various hominids, this is well forward of the back of the skull, showing unequivocally that the head was held upright, with the spinal cord extending almost straight downwards from it. The first skull found to possess this feature was of a child from somewhat more than 2 Myr, found in South Africa by the anatomist Raymond Dart in 1924. Dart was Australian, and it was perhaps partly in fun that he named the species *Australopithecus*, literally meaning 'Southern Ape'; but, as we have already said, it is now clear if it wasn't then that *Australopithecus* was not an ape but a hominid. Another indication of this was in its teeth. These were not the large, fighting teeth of apes with their attacking canines, but smaller and squarer. Obviously *Australopithecus* did not forage with its mouth but with its hands, left free by the upright gait. Yet the teeth also suggested that it was eating meat – raw, for it did not yet have fire – in the pursuit and cutting of which the hand-user had no alternative but to make extensive use of weapons and stone tools.

The story begun by Dart's discovery moved cautiously at first, but accelerated in the 1950s and 1960s, particularly due to the finds of Richard Leakey (Louis's son) in Olduvai Gorge, Tanzania, and then in the basin of Lake Rudolph, towards the northern end of the Rift Valley. Bronowski saw it as one of the great stories of modern science, comparable in its excitement and significance – and in its controversies! – to those of physics up to about 1940 and biology from the start of the 1950s. What is more, had he but known it, the rate of progress, both from new fossil finds and by the early application of methods from molecular biology, would increase yet further in the decades after he wrote.

One of the developments has been to identify the creatures of 4.5–5 Myr ago as *Australopithecines* too. Smaller-brained and skeletally more ape-like than Dart's discovery, these are termed *Australopithecus aferensis*, while their slightly smaller-bodied but larger-brained successors, found by Dart, have had their name refined to *Australopithecus africanus*. A variant now dated later than *africanus* (Cordain et al 1998) was *Australopithecus robustus*. The tooth-shape and heavy jaws of *robustus* suggest that it had adapted to eat large quantities of poor-quality plant food, in the drying savannah; this is now considered to have been a retrogressive adaptation, which did not develop further. The future would lie instead with the form of *Australopithecine* which could refine the tool-use necessary for an unarmed creature to kill prey and so return, after many millions of years, to meat-eating.

The advantages of so doing, to *africanus* and its successors, were both nutritional and social . . . and, consequent upon the social, intellectual as well. Nutritionally, the value of a kilogram of meat, with its high protein content, was many times greater than that of a kilogram of even the richest plant food and – as the heavy jaws of *A. robustus* indicated – most of the plant food on the savannah was far from rich. Socially, the collaboration which a weak and rather slow creature required, if it was successfully to hunt animals, many of which were far stronger and all of which were faster, was an immense and invaluable challenge. This challenge gave selective advantage to an ever-enlarging brain, with its consequent abilities to collaborate, communicate, and develop better tools and weapons. It also favoured monogamy and reinforced the production of only one baby at a time (though this had begun in the trees, where the baby had to be carried hanging on to its mother). Monogamy meant that mutual trust and support developed, and the males could go off together hunting, whereas the 'alpha male' of an ape colony would not have risked leaving his harem. Finally, in positive feedback on the other operative factors, the higher calorific density of meat would assist in energizing the highly-demanding large brain. So it was that creatures embodying such interacting adaptations survived better than their rivals.

The result of such competitive influences shows in the fossil record as the first hominid with 'man' in its Latin title: *Homo habilis*, the 'handy man', from about 2 Myr ago, went beyond using appropriately-shaped stones as tools by shaping the stones found into better ones. Quite soon after *habilis*, however, came *Homo erectus*, 'upright man', who had at least as much skill together with more bipedal athleticism *and* a stature comparable to that of modern humans. The earliest fossils of *H. erectus* have been dated at about 1.7 Myr.

Running

We have noted that foot-bones tally with the position of the foramen in indicating the upright posture from which *H. erectus* has been named. Berrill had some comments on this point which are still interesting:

> 'The great apes that share the present with us [chimpanzee, gorilla and orang-utan] all have legs . . . too short for fully effective walking. . . . In the[se] three large apes the tarsal bones of the foot, those numerous small bones which lie behind the metatarsals and form the instep, have undergone a conspicuous shortening. The shortening appears to be the direct result of weight of a large animal . . . completely adapted for arboreal life. In this kind of foot the body weight is thrown onto the front tarsal bones and in order to carry it better the bones have become compressed, in effect almost as if they had been crushed! The interesting point is that the gibbon foot does not show this and neither does ours; and the conclusion drawn is that our early ancestors must have abandoned the trees and taken up bipedal locomotion exclusively at a stage when they were no larger or heavier than the modern gibbon, and that they increased in bulk after they had assumed a truly erect posture, using the heel for support of the body weight and thus relieving the tarsal bones. It is certainly a far-reaching conclusion to put on to a few bones, but nevertheless it may be true. And it suggests that the gorilla, for instance, which as an adult is almost as fully grounded as we are, has left its elevated abode too late to make a satisfactory job of the necessary transformations.'
>
> (Berrill 1955, p 54–55)

Berrill actually suggested that humanoids and gibbons left the trees at about the same period, and indeed might have had a common stem. This is at odds with more recent thought. But that we came down to earth at rather similar *weights* is all his evidence actually indicates, and this remains a tenable proposition: the *Australopithecines* from whom we have descended were barely more than half our height, and so something like 1/3 our weight, which is probably light enough to support his proposition. On adjacent pages Berrill reflected further on 'the supporting heel and the sprinting foot', thus:

> 'Running for your life . . . . is more than a pair of spring-like feet with bones all aligned in the direction of travel. An ape scampers, a man does not. He runs with great extension of his legs, finishing each stride with a real drive; and in modern man the muscle which finishes swinging back the thigh in this final thrust is the powerful and massive buttock. All the swelling curves of thighs and calves that give such pleasure to the human eye are the products of a desperate existence, of a need to run like the wind at times or else fail to run at all. Buttocks and broad pelvic bones swung into serviceable position mark us off from other creatures as strikingly as any other features we possess. The way a man walks is the way only a man walks . . . . Carrying the body load poised alternately on the top of one thigh bone [then] the other has required a lot of practice!'
>
> (Berrill 1955, p 56–57)

The frequency of low back pain and the liability to knee-damage in modern humans are indications that the skeletal adaptations involved in becoming upright have not come easily; but life offers few gains which exact no cost.

Writing 50 years after Berrill, Bramble & Lieberman (2004) have taken his kind of argument forward, in particular using more advanced biomechanics, to contend that it was in distance running, not sprinting, that early humans stood out most notably. Other primates can occasionally sprint for short distances at speeds similar to ours, but no other primates (and only a minority of other mammals) can run continuously over long distances. If scaled to body mass, our speeds even compare favourably with those of horses in their equivalent gait, trotting – a biped has no way of galloping so comparison with *that* quadruped speed would not be helpful. 'Human legs have many long spring-like tendons connected to short muscle fascicles that can generate force economically' during running, but give little benefit in walking, which is essentially stiff-legged. (If the idea of energy return from tendon elasticity is unfamiliar, a particularly lucid source is Alexander (1988).) Bramble & Lieberman point out that this feature sits uncomfortably with the interpretation put by many researchers on the evolution of an essentially human body shape as having enhanced walking performance in open habitats.

Like Berrill, the two recent authors also give detailed consideration to the anatomy of feet, but here too their emphasis is on endurance running more than on sprinting. And they give weight also to hominid leg length, which benefits both modes of progression, noting that 'Long legs relative to body mass, typical of most specialized cursors, first appear unequivocally in hominids 1.8 Myr ago with *H. erectus*, whose relative leg length ... is possibly up to 50% greater than in *Australopithecus* ...'. Other features of the human skeleton suited to distance running (Fig. 1.3) are the greater space between rib-cage and pelvis than in other primates, which favours flexibility, and the broader shoulders, which enhance the ability even of quite light arms to provide counterforces to the leg movements during running. Like Berrill, Bramble & Lieberman place emphasis on the buttock muscle, *gluteus maximus*, 'whose increased size is among the most distinctive of all human features', and which 'is strongly recruited in running at all speeds but not in walking on level surfaces'. Among other features seeming to point to endurance running in hot climates as a significant selective challenge in human evolution, Bramble & Lieberman note our almost hairless skin and highly developed sweat glands, which can produce more sweat per unit surface than those of any other mammalian species. Unlike apes we also breath through our mouths during major exertion, which enhances heat-loss from the lungs. Overall, as Cordain et al (1998) also note, our maximum rate of heat dissipation is five times that of the hairy primates. This capacity is rarely fully utilized in walking, but is essential for running long distances in hot climates. After reading Chapter 3, you may wonder whether the histo- and biochemical properties of our muscles also differ from those of contemporary great apes in the respects which would show us to be the better endurance performers. At the time of writing this question does not seem to have been answered with sufficient precision, but one hopes it soon will be.

Before leaving the theme of human athletic capabilities let us recognize that, whether or not we are notable for even one specialized ability, we are unrivalled in versatility. The diversity of our sports is a reflection not only of our mental but our physical multi-competence. Imagine a horse attempting archery, a seal squash, a lion swimming, or an elephant gymnastics – and then ask any of them to climb a tree!

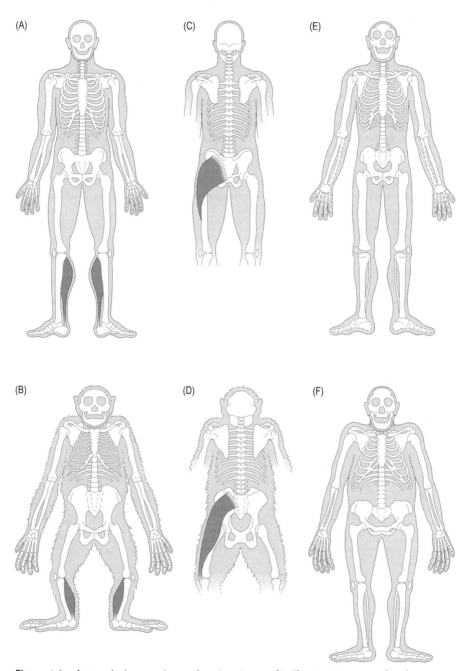

Figure 1.3 Anatomical comparisons of modern human (A, C) with chimpanzee (B, D), *Homo erectus* (E) and *Australopithecus afarensis* (F). Human features beneficial to endurance running include long, straight legs, flexible waist, broad shoulders, free-moving neck, large buttocks with broad, strong gluteal muscles, and long, resilient Achilles tendon. Contrasting chimpanzee features are bent legs, massive pelvis restricting waist movement, very long arms yet narrower shoulders, short neck, narrower buttocks and short Achilles tendon. *H. erectus* closely resembles the modern human in these respects, whereas *Australopithecus* has still much in common with the chimpanzee. After Bramble & Lieberman (2004).

Migrations

Homo erectus, having arisen from primates who had returned to Africa after a period elsewhere, in turn spread out again from Africa to Europe and Asia. By ~700 000 years ago *erectus* was in Java, by 400 000 in China and northern Europe. (The famous 'Peking man', from 350 000 to 400 000 years ago, was of this species.) There *erectus* had to face the first of the recent Ice Ages. These were the culmination of a remarkable climatic change which had followed many million years of temperate conditions in these latitudes, and the start of which had driven the great apes back to Africa. The ability to light fires has already been mentioned; its importance in surviving cold, along with that of obtaining and wearing animal skins, is obvious. In this and many other respects intelligence was advancing exponentially. Brain size of primates in the line which led to humans doubled in the period from 11 to 1 Myr, but it has doubled again between 1 Myr and now (Fig. 1.4).

The last examples of *Homo erectus* are now considered to have survived in Indonesia till at most 50 000 and perhaps as recently as 25 000 years ago. Meantime, there were many branches from the *H. erectus* stem. Those with the largest brains, high foreheads and almost vertical faces are designated *Homo sapiens,* and appeared probably a little less than 200 000 years ago. The well-known 'Neanderthal man', widespread in Europe and Asia until 30 000 years ago, was heavier and stronger than modern humans, with a brain which was actually slightly larger too – although probably no more than required to control the larger muscle mass. At the other extreme, another very recently discovered derivative of *H. erectus,* inhabiting the Indonesian island of Flores till just 13 000 years ago, was barely more than a metre high (Wong 2004). But none of these were truly modern humans, whom some scholars in this speciality have granted the presumptuous label *Homo sapiens sapiens* – 'Wise,

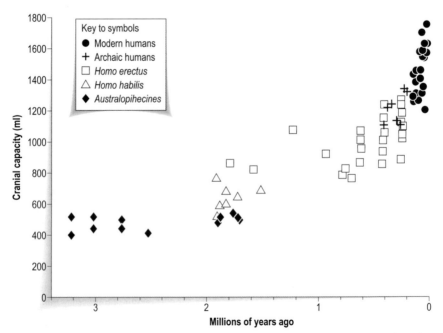

Figure 1.4   Increase in brain size in the last 3.2 Myr. After Figure 1 of Cordain et al (1998).

wise man'. Whether or not it is actually wise to adopt such a boastful designation, all who read this book, and those who wrote it, are of this species. We arrived in Europe some 40 000 years ago, living alongside the Neanderthals who had been there for the previous 160 000 years, and in some unexplained way displaced these stronger and apparently equally intelligent relatives in only a few thousand years.

However, many substantial points are still debated. One question is whether Neanderthals were a subspecies of *Homo sapiens*, to be termed *H. sapiens neanderthalensis* or a separate species, simply *H. neanderthalensis*. The fact that the fossil record offers no evidence of interbreeding between Neanderthals and early modern humans, despite locations in which they coexisted and others in which they replaced each other more than once, is one support for the now-standard view that they were a different species (Stringer 1990).

An even more major matter of debate concerns the manner of emergence of early modern humans (irrespective of whether we may simply name them *Homo sapiens* or must call them *sapiens sapiens* to distinguish them from Neanderthals). One view, the 'multi-regional model', is that separate evolutions from *H. erectus* occurred in different parts of the world since *erectus* began its migrations some 700 000 years ago, with traits appropriate to the particular environment, and these resulted in the various 'races' of *H. sapiens*. At the other extreme is the 'monogenesis model', according to which *H. sapiens* emerged just once and spread from its first site by migration. If so, the site was – yet again! – in sub-Saharan Africa, so the popular name for this is the 'African emergence' or 'Out of Africa' (OOA) model (see Starr & Taggart (2003) for a succinct summary and Stringer (1990) or Freeman & Herron (2004) for increasingly full ones). On this model, racial differences developed only after the migrants had settled in their new regions. The view is founded on the fact that the earliest *sapiens* fossils found in different places date from different times, which would fit a migratory pattern – the African ones of course being oldest (Fig. 1.5). If this is correct, the

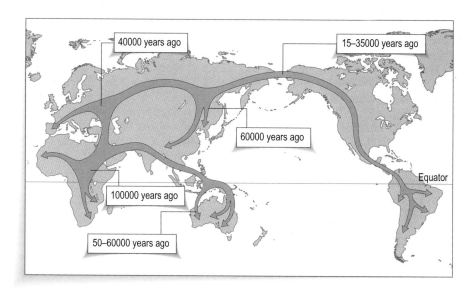

Figure 1.5   Dates when *Homo sapiens* colonized different parts of the world, based on fossil evidence. Arrows show the deduced dispersal routes, suggesting an African emergence ('OOA model'). From Figure 28.14 of Starr & Taggart (1998 edition), with permission.

Neanderthals were indeed a separate species, who emerged in Europe and migrated into western Asia a little before the early modern humans emerged in Africa, ultimately to migrate over most of the globe and displace the Neanderthals on the way.

At the time of writing, the balance of evidence seems increasingly to support this latter model. Intuitively, it would seem to require a remarkable coincidence for all the independent local modifications from *H. erectus*, adapting stature, body form, skin colour, facial characteristics etc. to the immediate environment, nonetheless to remain one species. (It is crucially important to realize that *races* are not species – all human populations can interbreed, whereas it is the definition of 'species' that one cannot breed with another.) However, proponents of the multi-regional model usually cover this point by suggesting that occasional inter-breedings have occurred and it is these which have prevented separate speciation.

More sophisticated evidence comes from the now-widespread application of molecular-genetic methods: these are sketched by Stringer (1990), and many are considered thoroughly in Chapter 4 of this book. Geneticists began by studying visible features such as eye colours and deeper yet accessible ones such as blood groups, but now can investigate the genes themselves. In particular, the small quantity of each cell's DNA which is carried on the mitochondria has many advantages in the pursuit of human origins. Mitochondrial DNA is handed down from mothers to their off-spring, without the equal and random admixture of paternal genes which complicate the biology of nuclear DNA. Mitochondrial DNA also undergoes more frequent mutations and copying mistakes than its nuclear equivalent. In circumstances where the mutations are, 'neither culled nor favoured by natural selection' (Stringer's words) 'the genetic similarities of organisms must be . . . directly proportional to the recency of their divergence from a common ancestor'. (A further assumption here is that the rate of mutation is constant over the period examined.) Neutral selection effects are assured by examining DNA which does not affect the phenotype – nick-named 'junk DNA'. The 'phylogenetic trees' in Figure 1.6 (A, B) summarize evidence from two DNA studies, the first mitochondrial, the second nuclear, which both support the concept of a monogenetic, African origin of all modern humans. The first of them also supports the earlier origin of Neanderthals.

We have noted that the human lines in Figure 1.6 (A) all diverge from a single point. In fact the DNA evidence (Cann et al 1987) is that, on the female side, this was just one individual, living in Africa ~170 000 years ago – 'Mitochondrial Eve' (mtEve). Unlike the Eve imagined by the author of Genesis, however, she would not have been the only woman breeding at the time: there were many others, but their *mitochondrial* DNA (mtDNA) has died out in the period since. By contrast, some of their nuclear DNA is likely to be present in modern people. So, while Mitochondrial Eve was the one maternal ancestor we all share, she was not the 'mother of us all' in every respect – just the mother of all our mitochondria!

To bring our story as far up to date as possible, let us finally refer to a study published just weeks before this book went to press. Macaulay et al (2005) have analysed mtDNAs from a large number of south east Asians, and interpreted the results in the light of the discovery of a pile of fish shells, >100 000 years old, on the coast of Eritrea. Taking this as evidence of early modern humans incorporating such food into their diets, Macaulay and colleagues suggest that dispersal from Africa took place across a narrow straight of the Red Sea called the Gate of Grief, and thence along a southern coastal route (along the whole of which shellfish could have been culled) all the way to south east Asia, finally crossing to Australia about 62 000 years ago (Fig. 1.7). Recent climatological evidence is that at that time most of Europe and

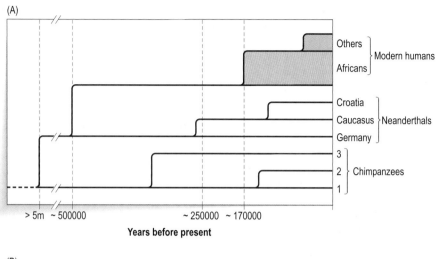

(A)

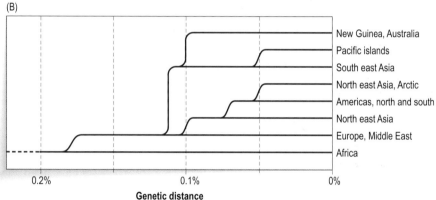

(B)

Figure 1.6 Phylogenetic trees based on (A) mitochondrial DNA studies of three chimpanzees, three Neanderthals and a total of several hundred humans, and (B) nuclear DNA regions coding for blood groups, immunological markers, etc. In the latter, 'genetic distance' is effectively proportional to the time since isolation of one group from another. (A) information from Figure 19.21 of Freeman & Herron (2004). (B) reproduced, with permission, and slightly modified from Figure 28.15 of Starr & Taggart (1998 edition).

northern Asia was desert, tundra, or covered in ice. However, the climate was improving, and about 50 000 years ago a group travelled from southern Arabia, through modern-day Turkey and thence into Europe. The similarity of this map to the equivalent areas of Figure 1.5, which was not based on either sort of DNA but on fossil finds, is encouraging. But a detail to which the mitochondrial DNA data point, which fossil bones could not even hint at, is that not more than three females may have been the maternal ancestors of the whole subsequent human race outside Africa. Note that this repeat of convergence into a very narrow stream of maternity occurred about 100 000 years after mtEve.

What plots like these cannot show is that the genetic variation within any one race of modern humans is scarcely any less on average than that between races – indeed, two individuals within one race *can* differ by more than two individuals of different

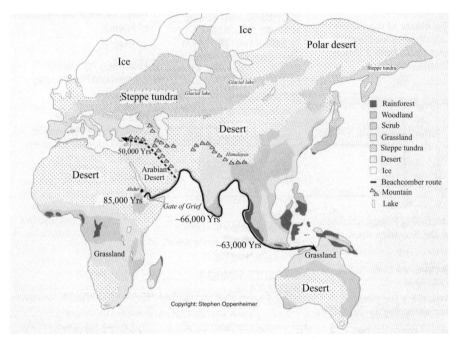

Figure 1.7 Map showing the migrations of *Homo sapiens* out of Africa, probably in search of food, as deduced from mtDNA studies reported or cited by Macaulay et al (2005). Climatic and vegetation data for the period of the main migration are also indicated. From Figure1.6 of Oppenheimer (2003), with permission; © Stephen Oppenheimer 2005.

races. Furthermore, any such statement is dependent on the choice of indicator, which must usually be a particular element of nuclear or mitochondrial DNA. In the latter instance, some distinctly counter-intuitive findings have been made: as an example, mitochondrial DNA studies have shown more diversity in one small region of east Africa than in most of Europe (Pitsiladis & Scott 2005). The most obvious inter-racial difference, skin colour, upon which so much tragic misunderstanding has until recently been based, is a simple function of the intensity of sunlight; near the Equator, this would cause severe burning of unclothed skin, and a high incidence of melanoma, if the incident rays (especially their ultraviolet component) were allowed to penetrate to the germinal layer unattenuated by protective pigment; in cold-temperate latitudes, by contrast, all possible sunlight must be allowed to penetrate or vitamin D deficiency will lead to serious ill-health. The genetic difference involved in this pigmentation-difference is very small. Ways to detect other genetic differences, within and between racial groups – those which affect physical performance of relevance to sport – will be the subject of Chapter 2. Nevertheless, the most important point to appreciate is that human beings are a rather homogeneous species, in keeping with the concept that they spread quite rapidly over the world from a single source.

The Lifestyles of *Homo Sapiens*

Homo sapiens did not at first live very differently from *Homo erectus* and the later differences from the Neanderthals were even less: in fact there is evidence that *sapiens* and the Neanderthals exchanged cultural developments, such as particular tools, even if they did not mate. Although we have stressed the development of hunting, because of its demands upon intelligence and co-operation, it is unlikely that any humans have been pure carnivores. Rather, all could be classified as 'hunter-gatherers', although the details of what they hunted and what they gathered varied substantially with local circumstances. Those living near water probably almost always 'hunted' fish rather than mammals or most birds, although the sea-coast dwellers might have been happy to catch a seabird when they could. As Macaulay et al recognize, if the shores were rich in shellfish even the process of fish collection would be one of gathering, not hunting. As for plant material, the range of fruit, berries, nuts and grains was very wide; roots also seem to have been quite extensively consumed, but leaves and green grasses were probably never the main component of human diets – we have neither ruminant stomachs nor the very long intestines of other herbivores such as horses, to allow us to benefit from these sources.

A variant upon opportunistic hunting of any prey which came near the tribe's home was to follow the herds in their recurrent seasonal migrations – the 'transhumance' way of life. This became particularly necessary in the cold regions, as the last Ice Age came and then departed. Bronowski (1973) wrote well about this, pointing out that it still existed at the time of his book among the Lapps of northern Scandinavia, who were dependent on the reindeer. This mode of living has some of the features of hunting, but some of herding, because the animals are not only pursued and intermittently caught but tended and to a degree cared for. It is thus half-way to animal agriculture. In warmer climates, such as the Mesopotamian basin, arable farming finally became a significant practice about 10 000 years ago. And, of course, in the last few hundred years, this has given way to the predominantly urban and industrial way of life in which we are now immersed.

THE CURRENT SITUATION

At this point our history must stop. It is widely remarked that selection now is affected at least as strongly by social forces as by raw biological ones; organized societies have, for a long time, cared for those who would otherwise have died, and given prominence and privilege to people with special skills and traits not necessarily associated with physical strength. There is still selection, although its mechanism is no longer straightforward. But even the agricultural period was too short to have much effect on our genetic make-up, and the industrial one has had almost none. It is considered (Cordain et al 1998) that 'the portion of our genome that determines basic anatomy and physiology has remained relatively unchanged over the past 40 000 years'. In any case agriculture was not exactly sedentary and nor was it fully predictable, so its physical demands were not so different from those of hunting and foraging, although its intellectual and social ones were.

It must therefore be concluded that, until the last 200 years, our forebears had been highly active for as long as we can discern. Whether they were mainly gathering or mainly hunting, two things were true of early humans and their anthropoid precursors: first, they were continually expending large amounts of energy (Fig. 1.8), and second, they would have had to cope with quite frequent periods of hunger, when the finds or kills were not forthcoming. Indeed, the hunter-gatherer stage was surely only the last in which this was true; the previous arboreal stage must have imposed such stresses to similar extents, at least as climates became drier and forced that stage towards its close. The arboreal richness which preceded this perhaps represented a

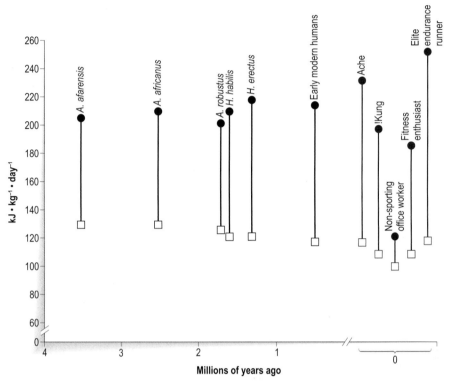

Figure 1.8   Estimates of hominid daily energy expenditures over the past 3.5 Myr. Open squares represent resting metabolic rates, filled circles total daily expenditures. Values for Ache Indians are elevated by the inclusion of ritual runners. Data mainly from Table 2 and Figure 3 of Cordain et al (1998).

brief respite, but before that the situation must have been much the same – intense activity, in the search for food, and substantial periods between when little or none could be found. So genes promoting physical activity on the one hand, and the conservation of excess intake as stored fat on the other, would both have been strongly selected for. In saying this, we do not necessarily mean that a gene would arise where there was none before, or even that one would be expressed which was silent before; more probably what was involved was the selection of a particular version, an *allele* of a given gene, with somewhat different effects from those of rival alleles.

Genes which helped us to withstand periods of shortage and near-starvation, between successful garnerings of fruit or kills of meat, were termed 'frugal' by Neel in the early 1960s. In a recent re-assessment, Neel (1999) emphasized in addition the fact that the musculature of our hunter-gatherer ancestors would have been very well conditioned – comparable to that of a highly trained modern athlete. Values of $\dot{V}O_{2max}$, for modern hunter-gather or transhumance populations on the one hand and non-athletic industrialized humans on the other, unequivocally support this point (Fig. 1.9), and trained muscle is muscle that is economical in its use of fuel.

Frugal genes and economical muscle both mean that today, in first-world societies where vigorous physical exercise is no longer necessary for immediate survival, we are liable to become obese unless we keep ourselves deliberately active. Metabolic, cardiovascular, respiratory and arthroskeletal pathologies are all inclined to follow.

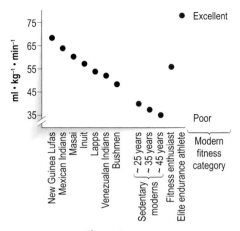

Figure 1.9 Maximum aerobic capacity ($\dot{V}O_{2max}$) data for contemporary hunter-gatherer and similar groups, compared with those for modern Western humans. Data mainly from Figure 4 of Cordain et al (1998).

We must respect our genes and the circumstances which selected them, or accept the consequences (Booth et al 2002, Cordain et al 1998).

KEY POINTS

1. Primitive bacteria seem to have originated on earth when it was about 15% of its present age (about 4.5 billion years), utilizing organic molecules produced by the energy of intense ultraviolet radiation. The atmosphere then contained negligible oxygen, so metabolism was entirely anaerobic.
2. Photosynthetically produced oxygen enabled aerobic metabolism to become established when earth was about half its present age. After this, aerobic bacteria, taken up by larger anaerobes, appear to have become the mitochondria of early eukaryotic cells. With earth ~75% present age sexual reproduction emerged, markedly increasing the rate of evolution. Multicellular animals followed fairly quickly, and tracks suggesting muscled movement were left 700–800 Myr ago (earth ~85% present age).
3. 'Explosive' animal development occurred slightly >500 Myr ago, leading to invasion of the land ~100 Myr later by fish with lobed fins which would evolve into legs. Mammals began nearly 200 Myr ago, but became dominant only after the dinosaur extinction 65 Myr ago.
4. Tree-dwelling favoured the evolution of primates, having binocular vision and prehensile forelimbs. A group of these lacking tails – the apes – emerged ~20 Myr ago in Africa, but left that continent for Eurasia, returning 7–8 Myr ago. Drying climate led to grasslands displacing forests and gave opportunity for some apes to go down again to the ground and become fully bipedal, as *Australopithecus* and thence *Homo* – who shows anatomical signs of having been best adapted for distance running.
5. In drying grasslands, hunting became a productive complement to vegetarian gathering, and the resulting stimuli to tool-use and co-ordinated group activity favoured brain enlargement. *Homo's* consequent adaptability led to successive re-invasions of Asia, and later of Europe, despite the return of Ice Ages there.

6. Modern humans are thus uniquely varied in their physical attributes, although inferior in every one of them to specialist species. Yet they retain the 'frugal genes' producing a metabolic make-up which results in diverse pathologies if physically active lifestyles are not continued, despite the fact that civilized environments no longer demand them for short-term survival.

Further Reading

The Sept 1978 issue of Scientific American, vol 239(3), was devoted entirely to evolution, and contains articles on every aspect from the chemical origin of life to the evolution of multicellular plants and animals. It is still well worth reading, although out of date on several details.

The first chapter of Astrand et al (2003) covers very similar ground to our own, but with different emphases. We have deliberately not quoted from this source, as it is likely to be readily available to readers of the present book. Note, however, that the 2003 treatment of this topic differs only slightly from that in the third (1985) edition, so it is significantly dated in certain details.

By contrast, an extensive and up-to-date textbook account of work in this field, which involves many debates and balancings of evidence from which we have tried to pick what seems the most probable story, is provided by Freeman & Herron (2004). See in particular their Chapter 19, on human origins.

There is also a rich literature for the general reader in this field; from it we can list only a very short selection. Most recently Palmer (2005) has surveyed the last 7 Myr of human evolution. Alternatively, in a more didactic vein, see Diamond (1992). A little more technically, Oppenheimer (2003) focuses on the use of mtDNA and its male-side counterpart, the Y chromosome, in studies of the dispersion of *Homo* across the globe from Africa. Finally, Dawkins (2004) explores the whole story of life on earth by running the clock backwards, so that he can start at the present and finish in the prebiotic seas – and teach one a great deal about both evolutionary and functional biology along the way.

References

Alexander R M 1988 Elastic mechanisms in animal movement. Cambridge, University Press

Astrand P-O, Rodahl K, Dahl H A, Stromme S B 2003 Textbook of work physiology: physiological bases of exercise. Champaign, Human Kinetics

Baba M L, Goodman M, Berger-Cohn J et al 1984 The early adaptive evolution of calmodulin. Molecular Biology and Evolution 1:442–455

Begun D R 2003 Planet of the apes. Scientific American 289:64–73

Berrill N J 1955 (1961) Man's emerging mind. London, Scientific Book Guild

Booth F W, Chakravarty, M V, Spangenburg, E E 2002 Exercise and gene expression. Journal of Physiology 543:399–411

Bramble D M, Lieberman D E 2004 Endurance running and the evolution of *homo*. Nature 432:345–352

Bronowski J 1973 The ascent of man. London, British Broadcasting Corporation

Cairns-Smith G 1990 Seven clues to the origin of life. Cambridge, University Press

Cann R L, Stoneking M, Wilson A C 1987 Mitochondrial DNA and human evolution. Nature 325:31–36

Cordain L et al 1998 Physical activity, energy expenditure and fitness: An evolutionary perspective. International Journal of Sports Medicine 19:328–335

Dawkins R 2004 The Ancestor's tale: A pilgrimage to the dawn of life. London, Weidenfield and Nicholson. (Phoenix paperback edition 2005)

Diamond J. 1992 The third chimpanzee: the evolution and future of the human animal. New York, Harper Collins

Fortey R 1997 Life: An unauthorised biography. London, HarperCollins

Freeland S J, Hurst L D 2004 Evolution encoded. Scientific American 290:56–63

Freeman S, Herron J C 2004 Evolutionary analysis. Upper Saddle River, Pearson Prentice Hall

Henderson LJ 1913 The fitness of the enironment. New York, Macmillan

Macaulay V, Hill C, Achilli A et al 2005 Single, rapid coastal settlement of Asia revealed by analysis of complete mitochondrial genomes. Science 308:1034–1036

Margulis L 1970 Origin of eukaryotic cells. New Haven, Yale University Press

Neel J V 1999 The 'thrifty genotype' in 1998. Nutritional Reviews 57: S2–S9

Neyt C, Jagla K, Thisse C et al 2000 Evolutionary origins of vertebrate appendicular muscle. Nature 408:82–86

Nicholls D G, Ferguson S J 1992 Bioenergetics 2. London, Academic Press

Oppenheimer S 2003 Out of Eden: the peopling of the world. London, Constable

Ovcharenko I et al 2004 ECR Browser: a tool for visualizing and accessing data from comparisons of multiple vertebrate genomes. Nucleic Acids Research 32:W280–W286. Online. Available: http//ecrbrowser.dcode.org

Palmer D 2005 Seven million years: the story of human evolution. London, Weidenfield and Nicholson

Pitsiladis Y, Scott R 2005 The makings of the perfect athlete. Lancet 366:S16–S17

Starr C, Taggart R 2003 Biology: the unity and diversity of life, 10th edn. Belmont, Brooks Cole. (8th edn, 1998, published by Wadsworth)

Stringer C B 1990 The emergence of modern humans. Scientific American 263:68–74

Wong K 2004 The littlest human. Scientific American 291:40–49

Chapter 2

Top-down studies of the genetic contribution to differences in physical capacity

Neil Spurway

CHAPTER CONTENTS

LEARNING OBJECTIVES:

After studying this chapter you should be able to. . .

1. Understand the terms 'heritability estimation' and 'path analysis'.
2. Discuss the use of twins in exploring the contribution of inheritance to human physical performance, and the limitations of this approach.
3. Have an awareness of what has been learned from wider family studies, but also of how the conclusions may be affected by the assumptions adopted to make the study possible.
4. Quote representative data indicating the strength of the genetic contribution to various performance parameters studied in European and North American groups.
5. Explain why the methods giving rise to such data cannot be applied to comparisons between races or other disparate groups.
6. Distinguish between 'top-down' and 'bottom-up' studies of genetic influences.

EARLY THINKING

Obviously we cannot say how long ago human beings first began to wonder, in some half-formulated way, about the relative influences on an individual's capacities, both physical and mental, of inheritance – the 'blood line' – and life history – environment and experience, including what we would now refer to as education and training. Certainly there are hints in the Old Testament, and in the literature of Ancient Greece.

However, the first attempts to formulate the question scientifically are universally recognized to have been those of Francis Galton, a cousin of Darwin, in mid-Victorian England. Somewhat in conflict with the self-improvement ethos of his age, Galton (1869, 1875 etc.) argued strenuously for a paramount influence of inheritance upon even the mature individual. He used and extended such statistical methods as were available in his time to analyse the differences between 'identical' and 'non-identical' twins, the former but not the latter being assumed to have the same genetics. Whether he made adequate enough use of this method to be called its founder has been both questioned (Rende et al 1990) and defended (Bouchard & Propping 1993; Spector 2000), but we shall see later that, even with more modern statistical techniques, twin studies have almost invariably pointed to the conclusion that genetic influences are strong, if not very strong.

Educationalists took the lead in mounting reaction against this view, pioneering work being done in the 1920s and 1930s. They were intuitively convinced that committed educational effort could take great strides towards overcoming misfortunes of inheritance as well as upbringing – of 'nature' as well as 'nurture'. The analogous question, in relation to physical performance, will occupy us extensively as this chapter develops. Meantime it must be noted that, when twin studies were first applied to human physical performance in the early 1970s, they used methods worked out by the educationalists of 50 years earlier.

TWIN STUDIES OF HUMAN MUSCLE AND PHYSICAL PERFORMANCE

Estimating Heritability

The first approach adopted, initially by educational researchers such as Merriman and Holtzinger, and two generations later by investigators of physical performance, was to compare 'identical' with 'non-identical' twins on the basis of very simplifying assumptions. Non-identicals are also known as 'fraternal' twins, despite the fact they may be of either sex or one of each! In explaining the assumptions we must also adopt the technical terms *monozygous* (MZ) for 'identical' twins (they originated by the division of a single fertilized ovum – a single *zygote*) and *dizygous* (DZ) for fraternals, who arose from two separately fertilized ova in the same womb.

Since the MZ twins have identical genetic constitutions (*genotypes*), it is assumed that any differences in their performances under some test which are not due to errors in the measurement can only be caused by differences in the environments they have experienced since their conception. By contrast, the DZ twins have genotypes no more alike than those of any other siblings. Nevertheless, their performances will be affected by their environmental histories, and the studies of them will be subject to measurement errors, just as for the MZ pairs.

Of course, one other assumption is that the zygosities of all the twins have been correctly assessed. Methods for determining zygosity, although better now, were already pretty good in the 1970s – and we may be confident that the organizers of every study excluded any cases which looked doubtful. So this error is unlikely – at worst not more than a 5% chance (Thomis et al 1998) – although it will be serious if it occurs. Two other potential errors, however, are considerably more probable; and these errors are not technical but fundamental to the simple additive model adopted. To demonstrate these points, let us state the model algebraically, in terms of variances between the members of twin-pairs. It is that:

$$Var_{DZ(total)} = Var_{DZ(gen)} + Var_{(env)} + Var_{DZ(meas)}$$
$$Var_{MZ(total)} = \qquad\qquad Var_{(env)} + Var_{MZ(meas)}$$

In these equations Var = variance, gen = genetic, and env = environmental. The first big assumption made was that the variances between members of twin pairs, due to environmental effects accumulated over the lifetimes up to the study, were the same for DZ as for MZ twins; if so, by subtracting the bottom line from the top one, the term 'Var$_{(env)}$' can be eliminated. The second assumption was that genetic effects within the pairs of DZ twins expressed themselves directly, without any interaction with the twins' environments – otherwise there would have had to be a further, interaction term in the DZ line. Making these assumptions, we may write:

$$Var_{DZ(gen)} = [Var_{DZ(total)} - Var_{DZ(meas)}] - [Var_{MZ(total)} - Var_{MZ(meas)}]$$

Finally, we express the variable Var$_{DZ(gen)}$ as a percentage; this is termed the *heritability estimate* (H$_{est}$), so:

$$H_{est} = 100 \frac{[Var_{DZ(total)} - Var_{DZ(meas)}] - [Var_{MZ(total)} - Var_{MZ(meas)}]}{Var_{DZ(total)} - Var_{DZ(meas)}}$$

The value of H$_{est}$ can vary between 0%, meaning that all the variation is environmentally caused, and a theoretical 100% (actually greater or less than 100% according to the influence of experimental errors) meaning that it is all genetic.

One essential statistical precaution must be noted before we proceed. Reasonably enough, the total variance found among the DZ twins must be considerably larger than that among the MZ for H$_{est}$ to be worth calculating; if the DZ variance is only a little larger, too many unconsidered errors are likely to have been substantial. The formal statistical condition embodying this requirement is expressed in terms of the 'variance ratio' (symbol F):

$$F = \{Var_{DZ(total)} / Var_{MZ(total)}\}$$

F must obviously be >1. The requirement is that it be so by an amount significant at a predetermined probability level (normally 5%) for the number of subjects involved.

The Trail Blazers

The above analysis was presented by Klissouras (1971), who lucidly spelled out all the assumptions involved. He studied 15 pairs of MZ and 10 of DZ male twins, aged 7–13 years; the sample is not large, but under-7s could not be expected to exert themselves consistently for the several minutes required by the performance tests, and over-13s were judged liable to have experienced less-uniform environmental influences. The main performance tests utilized were maximal aerobic power (usually referred to now as $\dot{V}O_{2max}$), maximum heart rate (HR$_{max}$) and maximal blood lactate (indicating anaerobic capacity), all measured as responses to treadmill running. Klissouras's conclusions, in this pioneering paper, were that all three variables were predominantly and strongly genetically determined – H$_{est}$ for $\dot{V}O_{2max}$ scaled to body weight (L·min^{-1}·kg^{-1}: F = 14, significance level 1%) was calculated at the extraordinarily high value of more than 93%, that for HR$_{max}$ (F = 7, significance level 1%) almost 86% and for anaerobic capacity (F = 5, significance level 5%) more than 81%. A visual illustration of the MZ/DZ difference can be obtained by plotting the readings of a given parameter in any one twin against those in the other, and then calculating correlation coefficients. This is done in Figure 2.1, for the $\dot{V}O_{2max}$ data; the only slightly weaker results for Klissouras's measure of anaerobic capacity, maximum blood lactate concentration, are shown in Figure 2.2.

Two years later Klissouras, with colleagues (Klissouras et al 1973), extended this form of analysis to 39 twin pairs, of both sexes and to ages up to 52 years, fully supporting his earlier conclusion that the genetic contribution to the differences

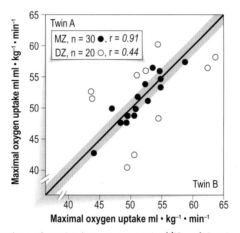

Figure 2.1 Intrapair values of maximum oxygen uptake ($\dot{V}O_{2max}$) for the indicated numbers of MZ and DZ twins. The diagonal line is that of equality for values of both members of a pair; shaded area represents magnitude of measurement error, estimated as the standard deviation of duplicate readings. Ratio of variance among DZ twins to that among MZ s (F) = 13.9. Reproduced from Figure 1 of Klissouras (1971) and used with permission.

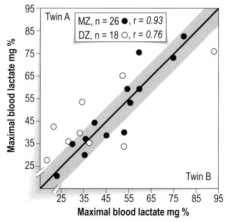

Figure 2.2 Intrapair values of maximum blood lactate concentration for MZ and DZ twins. F = 4.9. Reproduced from Figure 2 of Klissouras (1971) and used with permission.

between individuals in $\dot{V}O_{2max}$ was very high. As Galton had said 100 years earlier, although in his case the reference was to intellectual gifts not aerobic capacity, 'There is no escape from the conclusion that nature prevails enormously over nurture'. A substantially more recent study of 48 twin pairs, by Fagard et al (1991), comes to an almost equally strong conclusion when applying the same kind of analysis: $H_{(est)}$, calculated as above, for $\dot{V}O_{2max}$ expressed in $L \cdot min^{-1} \cdot kg^{-1}$, was 80%. Of course, such measures of whole-body performance parameters give only very indirect indications of muscle properties. However, Klissouras's approach was first applied to direct measures of muscle properties just 6 years after his first paper.

Komi et al (1977) took muscle biopsies from the lateral vasti of 31 twin pairs (15 MZ and 16 DZ) of both sexes, and did basic histochemistry to determine the relative percentages of fast and slow fibres. (If this fast/slow distinction is unfamiliar to you, see the early sections of Chapter 3.) They concluded that the percentage of slow fibres was overwhelmingly genetically determined, H_{est} being 99.5% for males and 93% for females. (Note that these figures refer to the percentage *counts* of fibres, and say nothing about their relative sizes or metabolic capacities.) If generalizeable to the human race at large they would indicate that even the most intensive training regimes could only induce a small minority of fibres, if any, to change from slow to fast, or *vice-versa*, but would leave entirely open the possibilities of the two major groups ending up radically different in size, enzyme complement, or both. Indeed, we shall find, in Chapter 3, considerable evidence that the latter categories of change are much easier to bring about than substantial changes of relative fast and slow numbers.

However, these trail-blazing studies by Klissouras and Komi were to be challenged, methodologically as well as for their specific conclusions. Some of the challenges could be easily dismissed. In particular Howald (1976), after studying just 17 twin pairs, only six of them DZ, reported no significant influence of heredity on $\dot{V}O_{2max}$. However, he had disregarded the crucial requirement of equal environmental influences. Two of his pairs of MZ twins had been subject to palbably divergent experiences: when these were excluded from his analysis, H_{est} rose to 66%. Nevertheless, challenges from some other laboratories were more solidly based.

Before considering these, however, let us note three different grounds on which readers of the Klissouras and Komi papers themselves might have wondered whether the conclusions would prove generally reproducible. First, papers from each group embodied other data which one would have expected to show similarly high heritabilities, yet did not. Klissouras et al (1973) found a significant F ratio and high $H_{(est)}$ for vital capacity as well as for $\dot{V}O_{2max}$, but not for heart volume, maximum heart rate, maximum oxygen pulse, and other related parameters. Similarly Komi et al (1977) assayed for a battery of enzymes – myofibrillar ATPases, creatine kinase, myokinase, phosphorylase and several isozymes of lactate dehydrogenase – almost all of which would be expected to differ between fast and slow fibres (Ch. 3), yet none showed significant heritability despite the fast/slow ratio doing so exceedingly strongly. Second, for the case of muscle fibre percentage counts, sampling error itself (reviewed by Simoneau & Bouchard 1995, but including references prior to 1977) shows a variance in the order of 6%, so that a heritability indicator greater than 94% could not be credited for a full population. Finally, if one compares heritability values already available in the 1970s of parameters such as height, weight, girths, milk-yield and litter size (Table 2.1), which are measurable in humans and other well-studied animals with considerably greater precision than performance parameters and muscle characteristics one finds that relatively few came close to the 90+% range found by Klissouras and Komi in their studies. The 80% of Fagard et al (1991) is less disconcerting, and it is noteworthy that theirs was the largest sample. Nevertheless, a

Table 2.1   Heritabilities (to nearest 5%) of various readily-measured characteristics in a selection of accessible species. Data (all available by late 1970s) collected by Clarke (1956), Falconer (1989). The latter notes that the standard errors of the figures in his list ranged from about 2% to about 10%.

Species/phenotype	H_{est}
Human	
Height (different studies, different populations)	65–90%
Adult weight	70%
Birth weight	35%
Forearm length	80%
Forearm circumference	55%
Head length	55%
Head circumference	75%
Chest circumference	50%
Waist circumference	25%
Shoulder breadth	35%
Cattle	
Weight	65%
Butterfat	40%
Milk yield	35%
Mice	
Weight	35%
Tail length	40%
Size of first litter	20%
Poultry	
Weight	55%
Egg weight	50%
Egg production	10%

more recent tabulation (Frankham et al 2002) finds the mean H_{est} for size measurements of humans, domestic and laboratory animals to be 50%, with the equivalent for birds 57%. These authors also point out that extreme values, even greater than 100% or less than 0%, some of which contribute to the means they quote, can arise due to sampling variation in small experiments.

Clearly, we must be prepared to find lower estimates from more extensive studies, but recruiting much larger groups of twins becomes exceedingly hard. Other statistical approaches enable information to be gleaned from wider-ranging family studies, and even from studies of non-relatives. But it is also possible to reconsider the assumptions embodied in the simple, additive model applied so far in our accounts of twin studies. All three developments occurred.

Twin Studies from the Quebec School: $\dot{V}O_{2max}$ and Muscle Composition

In the two decades following the pioneering work of Klissouras, Komi and their respective collaborators, the most extensive series of investigations probing the contribution of inheritance to physical performance-capacity was made by Bouchard's team at Laval University, in the Canadian province of Quebec. Many of these were not twin studies, but we will start with some that were.

Bouchard et al (1986a) had the resources to measure $\dot{V}O_{2max}$ in 27 pairs of non-twin brothers, 33 pairs of male and female DZ twins and 53 of MZ; the age-range was 16–34 years. The authors calculated H_{est} for $\dot{V}O_{2max}$ expressed both in the direct way, per kg body mass, and per kg fat-free mass, having estimated body fat content on the basis of underwater weighing. Klissouras had already expressed $\dot{V}O_{2max}$ both ways in 1971 (his term for fat-free mass was 'lean body weight' and he deduced it from skinfold thicknesses) and the two values he found for H_{est} were not significantly different; however it may be relevant that his subjects were all pre-pubertal boys, and none of them had excessive fat (V Klissouras, personal communication, 2005). The H_{est} values arrived at by Bouchard et al were not only lower but much more divergent – 47% for the scaling to whole body weight and just 17% for that to fat-free mass. Since the fat-free mass is closer to the muscle mass, and muscle is the main user of oxygen in strenuous exercise, this divergence seems to be in the wrong direction. A further surprise came from their intraclass correlation coefficients, which were respectively 0.70, 0.51 and 0.41 for MZ, DZ and non-twin brothers. On the assumption which everyone else had made, DZ twins should not correlate significantly more closely than ordinary siblings. Bouchard and colleagues concluded that environmental influences common to both types of twin had inflated even *their* H_{est} values, and speculated that a true per-kg figure might be more like 25% than 47%. However this was a guess, albeit an informed one, so it is perhaps slightly unfortunate that it has been given considerable currency in the subsequent literature.

In the same paper, Bouchard's team measured two other whole-body parameters indicative of aerobic performance capacity – total work output during a 90-minute cycle ergometer test, and lactate threshold (LT). For the first of these, in particular, they found a much higher heritability of 72%, which they admitted that they could not reconcile with their conclusions about $\dot{V}O_{2max}$. We shall return to the LT later.

Another paper that year from the same laboratory (Bouchard et al 1986b) reported on a biopsy study of lateral vastus in 32 pairs of non-twin brothers, 26 DZ and 35 MZ twins of both sexes. Thus they were here responding to Komi in the same sense that their previous paper was a response to Klissouras, but this time their rebuttal was even more radical. After eliminating the variances attributable to differences of age and sex (both of which affect fibre type proportions yet neither of which is a heritable influence on muscle, in the sense at issue) they found F ratios equal or close to unity for fibre type proportions, and consequently concluded that there was no contribution of heredity at all to these parameters! Their figures for enzyme activities, by contrast, were significant in several instances. Heritabilities were estimated by two different statistical procedures (see next section), in addition to the one we have considered so far, but values for phosphofructokinase, oxoglutarate dehydrogenase lactate dehydrogenase, malate dehydrogenase and 3-hydroxyacyl CoA dehydrogenase ranged from 30 to 67% on one measure, 14 to 59% on another which tends to behave in similar ways, and were very high on the third. There were reasons for questioning the particularly high values obtained for the last three enzymes in this list, but the overall indications are diametrically opposite to those of Komi et al (1977), who had found extremely high heritabilities for fibre types but no significant values for enzymes. Beyond pointing out that the latter group's H_{est} values for fibre-type percentages were improbably high in relation to sampling variance, Bouchard et al offer no direct explanation for the disparity. Their sample was larger, covered a rather greater age-range and did not make separate calculations for the two sexes – instead

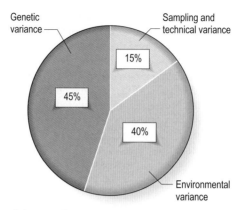

Figure 2.3 Estimates of the sampling and technical, environmental, and genetic variances for the proportion of type 1 fibres in human skeletal muscle. From Figure 1 of Simoneau & Bouchard (1995), with permission.

it factored out the effects of both the latter influences. Nevertheless all these together seem highly unlikely to account for the finding that fibre type percentage was entirely uninfluenced by genotype. Nor do Bouchard et al explain an internal feature of their own study, no less worrying than those we have noted above for the earlier investigators: the correlation coefficients among DZ twins, while almost identical to those of MZ twins for % type 1 fibres (hence the negligible H_{est} value arrived at), were substantially lower than for non-twin brothers in respect of half the enzymes looked at. Neither result seems reasonable.

Although the subsequent publications from this group consistently concluded that genetic influences were smaller than those estimated by Klissouras and Komi, their views on muscle were never quite as extreme again. In fact Simoneau & Bouchard (1995), taking account of a mouse study (Nimmo et al 1985) indicating that genetic factors accounted for about 75% of the variation in proportion of slow fibres in that animal's soleus muscle, reconsidered their own 1986 data. Placing more emphasis on less dismissive heritability estimators (below) they concluded that 'the genetic variation component for the proportion of type 1 fibres in human muscle is of the order of 40 to 50%' (Fig. 2.3). They did not comment on why they had been so much more radical 9 years earlier.

Other Heritability Estimators

There are more ways of estimating heritability than the one with which we began this chapter, which had been adopted by Klissouras from 1920s educational researchers such as Holzinger. This section presents derivations of two other methods, which you will encounter if you want to study the literature in detail. If you have no such ambition, it is safe to skip to the quote from Clark at the end of this section (p 35).

To begin the further derivations, let us express Klissouras's algebra in more concise terms than before, by writing:

$$h^2 = (\sigma^2_{DZ} - \sigma^2_{MZ})/\sigma^2_{DZ}$$

Here, h^2 is the accepted modern symbol for a heritability estimate, differing from H_{est} only in having a value between 0 and 1, not between 0 and 100; and σ^2 (standard deviation squared) is the variance of the sample indicated by the suffix, *after subtraction of the error of measurement*. (Since measurement error has always to be subtracted, formulae can be written more economically by assuming this has been done.)

The formulation above was first put forward by Clark (1956) – a short, lucid paper with many helpful comments on twin studies. However, another way of saying almost exactly the same thing is in terms of intra-class correlation coefficients, r:

$$h^2 = (r_{MZ} - r_{DZ})/(1 - r_{DZ}).$$

This is commonly known as the Newman formula, he having co-authored a textbook with Holzinger in the 1930s. As Clark shows, it is virtually equivalent to the Holzinger/Klissouras formulation if:

$$r_{MZ} = 1 - \sigma^2_{MZ}/\sigma^2_T$$
$$r_{DZ} = 1 - \sigma^2_{DZ}/\sigma^2_T$$

(where σ^2_T is the total variance for all twins, both mono- and dizygous) because these expressions imply that:

$$h^2 = (1 - \sigma^2_{MZ}/\sigma^2_T - 1 + \sigma^2_{DZ}/\sigma^2_T)/(1 - 1 + \sigma^2_{DZ}/\sigma^2_T)$$

in which the figures 1 delete each other and we can multiply throughout by σ^2_T to arrive back at the expression $h^2 = (\sigma^2_{DZ} - \sigma^2_{MZ})/\sigma^2_{DZ}$. So the step we must justify is the claim that $r_{MZ} = 1 - \sigma^2_{MZ}/\sigma^2_T$, or:

$$r_{MZ} = (\sigma^2_T - \sigma^2_{MZ})/\sigma^2_T$$

Now σ^2_{MZ} is the sum of variance due to error and variance due to different environmental effects on the monozygous siblings. So $(\sigma^2_T - \sigma^2_{MZ})$ represents the variance between different pairs of monozygous twins, due to the genetic differences between them. Expressed as a fraction of σ^2_T this gives an acceptable rendering of the intra-class correlation coefficient, r_{MZ}. Similarly for r_{DZ}.

So now we have two ways of estimating heritability. Each is appropriate if we consider the fundamental definition of the term:

Heritability is the Proportion of the Total Variance in the Phenotype Attributable to Genetic Differences.

Statisticians call this 'broad-sense heritability'. Often, however, it is more feasible to consider only the additive genetic variance, as in the Klissouras formulation with which we began. This is termed the 'narrow-sense heritability'. Since the forms of interaction which cause departures from the simple, additive condition – gene-gene and gene-environment interactions, plus dominance effects of one form of a gene (one 'allele') over another – can each be analysed only on the basis of more detailed knowledge than exercise scientists usually have of genetic effects, whether on whole-body parameters such as VO_{2max} or muscle parameters such as fibre-type percentages, we are concerned mainly with narrow-sense heritabilities here.

One more formula, due to Falconer (1989) is commonly cited in human performance literature:

$$h^2 = 2 (r_{MZ} - r_{DZ})$$

(Note that r, unlike σ, is a 'standardized' variable, lying between 0 and 1, so this formula, like that of Clark, gives h^2 values in the 0 – 1 range.)

Table 2.2 Shares of the heritable variance predicted for different relatives, on the assumptions that the phenotypes of interest are affected additively by many genes, distributed widely through the non-sex chromosomes - technically described as 'non-interactive polygenic autosomal inheritance'.

Relatives	Genetic variance shared
'Identical' (MZ) twins	1
'Fraternal' (DZ) twins	$\frac{1}{2}$
Normal siblings	$\frac{1}{2}$
Parent and offspring	$\frac{1}{2}$
Half siblings	$\frac{1}{4}$
Cousins	$\frac{1}{4}$
Adopted siblings	0

Falconer's formula follows from first principles if we consider the shares of the heritable variance which would be predicted for the different types of sibling (Table 2.2). DZ twins, like ordinary siblings, would be expected to share half the genetic influence but all the common environmental influences with MZ twins. Writing c^2 for the variance due to these common environmental factors, the predicted intra-class correlation between the dizygous twins is:

$$r_{DZ} = h^2/2 + c^2.$$

But

$$r_{MZ} = h^2 + c^2$$

therefore

$$r_{MZ} - r_{DZ} = h^2/2$$

so

$$h^2 = 2(r_{MZ} - r_{DZ}).$$

Finally, we can introduce a term e^2 for the non-shared environmental influences. As h^2, c^2 and e^2 all represent proportions they must add up to unity:

$$h^2 + c^2 + e^2 = 1$$

i.e.

$$2(r_{MZ} - r_{DZ}) + [r_{MZ} - 2(r_{MZ} - r_{DZ})] + e^2 = 1$$
$$r_{MZ} + e^2 = 1$$

So

$$e^2 = 1 - r_{MZ}$$

This derivation is taken from Purcell (2000), who adds, 'This conclusion is intuitive: Because MZ twins are genetically identical, any variance that is not shared between them (i.e. the extent to which the MZ twin correlation is not 1) must be due to non-shared environmental sources of variation'. (Purcell's whole treatment, a minimally technical, 44-page outline of statistical methodology written for final-level students of behavioural genetics, applies equally to the genetics of physical capacity. It is recommended.)

We have now presented three different expressions for h^2, each trying to encompass the definitions of broad or narrow-sense heritability in manageable algebra, but each doing so with the aid of somewhat different assumptions and simplifications. This means that only rarely will the figures given by any two of them coincide; for all three to do so is almost inconceivable. Table 2 in Fagard et al (1991) and even more so Table 1 in Klissouras (1997) amply illustrate this. Differences in the second decimal place between two h^2 values, even when arrived at from the same formula, can be effectively disregarded. Indeed many authors nowadays are content to cite h^2 figures in very broad terms, such as 'under 0.10', '0.25–0.5', etc. But if a significantly non-zero value emerges at all, especially from more than one of the formulae, investigation of the role of inheritance is worth going on with. Much of the rest of this book exemplifies just this point.

Any reader wishing to pursue the subject of heritability estimates beyond the references already given should start with Kang et al (1978) and could helpfully then move on to Christian et al (1995) and Christian & Williams (2000). (The latter two references provide some of the reflective follow-up anticipated in the first paper, which did not in fact appear at the time.) Text books of quantitative genetics, notably that by Falconer (1989, or more recent editions co-authored by Mackay) will provide helpful background, but none focus on h^2 calculations as sharply as Clark (1956) and the above three references.

However, it is appropriate to end this section with one more caution. It is that, while high values of h^2, from suitably conducted studies, always indicate strong genetic influence, low ones do not necessarily indicate its absence. In Clark's words:

> 'The statistic h^2 is an estimate, not of the extent to which a trait is genetically determined, but of the proportion of the variation in the trait which is genetically determined. If all of the genetic factors responsible for a character are identical in every individual in some population, the genetic component of the variance will be zero in that population – even if the genetic factors almost completely determine the character.'
>
> (Clark 1956, p 53)

Heritability of Strength and Anaerobic Power

Although aerobic performance was the first topic to be investigated quantitatively from the 'nature versus nurture' standpoint, it tells us more about cardio-respiratory function than about skeletal muscle. Among human performance tests, strength and anaerobic power are much more indicative of muscle properties.

On the matter of baseline strength, as with fibre type percentages, we begin with Komi and colleagues who first published on the topic in 1973. Their mature results were presented by Karlsson et al (1979). By then the group had tested 15 MZ and 16 DZ twins (both sexes) for a number of experimental indicators of muscle strength and power, such as isometric knee-extension force, integrated electromyogram and Margaria's stair-climb sprint, together with the battery of enzymes assayed earlier by the same group (Komi et al 1977). Only muscular power, as demonstrated by the stair-climb, showed a significant genetic component. The lack of heritability indication for the other performance measures was in keeping with that for muscle enzymes. However, it contrasted to an extreme degree with that for fibre type percentage.

Other early twin studies, reviewed by Bouchard & Malina (1983), produced much higher heritability estimates for performances lasting not more than 20 seconds. In particular, the estimated genetic contribution to sprint running ranged from 45 to 90% – much more compatible with the Komi group's conclusions on fibre type percentages than on enzymes or most functions.

A strong mid-1980s study of anaerobic performance was that of Simoneau et al (1986). They measured total work output (scaled per kg body weight) during 10 seconds of maximal cycling exercise in every kind of sibling from adoptees to MZ twins (both sexes). F ratios of between-sibship to within-sibship variances (which indicate the degree of similarity between siblings) were about 2, 4 and 9 respectively for non-twin biological siblings, DZ and MZ twins – even the non-twins' value being significant – but were not significant for the adopted siblings. In the same sequence, intra-class correlation coefficients were ~0.4, ~0.5 and ~0.8 respectively, indicating high levels of familial resemblance with substantial genetic components: h^2 estimates ranged from 0.44 to 0.92, depending on the calculation method. Although studies using twins have a marked tendency to produce higher heritability estimates than broader population studies, for such high values to come from the Quebec school was striking.

A test traditionally regarded as being at the interface of aerobic and anaerobic performance (although see Spurway (1992) for a critique of this interpretation) is running speed at a blood lactate concentration of 4 mmol L^{-1}, a value which approximates the onset of continuous blood lactate accumulation throughout the course of the exercise. Klissouras (1997) briefly reports a twin study giving intraclass correlations of 0.83 for MZ and 0.54 for DZ, with F ratio ~5 ($P<0.01$), leading to an h^2 of 80% according to the Holzinger/Clark formula, though rather lower following Newman or Falconer. In the same study both maximum power and anaerobic capacity (the latter assessed as power output in 30 seconds), gave F ~7 ($P<0.001$) and h^2 (Clark) 0.86. Returning to his original interest, $\dot{V}O_{2max}$, in this more recent study Klissouras and colleagues found for its absolute value $h^2 = 0.87$ (F ~7) and if scaled to lean body weight $h^2 = 0.75$ (F ~4).

Responses to Training

People involved in sport have long suspected that individuals differ in their susceptibility to training. Prud'homme et al (1984) were the first to provide evidence that this difference has a substantial genetic component. After 20 weeks of endurance training, the increases of $\dot{V}O_{2max}$ found in 10 pairs of MZ twins varied from 0 to more than 0.75 L·min^{-1}, but the correlation between the twins of each pair was strong (Fig. 2.4): as the F ratio indicates, the gains showed almost eight times more variance between pairs than within pairs. However, the greatest gains in both groups were made by individuals who started with the lowest $\dot{V}O_{2max}$ levels, and Klissouras (1997) argues on this and other grounds that the case for aerobic trainability being highly heritable can be questioned. Bouchard et al (1990), discussing their group's previous results, had already written that 'the major causes of human variation in the response to training appear to be . . . the pre-training status of the trait considered, and perhaps a genetically determined capacity to adapt to exercise training' – a distinctly tentative claim. Nonetheless, further analysing the 1984 data they concluded that, even after adjustment for pre-training level, 'the sensitivity of maximal aerobic power to endurance training is largely familial and most likely genetically determined', which seems to challenge the 'perhaps' in their previous statement!

Several other indicators of aerobic trainability, investigated in the few years following this 1984 observation were reviewed by Bouchard et al (1992). The most

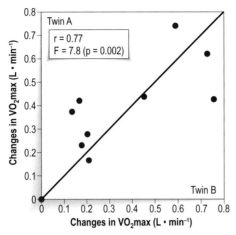

Figure 2.4 Intrapair values for increases in $\dot{V}O_{2max}$ after 20 weeks' endurance training in 10 pairs of MZ twins. Reproduced with permission from Figure 2.2 of Bouchard et al (1992), which used data from Prud'homme et al (1984).

Table 2.3 Evidence for gene-physical activity interactions in responses to exercise training, summarized by ratios of between-genotype to within-genotype variances. Data from Table 7 of Bouchard et al (1992).

Phenotype	Approximate F ratios
Aerobic performance	
90-min work output	10–12
$\dot{V}O_{2max}$	6–9
Maximal O_2 pulse	6–10
Submaximal power output	2–4
Anaerobic performance	
90-sec work output	8–10
10-sec work output	2–3
Muscle metabolism	
Muscle fibre type composition	1–2
Muscle oxidative potential	2–5
Systemic metabolism	
Lipid substrate oxidation	2–5
Lipid mobilization	5–10

marked difference seen between 'responders' and 'non-responders' to training, albeit that the study involved only six twin pairs, was in 15 weeks' training for a 90-minute maximal cycle ergometer effort: the F ratio here was about 11 and the intraclass coefficient for twin resemblance in the response reached 0.83. The Quebec school's evidence for trainabilities of other functions related to aerobic performance are among those indicated by F ratios in Table 2.3.

Anaerobic trainability showed genotype dependence in the Bouchard group's investigations also. The dependence was only slight for 10 seconds maximum power bursts but an anaerobic endurance programme (maximum work output in 90 seconds) produced an F ratio ~9. Aspects of genetic involvement in strength training were investigated during this period too. The muscle enzyme adaptations again varied between twin pairs significantly more than within pairs, though there were no complete non-responders and F ratios only varied between about 2 and 5 (Table 2.3). Changes in the relative numbers of type 1 and 2 fibres were small.

The strength-training theme was taken up more directly 8 years later, in a beautifully-executed study of elbow flexion training among 25 MZ and 16 DZ male twins, mainly in their early 20s, by another group (Thomis et al 1998). Their highly sophisticated methodology will be considered later; at this point we only outline their results. They found that three strength-training parameters, one-repetition maximum (1RM) for a full biceps curl, isometric elbow-flexion torque at 110° elbow angle, and concentric moment at an angular velocity of 120 $°·s^{-1}$, showed significant indications of genetic influence, *independent* of the genetic influences operating on the baseline states. For these three parameters, about 20% of the variation in post-training performances was explained by the training-specific genetic factors, although other factors had explained higher proportions of the variance of the various pre-training phenotypes ($h^2 = 0.77$ for the most strongly influenced parameter, 1RM, but only 0.30 for the one under least genetic influence, concentric contraction). However, other strength-parameters, notably concentric moments at other velocities and all eccentric moments, showed no significant evidence of genetic effects on their training responses. By contrast, baseline cross-sectional area of upper-arm muscles – changes in which would barely have started in a 10-week programme – showed $h^2 = 0.85$.

Direct quantitative comparisons between these findings by Thomis et al and those of the Bouchard group are hampered by the fact that Bouchard et al were not regularly quoting h^2 values by the time of their trainability studies, and Thomis et al cite intra-pair correlations for all exercises tested on MZ twins but only for 1RM in the case of DZ twins. This test, however, was the one which gave the greatest indication of genetic influence on trainability, and even its F ratio is only just above 2 – if, indeed, it is worth calculating at all, because r_{DZ} did not quite reach significance (Fig. 2.5). Other indications are in the same direction, namely that responsiveness to aerobic *training* is under stronger genetic influence than that to strength and burst power training, but – contrary to Klissouras and Komi, and instead assuming the subsequent consensus to be more nearly right – the strength and power *baselines* are more heritable than the aerobic ones.

Complicating Factors in Twin Studies

We have stressed several times that to make genetic analysis feasible many simplifying assumptions have to be made. The great majority of the findings considered so far – including all for which we have discussed the methodology – have been from studies of twins. Crucial to every twin study is the assumption that the variances between MZ and DZ twins due to within-pair environmental differences are not significantly different. Clark (1956), Heath et al (1989) and Klissouras (1997) make a number of points about this, some of which we summarize now. To start with, most people would suspect that the post-natal environments of MZ twins are actually more similar than those of DZs, and there is some objective evidence to that effect: during childhood and youth they are more likely to be treated alike, by both family and the wider society. However, it is crucial to appreciate that only the 'trait-relevant' environments matter:

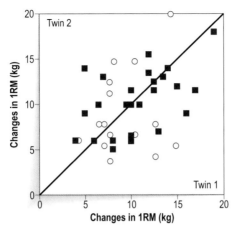

Figure 2.5 Simplified plot summarizing intrapair resemblances of inceases in 1RM load after 10 weeks' strength training, in 128 MZ and 143 DZ twins. Correlation coefficients r_{mz} = 0.49, P <0.01; r_{DZ} = 0.22, not significant; F = 2.2. From Figure 3 of Thomis et al 1998, with permission.

two little girls may be dressed alike, but this will not affect their muscle development unless it indirectly makes them more likely to be offered the same exercise opportunities. Furthermore, it is only if the MZ twin pairs are *passive recipients* of more similar treatments than are DZ twin pairs, as in the instance just hypothesized, that problems will arise. If an environmental similarity is selected or created by the MZ twins, as a part or total consequence of genetically determined traits, then it is an expression of their genetic similarity not a confusing factor. Thus analysis of whether or not the post-natal environments of MZ twins in a study have been materially more similar than of the DZs would often be extremely hard, if not impossible.

A further complication is that the pre-natal influences almost certainly bend the other way. One particularly important reason is that MZ twins usually share a single placenta, and it is rare for them to get exactly equal nourishments from it. Weight differences at birth, resulting from such causes, are commonly made up afterwards, but the possibility of lasting differences in muscle biology and performance potential should not be dismissed. With so complex a picture, there is usually no alternative to the assumption that pre- and postnatal effects have cancelled out, making an equal-environments model permissible. But if the MZ twins studied really have, on average, had more similar experiences, the heritability estimates computed will be inflated. This is likely to be a major reason why estimates from other study designs are usually lower. Appreciating this, many authors now interpret high values of h^2 as indicating a strong 'familial' influence, but not necessarily an entirely genetic one.

Another assumption, made in virtually all work up to about 1990, was that no gene–environment interaction occurred. However, Bouchard et al (1990) point out that if heredity has a role in trainability, this *is* a 'genotype–environment' interaction, in the formal sense. Although in everyday usage the environment is that which surrounds us, from the standpoint of genetic analysis it is all that is not the genotype – the totality of 'nurture', as against inherited 'nature'. Perhaps the most helpful way to think of it, in this all-embracing sense, is as the environment, not of the whole individual, but of the individual's genes.

In explaining the concept of interaction, however, Bouchard et al revert to using 'environment' in the more limited everyday sense, adding 'lifestyle factors' to make up the necessary generality: 'Genotype–environment interaction refers to a situation in which the sensitivity of the individual to the environment or to given lifestyle factors depends on his or her genotype. This effect is *an interaction above the main linear effect of the genotype and of the environment–lifestyle components*' (our italics) – an effect 'resulting from individual differences in the response to existing environmental and lifestyle conditions or to changes in such conditions'. If the effects of training varied randomly they would be a linear addition to the genetically and historically determined baseline state. As in fact they appear to depend quite strongly on the genes, that implies an interaction.

Further consideration of genotype–environment interaction must be postponed until path analysis has been introduced.

STUDIES OF WIDER FAMILY GROUPS

Basics of Path Analysis

To derive information about the relative roles of inheritance and environment from non-twin relatives required statistical methods different from the classical heritability estimation. A major advance was the adoption of path analysis. This is a class of procedure, not a specific formula, so it cannot be effectively presented in the same way as the older-style heritability analysis. To carry out such a procedure one first constructs a 'path diagram' of the presumed interactions between the variables, then performs a multivariate regression analysis, or series of analyses, to evaluate these interactions between each pair of the variables in turn. In this and the following section we introduce the methodology for those of you who want to study the literature in detail. As with the earlier section, '*Other heritability estimators*', if you don't anticipate doing this you can safely skip to '*Some findings from path analysis*' (p 45).

The principles are well outlined by Purcell (2000, pp 359–371): 'Path analysis provides a visual and intuitive way to describe and explore any kind of model that describes some observed data'. 'Paths, drawn as arrows, reflect the statistical effect of one variable on another, independent of all the other variables – what are called *partial regression coefficients*'. The variables can be either measured traits or 'latent' (i.e. potential) variance components; these are usually diagrammed as boxes and circles respectively. Path analysis does not necessarily assume the additive model essential to the approaches considered until this point. Nevertheless, to introduce the new idiom let us follow Purcell in illustrating how the situation already discussed, the 'ACE model' for twins, would be represented (Fig. 2.6). (Readers of this book need to take care over an ambiguity! Here 'ACE' stands for Additive genetic variance + Common environmental variance + Environmental effects not common to all groups. Elsewhere the same three letters indicate angiotensin-converting enzyme. The context will always make clear which is meant.)

Quoting Purcell again, with reference to Figure 2.6, 'The curved, double-headed arrows between latent variables represent the covariance between them. The 1.0/0.5 on the covariance link between the two *A* latent variables indicates that for the MZ twins, this covariance link is 1.0; for DZ twins, 0.5' (cf. Table 2.2). By definition, the common environmental variance has covariance 1.0 while effects which are not common have zero covariance. The little double-headed arrow loops against each latent variable indicate that these variables are assumed, in path analysis, to have variance 1.0. However, the path coefficients *a, c, e*, representing the strengths of the effects, are estimated by trial-and-error fitting to the data. This has an outcome mathematically equivalent to the previous procedure of allocating variances less than

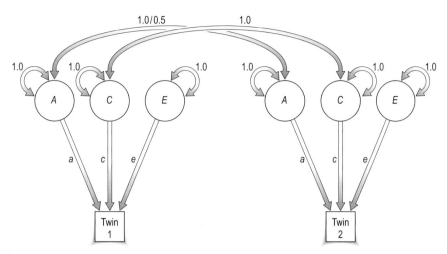

Figure 2.6 Path diagram representing a simple 'ACE' analysis. From Figure A9 of Purcell 2000, with permission.

1.0 (σ^2_A, σ^2_C, σ^2_E) to the variables themselves, because 'the covariance between any two variables is represented by tracing along all the paths that connect the two variables' and multiplying 'all the path coefficients together with the variances of any latent variables traced through. We sum these paths to calculate the expected covariance'. Finally, 'When we trace the two paths between . . . twins, we get (a × 1.0 × a) + (c × 1.0 × c) for MZ twins and (a × 0.5 × a) + (c × 1.0 × c) for DZ twins. That is, $a^2 + c^2$ for MZ twins and $0.5a^2 + c^2$ for DZ . . . as before'.

An early and well-expounded deployment of path analysis in exercise physiology was by Fagard et al (1991), in their study of whole-body performance parameters such as $\dot{V}O_{2max}$. Like Purcell, they have us hasten slowly, by actually representing in the new symbolism an additive, ACE model (Fig. 2.7). This diagram puts MZ and DZ twins in two separate plots and takes as read the unity self-covariance which was represented by small double-headed arrow loops in 2.6. For any pair of twins, T1 and T2, the relevant data about the Phenotypes (values of the performance parameter under investigation) are in the boxes, and the potential influences of genes (acting only Additively, not interactively), Common (shared) environmental factors and unshared Environmental factors are circled. The paths of these influences (single-headed arrows) are labelled c, e, for obvious reasons but h rather than a because the variance due to additive genetic influences is the heritability with which we are familiar, h^2.

Path analysis has thus been introduced by instances in which it is employed to tackle problems which could also be handled, albeit less flexibly, by heritability estimation. But it is not limited to these. Instead, various possible models can be tested in path-analytic terms, so that the one which fits best with the observed variances – or, more often, the simplest which does not fall significantly short of the best fit – can be selected. An extended process of trial and error may be involved, but this is the kind of thing which computers make possible to an extent that could not be contemplated in earlier generations. Thus the path-analysis/computer combination has the effect of freeing investigators to explore a range of models (different influences, and different strengths of particular influences), with and without the simple additive assumptions to which H_{est} and h^2 calculations were effectively tied.

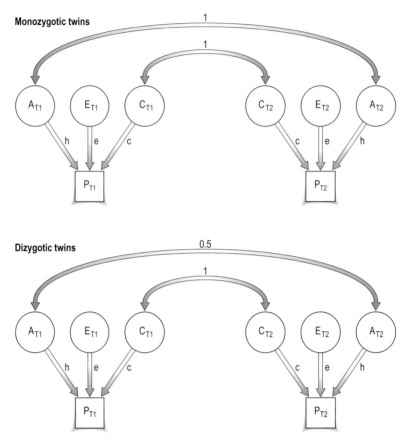

Figure 2.7 Path diagrams for ACE analysis of performance parameters in MZ and DZ twins. Substantially modified from Figure 1 of Fagard et al (1991).

More Complex Path Analyses

We shall give four examples, of increasing complexity. Early uses of path analysis in exercise studies were made by the Quebec group. An investigation of physical activity by Perusse et al (1989) will represent them in this section. To keep the number of variables within bounds their model assumed, as narrow-sense heritability estimates do, that genetic and non-genetic factors are additive and the kinds of mechanism which would lead to consistent departures from linearity (gene-gene and gene-environment interactions) can be neglected. But it does include a term for the degree of departure from the 'mid-parent genic value' – the mean of the two parental phenotypes. Crucially also, it allows for cultural factors in addition to genetic ones to be transmitted between generations, as well as for the environmental factors which are not transmitted. The algorithm enables the investigators to explore by trial and error, with their computer, which combination of values for the path coefficients and other parameters best fit the observed results. Technically therefore it is a 'maximum likelihood' method, as are all the examples which follow.

An important paper by Thomis et al (1998), results from which have already been described, compared two bivariate models of the effects of strength training on twins

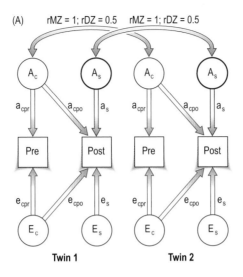

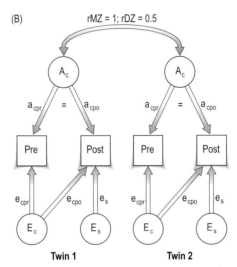

Figure 2.8 Path diagrams for investigation of genetic component of responses to strength training. From Figure 2 of Thomis et al (1998), with permission.

(Fig. 2.8). The rectangles represent the relevant pre- and post-training 'phenotypes' (performance data). In the circles, A are additive genetic influences and E are environmental ones; suffixes indicate those that are common to the pre- and post-training situations and second factors which operate during training but not otherwise so that they affect only the post-training phenotypes and thus constitute genotype-training interactions. The path coefficients a and e represent the strengths of the additive genetic and environmental effects respectively. Selection of the optimum model (called the 'most parsimonious' because it involves the fewest non-zero values for path coefficients providing adequate fit to the data) is done by comparison of the goodness of fit achieved using each of the variants. Model A is the full model and Model B a reduced version, representing the null hypothesis that there is no training-specific genetic factor (no A_s), and the pre-and post-training phenotypes are influenced by the same genes in the same proportions ($a_{cpr} = a_{cpo}$). If Model A fitted the data better than Model B, genotype-training interaction was present. This in fact proved to be the case for several performance criteria, but not for all.

A further example is a Finnish study of women in their 60s and 70s (Tiainen et al 2004). These authors measured isometric strength in three different body locations – hand grip, knee extension and ankle plantar flexion – and wanted to investigate not only the degree of genetic influence on each of these separately but also whether they shared a genetic effect. Figure 2.9 reproduces both the theoretical model with which they began (top) and the most parsimonious one which adequately fitted the data (bottom). The symbolism used should be self-evident, except perhaps for suffix *s*,

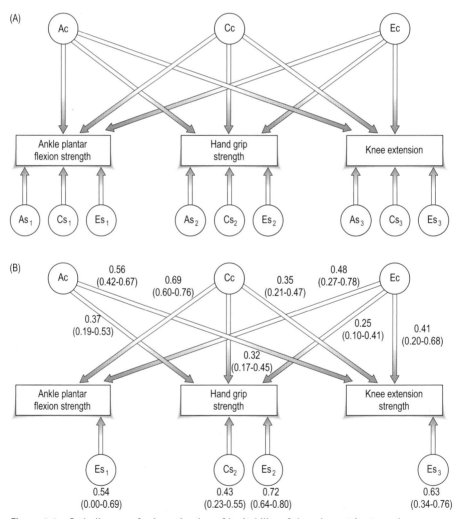

Figure 2.9 Path diagrams for investigation of heritability of three isometric strength parameters in older female twins. From Figures 1 and 3 respectively of Tiainen et al (2004), with permission.

which here indicates influences specific to the particular function, as against those which they experience in common. The parsimonious path diagram indicates that plantar flexion was under insignificant genetic influence, but there was a common influence on hand grip and knee extension strengths. Non-genetic familial effects (Cc) as well as environmental influences (Ec) were common to the performances of all three muscle groups.

As a final example, one of the most complex path-analyses in the physical performance literature had been applied in 1996 by the Belgian-American team from whom we have already taken Figure 2.8. As a final stage of an extended project, which had previously extracted all the information it could from fairly simple models, Maes et al (1996) wanted to allow for the interactions of genetic and cultural transmissions between parents and twins, and to take account of two possible mechanisms not allowed for in the other investigations we have described, namely a set of genes specific to one sex, and dominance of some genes over others. Figure 2.10 is the remarkable model they produced. The square boxes are the individual phenotypes of mother and father (P_{Mo}, P_{Fa}) in the upper row, and of their twin children (P_{T1}, P_{T2}) in the lower one. Circle A represents genes expressed in both sexes while B signifies genes expressed only in males. A similar division, known as a 'Cholesky decomposition', is applied to common environmental effects (C, D) and dominance factors (K, L). Specific environmental effects are estimated separately for males (E) and females (F). Cultural transmission effects are the paths in the middle of the diagram; these too may be either gender-common (m, p) or male-specific (n, o). Non-parental environmental influences shared by the twins have labels g and j. Parameters a-f, k and l, with suffixes for male and female where necessary, indicate the strengths of genetic and environmental effects, while at the top of the diagram p, q, r, s, t, u, v, w, x, y, z represent genotype–environment and other covariances and residual variances – all these being assumed to be equal across generations. Pale grey lines represent genetic transmission parameters from parents to offspring (fixed at 0.5) and assortative mating between the parents (i) which generates covariance between the latent parental variables. Finally, pale grey lines at the bottom of the diagram represent correlations between the dominance effects in the children; these are fixed at 0.25. It is perhaps not surprising that 10 authors were needed to handle this model!

Some Findings from Path Analysis

On the basis modelled in Figure 2.7, Fagard et al (1991) found for their 29 pairs of MZ and 19 DZ male twins, aged 18–31 years, genetic variances of 91% for weight, 83% for skinfold thickness and 50% for height. They speculated that the reason why the latter was so much the lowest of the three figures was the assortative mating effect that tall men tended to marry tall women, and conversely. This gives even DZ twins a substantial tendency to follow their parents' height and reduces the proportionate difference between them and MZ twins, from which the genetic component of variance is deduced. As noted near the beginning of this chapter, H_{est} for $\dot{V}O_{2max}$ per kg body weight was 80% by Clark's formula; in absolute terms (i.e. not scaled to body weight) it was 78% by that formula, and 77% by the most efficient path analysis (in which c^2 was taken to be 0). Even factoring out weight, skinfold thickness and sports activity only reduced this to 66% – a figure which makes an interesting comparison with the 25% guesstimate for $\dot{V}O_{2max}$ per kg by Bouchard et al (1986). It compares interestingly also with conclusions from non-twin studies, which we shall now consider.

As some of the instances in the previous section imply, one of the advantages of path analysis is that it can be applied to studies of family members less close than

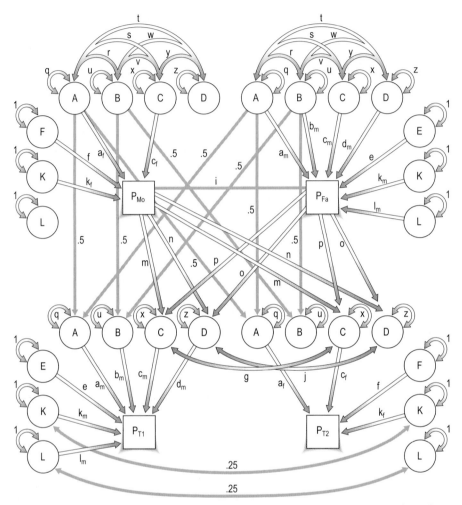

Figure 2.10 Path diagram for investigation of mixed genetic and cultural transmission using data from twins and their parents, allowing for sex differences in genetic and environmental effects. From Figure 4 of Maes et al (1996), with permission.

twins, such as parents and children, and other relatives by descent – of whom, of course, far larger numbers are available, and from whom additional types of information can be gleaned. It can even be structured to take account of adopted siblings; these are, as it were, the opposite of MZ twins, being subject only to environmental influences, without any shared heredity. (Opportunities for prospective parents to choose babies like themselves – which might be termed 'assortative adoption' – are extremely limited in most societies.) Perusse et al (1987) studied 1630 subjects living in 375 Quebec households, involving a total of nine different kinds of relative. They did not find it possible to subject all these people to $\dot{V}O_{2max}$ tests, instead utilizing physical work capacity at a heart rate of 150 beats·min^{-1} (PWC$_{150}$). Their analysis of these data led them to conclude that about 80% of the age-, gender- and weight-adjusted variance was associated with non-transmitted effects, and the remaining 20% attributable to cultural and lifestyle inheritance. Thus no genetic effect at all was identified! In assessing this result it is important to note that Fagard et al compared PWC_{150} with $\dot{V}O_{2max}$ in their study of a much smaller yet at the same time much tighter-knit group. They also found that PWC_{150}, after adjustments for the same complicating factors, reflected only a non-significant hereditary component. One has to suggest, therefore, that the assessment of power output at a given heart rate has, by some mechanism not yet identified, obscured the genetic contribution to that fitness.

Utilizing again as subjects almost all the people who took part in the 1987 investigation, Perusse et al (1989) examined not another physiological function but frequency of physical activity. They concluded that non-transmissible environmental factors were the major determinants of activity but 29% of the average influence within their large sample of people could be attributed to genetic factors, and 12% to transmitted cultural ones. Those of us who crusade for more physical activity might have hoped for the opposite ratio!

Of the five papers chosen to illustrate increasingly complex methodologies in the preceding two sections, we have just considered the findings of Fagard et al (1991) and of Perusse et al (1989), while those of Thomis et al (1998) were extensively recounted earlier in the chapter. The interest of Tiainen et al (2004) is, firstly, that it extends the subject range (previously confined to young adults, and to children plus their parents) to senior citizens; and secondly that it compares three muscle groups for shared and independent influences. The detailed quantitative findings, however, are likely to be of greater interest to practitioners than students, and will not be expounded here.

By contrast, the remaining paper, by Maes et al (1996), must be considered in detail. We have already seen that the analytic procedures used in this study were highly sophisticated. Equally impressive was the tally of 105 either-sex twin pairs, all 10 years old (and so pre-pubertal) plus at least one parent in each case (97 mothers, 84 fathers), from all of whom they were able to collect extensive anthropometric and performance data. Even the zygosity determination set a new standard, because it had been initiated when the twins were born and so included placental and fetal membrane details; determination of a range of blood groups (itself now regular practice in zygosity studies) had utilized umbilical blood and thus been non-invasive. Data were analysed twice – first using the twins alone, so that the results could be compared with other twin studies, and second as twin-parent analyses, which enabled cultural and assortment effects to be detected and comparisons to be made with other parent-offspring studies. (It was the final stage of the latter analysis which utilized the model reproduced in Fig. 2.10.)

In the twin-only analysis, inclusion of parameters for genetic dominance or interaction between twin phenotypes did not significantly improve the fit of models to data. Even the common environment factor (the 'C' in the ACE model) was only necessary for running speed and flexibility; gender heterogeneity was located in this component, suggesting that the differing social expectations and play choices of the two sexes were the differentiating influences – remember that these were *pre-pubertal* children! The genetic component was left accounting for only 23% of total running-speed variance in the boys and 33% in the girls; for flexibility the equivalent figures were 38% and 50%. In relation to other characteristics the AE model, sometimes even with equal parameters for the boys and the girls, gave the best fits, with genes accounting for ~70% variance in strength tests such as the bent-arm hang, and at least 80% for body fat, estimated from skinfolds. The most surprising and unexplained sex-difference, however, was for $\dot{V}O_{2peak}$ (the less exacting approximation to $\dot{V}O_{2max}$ testing, widely adopted in work with children). 85% of the $\dot{V}O_{2peak}$ variance was explained by genetic factors in the girls, yet there was no evidence of a genetic factor in the boys! The contrast with Klissouras's (1971) figure of 93% for boys of 7–13 years could not be more striking, yet remains totally unexplained.

When parental data were embodied in the analysis, many considerations arose. One of the first was that parent–child correlations were generally lower than DZ correlations, making it unlikely that cultural transmission was significant. Another striking aspect was that there were highly significant positive husband–wife correlations for several measures, including running speed, trunk strength and VO_{2peak}, indicating a considerable degree of assortative mating. However, spouses correlated negatively (although less strongly) for skinfolds; apparently, in this sample of nearly 100 couples, plumper men had tended to attract or be attracted by slimmer women, and *vice-versa*. In an instructive comparison with other findings in the literature, Maes et al note that, while their twin correlations are relatively high, especially for path rather than heritability analyses, their parent–offspring correlations are lower than in other studies. They suggest that the narrow age-range of their twins, and the large difference in age between the twins and their parents, may explain these differences: age-related variation would express itself as reduced detectable transmission.

Equally instructive is that the findings of Maes et al for twins tally well with those of Fagard et al (who had worked a few years earlier in a different department of the same Belgian university) yet diverge severely from the much lower figures of the Quebec school (e.g. Perusse et al 1987) and some other groups we have not discussed. Maes et al make the important point that their own principal method of path analysis, based around the ACE model, is fundamentally akin to Fagard's, whereas the other groups used models known by the acronyms TAU or BETA, which have different characteristics. The latter models allow variances to be partitioned into transmissible and non-transmissible components, but not into genetic and environmental: instead 'the transmissibility includes both heritability or biological inheritance and cultural inheritance'. This points up the fact that the choice of path-analytic procedures is a matter for judgement and preference – as much art as science.

In one more comment on analytic methods, Maes et al discuss the widespread practice of scaling performance parameters such as VO_{2max} and anaerobic power per unit body weight or fat-free mass. Their own results, as quoted above, were not scaled; when they did try scaling their VO_{2peak} data, lower heritability estimates resulted. They cite a classic paper (Tanner 1949) which shows that such scaling is less justified than superficially appears, and may result in misleading statistical conclusions. More recent arguments have underlined the need for caution in this respect (e.g. Winter & Nevill 1996).

Finally, Maes et al divide their motor tests into a group considered to relate principally to health (including trunk strength, VO_{2peak} and flexibility) and others related more to performance (including explosive strength, speed and balance). A suggestion in the earlier literature that performance-related characteristics were more determined by genetic factors than health-related ones was not supported by their findings.

One More Method

A further statistical method, the 'Quantitative Transmission/Disequilibrium Test' (QTDT), which may be regarded as a potentially important development out of path analysis, has recently been introduced by the Leuven team (Huygens et al 2004). In this paper the authors used it to place upper bounds on the heritabilities of skeletal muscle mass and strength parameters, valuably supplementing the previously rather few figures available on these aspects, which are central to the theme of this book. Their study was a large one, involving 748 pairs of young-adult male siblings. Maximal isometric strength measures of knee, trunk and elbow flexions and extensions had upper-limit values equivalent to h^2 values of 0.82–0.96. Concentric contraction strength measures, on an isokinetic dynamometer, gave only slightly lower figures (0.63–0.87). Indicators of muscle mass revealed very high transmissions (>0.90 or '90%'), and fat-free body mass, treated as an underlying factor, was the primary determinant of knee and trunk strengths. While it is imperative to note that these were upper bound figures, they are intriguingly much nearer to the kinds of figure produced from small-sample twin studies in the 1970s (although for different parameters) than from many in the intermediate period. The significance of this point will no doubt be extensively debated.

TAKING STOCK

Collected Figures

We have surveyed about 35 years of work, from which the first impression must be the widely varying conclusions about the extent – even, at times, the existence – of genetic influence on muscle properties and physical performance. Table 2.4 lists the heritability estimates quoted in this chapter. Estimates for other performance measures have been tabulated by Maes et al (1996), Klissouras (1997), Thomis et al (1998), Beunen & Thomis (2004) and Huygens et al (2004). Extensive information with similar implications, but expressed in terms of interclass correlation coefficients or F ratios instead of h^2, can be found in the various reviews by Bouchard and colleagues, notably Bouchard et al (1992) and Bouchard & Perusse (1997).

For the purposes of the rest of this book, the fundamental point is that all these parameters show sufficient indication of genetic influence that the mechanisms involved can fruitfully be pursued. Nevertheless, where there are several estimates for a given parameter, the divergence between the largest and smallest figures cannot comfortably be ignored.

Some of this variation must be attributed to the different samples of people studied. Careful investigators have always recognized that a heritability estimate is only applicable to the population actually sampled. Whether it is correct for that population will depend on whether the sample was representative, as well as on all the factors to be considered below. But whether it applies to a different population is a further question, which can only truly be answered by a separate study, because the environmental influences in a Canadian city, even if they are the same for MZ and DZ twins there, will be different from those in a Finnish or Greek city, let alone among the farming communities of Kenya or the Sherpas of Nepal. Equally likely is that the different genetic make-ups of these populations would lead to their responding differently to the *same* environment.

The next problem, just as applicable when comparing two studies of the same population as studies from two different ones, is that of sample size to which we have had to refer several times already. Every investigator would like to be able to include many more subjects than are practicable, but several though not all the studies we have cited were of very small samples. A basic element of good practice in this respect would be to publish the confidence limits of correlations and heritability estimates, yet this statistical discipline is often disregarded. However, the confidence limits themselves will inevitably be too narrow, because many other factors than limited

Table 2.4 Heritability estimates cited in text. NS – not significant

Parameter	Authors	Date	Heritability
$\dot{V}O_{2max}$	Klissouras	1971	93%
	Fagard et al	1991	80%
	Bouchard et al	1986a	47% (?~25%)
	Klissouras et al	1997	75–87%
$\dot{V}O_{2peak}$	Maes et al	1996	NS–83%
90-min work capacity	Bouchard et al	1986a	72%
30-sec work capacity	Klissouras et al	1997	86%
10-sec work capacity	Simoneau et al	1986	44–92%
Max anaerobic power	Klissouras et al	1997	86%
Sprint speed	Bouchard & Malina (review)	1983	45–90%
	Maes et al	1996	23–33%
Arm strength	Thomis et al	1998	77%
	Maes et al	1996	70%
	Huygens et al	2004	Up to 90%
Leg strength	Huygens et al	2004	Up to 70%
Trunk strength	Huygens et al	2004	Up to 77%
% type 1 fibres	Komi et al	1977	96%
	Bouchard et al	1986b	NS
	Simoneau et al	1995	~40–50%
Muscle enzymes	Komi et al	1977	NS
	Bouchard et al	1986b	30–67%
90-min trainability	Bouchard et al (review)	1992	+++
90-sec trainability	Bouchard et al (review)	1992	++
10-sec trainability	Bouchard et al (review)	1992	±
Enzyme trainability	Bouchard et al (review)	1992	+
% type 1 trainability	Bouchard et al (review)	1992	NS

sample-size are operative but cannot be estimated quantitatively: differences of age and gender are obvious, but not all their effects may be recognized; social differences, between and within societies, almost certainly have stronger and more diverse influences than can easily be appreciated, let alone given proper quantitative weight. And so on . . .!

There will also be errors of technical origin. In twin studies, the crucial matter of zygosity may not always be correctly determined. In any case the performance or muscle property being analysed will always embody some measurement error. Probably these are in most instances the smallest sources of difference between conclusions, but one cannot be sure.

Certainly, the assumptions made in the analysis of the data are critical, and have differed widely. But note first that the same assumptions may be a source of much greater error in one study than another: the equal-environments assumption in two different studies of, say, 30 twin pairs would be a case in point. Another example is the assumption in all twin-based heritability studies that there is no gene-environment interaction: we have already seen some reason and will see more to think that this may be more misleading in better trained subjects, but other kinds of gene-environment interaction may so far have gone unnoticed. The one point on which we can be sure is that all traditional heritability estimates are upper bounds, but will exceed the true figure by much greater extents in one instance than another.

As to the differences between assumptions, clearly path analysis allows more flexibility than older-style heritability estimation, and enables data from non-twin relatives and even non-relatives to be utilized. But assumptions are embodied in the different ways of conducting path analysis, and the wider the scope of the survey, the more divergent the outcomes of these different methods are likely to be. Within one fundamental approach – an ACE-type approach or a BETA one, for instance – it is possible to run one's analysis many different times, and study the effects on goodness of fit of including or excluding various possible influences, or giving them different weights, but no team to our knowledge has yet compared two entirely different approaches to the same data – i.e. to pursue our example, analysing the data by both ACE and BETA algorithms, and publishing the two outcomes side by side. Such comparisons could be highly illuminating!

However, it is a school pupil's error, though one all too often repeated in the media, that science is good only when it has achieved certainty. In fact, as we tackle more complex problems, whether in particle physics, meteorology or human genetics, the possibility of even coming near to certainty recedes. Science begins with the recording of simple observations and the making of basic measurements, and at this level there is not much scope for differences of approach. But as its ambition extends into harder and more complex problems, the contributions of the investigators' minds become much greater. We should not be unhappy with this – there is no other way. What we *can* ask is that researchers reporting their work should be at pains to spell out clearly what assumptions and models are involved. If there is a valid criticism of the literature in this field, it is that such spelling-out is often skimped. Both pressure to publish, and the desire of editors to keep papers as short as possible, contribute to this. The beginner entering the field must be alert to the problems from the outset, and strive to cultivate, as early as possible, sufficient understanding of the various methods to weigh up their conclusions for her- or himself.

GENE ACTION
What Do Genes Do?

The grossest misunderstanding of a percentage heritability estimate of X% is to think that it means that X% of the characteristic at issue is determined by genes, and the rest by environment. 'It would make no sense at all to say that of someone's height of five feet eleven and a half inches, five feet two were the result of her genes and the other nine and a half inches were put there by the food she ate' (Lewontin 1993). By the same token, as Klissouras (1997) points out, even if the Komi group's finding, that 96% of the influence on the percentage of Type 1 muscle fibres is genetic, were proved generally applicable to the Finnish population, that would not mean that 96% of a Finn's Type 1 fibres were determined by inheritance, and 4% by environmental influences. In fact, it is hard to imagine a more total misunderstanding than this would be. To see the error, it is probably helpful to argue in two steps. First, if it were the case that in every separate Finnish person 96% of the influence was genetic, that would mean that 96% of *the influence on every fibre's type* was genetic and 4% of it environmental – not 100% of the influence on 96% of fibres. But second, a heritability figure is a *population* statistic, an estimate of the extent to which heredity affects the variation of the attribute concerned in the population sampled. Within that population, individuals may be more or less strongly influenced by inheritance.

Just as importantly, it must be stressed that few, if any, genetic effects are totally deterministic. The nearest are the few instances where a single gene is responsible for the phenotype. An example often quoted is sickle cell anaemia: here the expression of sickle-shaped red blood cells cannot be avoided, but is fortunately not fatal. Another instance is Wilson's disease, a genetic defect preventing its sufferers from detoxifying the minute traces of copper absorbed from food, which is fatal if not treated. Yet people with this defective gene can lead a perfectly normal life . . . 'by taking a pill that helps them get rid of the copper', as Lewontin (1993) put it. The 'environmental' change represented by the drug's presence in the blood stream radically alters the effects of the gene. In any case, none of the muscle or performance properties with which we have been concerned has yet been shown to depend on a single gene, let alone in so radical a way as in these medical disorders. We are dealing with quantitative differences in potential between people who all have the genetic endowment to be reasonably healthy in a normal human environment without taking any special steps. In this circumstance, even more clearly than in that of Wilson's disease, genetic make-up does not determine phenotype, only the potential for expression of that phenotype in response to a particular lifestyle and environment. Thus it is common nowadays to find commentators warning that the traditional way of formulating the 'nature/nurture' dichotomy was dangerously over-simplified: 'nature' operates one way under one particular 'nurture', but may operate in quite another way with different nurture.

Genes and Sport

In the context of physical performance Klissouras put the above point vividly:

'No genes can operate in a vacuum, nor [can] phenotypes .. develop and be actualized without the action of environmental forces. Thus, when it is stated that VO_{2max} is highly heritable, what is really meant is that after individuals have reached the upper limits of their VO_{2max}, with appropriate training, there will still be a wide interindividual variability which is genetic in origin. The levels of absolute individual ceilings [are] reflection[s] of the actualized genetic potential of these individuals. . . . . Apparently training does contribute significantly to the development of VO_{2max}, but cannot contribute beyond a ceiling set by the genotype. Superior performers in aerobic sports are endowed with a higher genetic potential for VO_{2max}. However, this genetic potential is not a passive possibility but an active disposition realized through .. prodigious effort. The realization of the .. potential does not occur instantly. As Bromfenbrenner (1993) eloquently put it, "this dynamic potential does not spring forth full-blown like Athena out of Zeus's head from a single blow of Vulcan's hammer. The process of transforming genotypes into phenotypes is not so simple or so quick".'

(Klissouras 1997, p 4)

Where do Genetic Effects Show Most?

It follows from that passage that studies on the general population are likely to obscure the full extent of inter-individual genetic differences. There are two reasons: first, most people are largely sedentary, so would not show any of the training-dependent effects; second, the varying influences they are under will be difficult to represent adequately in a statistical analysis. Genetic differences are likely to be seen to best effect in people who have challenged their inherited capacities most strongly – for our purposes, therefore, in the most highly trained subjects. We see them at their least ambiguous in an Olympic final. Everyone who gets this far has been socially selected and personally trained to very near his/her genetic limits. Although one coach may be fractionally better than another, and one athlete fractionally luckier, the difference between first and last place is likely to be decided more by genetic potential than by anything else.

On these grounds, Klissouras has argued that twin *athletes* are the ideal subjects for evaluation of the relative powers of genes and environment to influence performance, and has initiated with colleagues a twin register for sports scientists to facilitate such research.

One Gene or Many?

Almost certainly no property with which we are concerned in physical performance is affected by one gene only – one gene, that is, with two different forms (or *alleles*). The great experiments of the Abbé Mendel, the rediscovery of which at the turn of the last century provided the foundation for modern genetics, were of that form. The heights, pod-colours, flower positions and colours, and other properties of the peas Mendel studied were each single-gene phenotypes. So are a small number of human heritable diseases as we noted on p 52. But most phenotypes are *polygenic*, influenced by many genes. We hope, rather than know, that the effects of these many genes are additive, not interactive in any of the more complex ways acknowledged as possible earlier in this chapter. Almost certainly the nearest exercise physiologists are likely to get to single-gene effects are instances similar to that of eye colour, in which the presence of the blue or brown allele of the principal gene can almost always be recognized, but the exact colour of each person's iris is affected by many other fine-tuning genetic influences. At present, however, even this is just a speculation – we do not yet know of any performance attribute on which a single gene has the predominant influence. The wise starting assumption is that all the phenotypes of interest to sport and exercise scientists are radically polygenic.

TOP-DOWN AND BOTTOM-UP

This chapter has been concerned with studies of the physiological and anatomical characteristics of groups of human beings, aimed at deriving indications of the relative importance of heredity on the one hand, and environment in its broadest sense on the other, in the development of that characteristic – that phenotype. What such studies cannot do is to define either the chromosomal location of any gene involved or the protein whose expression it controls. Regarding genes as at the bottom of a chain of influences and the whole human being as at the top, this latter approach is widely known as the 'bottom-up' approach, whereas what we have been considering in this chapter has been 'top-down' (Fig. 2.11). Alternative names are 'measured genotype' for bottom-up, and 'unmeasured genotype' (top-down). The first of these terms does not imply that the whole of the genotype will be measured in any single investigation, but technology already available allows checking for 100 000 gene variations in an overnight experiment.

Bottom-up methods figure substantially in the second half of this book (Chapters 4–6). The sequence of chapters reflects that of research. There would be no point in looking for the location or properties of a gene that influenced an aspect of the

Top-down

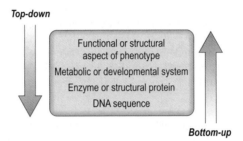

Functional or structural
aspect of phenotype
Metabolic or developmental system
Enzyme or structural protein
DNA sequence

Bottom-up

Figure 2.11   Diagrammatic representation of the comparison between 'top-down' (unmeasured genotype) and 'bottom-up' (measured genotype) strategies for investigation of genetic contributions to human performance.

phenotype which was in fact entirely determined by environmental factors. Notice, however, that all the top-down methods we have considered apply to the search for genetic differences *within a population, not between populations*: compare Clark's comments (p 35) and Box 2.1, on racial differences exemplified by East African runners. So researchers attacking such topics have done so on the basis of informal rather than formal top-down genetics. But top-down must come first, whether formal or not.

Hybrid Methods

A number of investigations which would be considered to come into the bottom-up category nevertheless make considerable use of techniques familiar in top-down work. One instance is the study of *quantitative trait loci* (QTLs). The term refers to the locations on the chromosomes of genes influencing a quantitative (as against an all-or-nothing) phenotypic trait. A minimum of two generations is required, and the greater the variance in the characteristic concerned the better for the investigation. Originally applied to animals, which could be selectively bred and cross-bred (Bouchard & Perusse 1997), the method even then had ample relevance to human studies because there is what is termed 'a high degree of homology' in the genomes of all mammalian species – that is to say, in the great majority of instances a gene influencing a particular phenotypic trait occurs in the equivalent ('homologous') location in every mammal including, of course, the human. More recently, however, QTL mapping has been performed directly on human subjects. This was first made possible by the HERITAGE Family Study, an extensive two-generation survey of families living near any one of five laboratories in the USA. A range of cardiovascular, metabolic and hormonal responses to aerobic exercise has been measured in the volunteers' initial, sedentary states and again after a standardized 20-week aerobic training programme. DNA was sampled from lymphoblasts and analysed, by methods outlined in Chapter 4 for genomic markers on each of the 22 non-sex chromosomes (autosomes). At the time of the report considered here (Bouchard et al 2000) 481 individuals, including 415 pairs of siblings, from 99 families had been fully documented. Multivariate analysis of variance, path analysis and heritability estimates were all deployed, and the results suggested the presence of genes associated with pre-training VO_{2max} on four different chromosomes and others associated with response to training on five.

Box 2.1

It is popularly accepted that certain ethnic groups have attributes which others do not. Some such impressions may be more myth than reality, but many are well founded. Bolivian Andeans are clearly selected for physical exertion under low oxygen partial pressure, people of West African descent seem particularly endowed for sprint and plyometric actions, while certain East and North Africans are particularly well adapted for middle- and long-distance running. At the end of the 2004 athletics season all world running records for males were held by men of 'black' African ancestry – distances from 100 to 400 m (including hurdles) by people of West African descent, and all from 800 m to the marathon by East or North Africans.

The especial prowess of a few relatively small highland tribes, notably the Nandi people of Kenya and the Oromos of Ethiopea, is a topic of vigorous research by teams from several countries, particularly Denmark, South Africa, Australia and the UK. Saltin et al (1995) were the first to establish some fundamental points, notably that – contrary to what might be predicted from the altitude at which they live – the Kenyans did not have higher $\dot{V}O_{2max}$ values than their Danish counterparts; nor were muscle properties significantly different among those similarly trained. Kenyan diet has been considered, but it is at best adequate, not exceptionally good (Christensen, 2004). The strongest candidate explanation for the African prowess is their physique; from Morocco to South Africa, 'black' distance runners are small, with particularly long, slim legs for their height. This enables them to run with exceptional economy, and thus maintain higher speed at given percentage of $\dot{V}O_{2max}$ than equally trained Caucasians (Noakes et al 2004). It also facilitates heat dissipation.

This raises the question why they have this physique, and a substantial genetic component immediately suggests itself. Furthermore, speculations can readily be formulated about lifestyle and social factors which could have offered strong selective advantages to those both physically and psychologically adapted to endurance – although whether such factors could have acted long enough to produce a significant effect is more doubtful. Certainly, attempts to isolate any genes involved have so far met with very limited success (Scott et 2004). The puzzle is therefore only partially resolved. At the time of going to press, the most convenient source for a wide range of information is the November 2004 issue (vol 1, part 4) of *Equine and Comparative Exercise Physiology*, which includes many of the papers cited above, plus an overview by one of us (Spurway 2004).

To conclude this box, however, note that a heritability study of Nandi or Oromo twins would probably give a very low figure for h^2. The reason is that if there are genes which make for their distance-running aptitude, not only all MZ, but all DZs too, probably share most or all of them. (This is the point made by Clark, in the quotation on p 35.) The logical impossibility of finding a pair of DZ twins, one of whom was of successful-runners' ethnicity and the other of 'ordinary' inheritance, would be necessary to s how that the former had propensities the latter lacked! And similarly with wider f amilial studies.

That is why we say in the main text (p 54) that the judgement, that genetic differences between different populations may help to explain their divergent physical performances, must be informal rather than formal. However, this perhaps sounds negative. A positive way to put the matter is that, where differences are obvious, formal statistical methods are not required. By contrast, where they are needed, they are happily available.

Rather similar combinations of top-down and bottom-up methods in the context of strength are exemplified by the work of Tiainen et al (2004), referred to earlier, and (Beunen & Thomis, 2004). Other examples, in connection with aerobic performance, were summarized by Hagberg at al (2001).

A CHALLENGE TO READERS

To conclude this chapter, let us recall the passage, from the Quebec laboratory, which we cited in the Preface:

> 'The greatest challenge at this time is to improve understanding of the potential of genetic and molecular medicine among the physical activity scientists, to train a new generation of these scientists to undertake these genetic studies, and to establish several competing centres of excellence where such investigations would be carried out routinely. Too few physical activity scientists and laboratories are involved in genetic and molecular biology research . . . Corrective measures and coordinated efforts are needed to explore the current revolution in the biological sciences, particularly in DNA technology and the study of the human genome.'
>
> (Bouchard & Perusse 1994, pp 115–116)

The situation has improved a little since this was written, but the scope for further development is great. Why not make it your business to respond?

KEY POINTS

1. Initial studies of the role of inheritance compared monozygous (MZ) with dizygous (DZ) twins, regarding the greater variation between the latter as wholly due to their non-identical genomes. Conclusions were expressed as 'heritability estimates' (H_{est}, a percentage, or h^2, a figure between 0.0 and 1.0).
2. Early values of H_{est} for performance parameters such as $\dot{V}O_{2max}$, and for the proportions of types 1 and 2 fibres in skeletal muscle, were over 90%. These are now considered to be atypically high, probably due partly to chance in relatively small samples and perhaps also partly to systematic errors such as more equal environmental influences on the MZ than the DZ twins. More recent values are typically in the range of about 40–80%, although some very high figures have still been obtained for measures of anaerobic performance.
3. Results of twin studies may also be expressed without assumptions, as the ratio of DZ variance to MZ variance (F); this must significantly exceed 1 to indicate a genetic effect. High values, ~10, are reported for aerobic performance parameters, but much lower ones for muscle fibre composition and usually intermediate ones for metabolic properties.
4. A more flexible statistical approach, path analysis, allows a wider range of family members to be compared, with consequently much larger samples. Simplifying assumptions are still needed, but different ones can be compared for their influence on the fit of model to data. It is even possible to look for non-additive effects, such as gene-gene interactions and dominant alleles, which have to be assumed absent in simple twin studies; however, such analyses are complex.
5. Path analyses commonly, but not always, produce lower heritability estimates than twin studies. Nevertheless, wherever either form of 'top-down' investigation

indicates significant genetic effects, attempts to identify specific genes involved ('bottom-up' investigations) are worth considering.
6. Formal top-down methods apply to the study of relatives. Unrelated groups cannot be compared this way, but where their performance capabilities obviously differ, as in the example of Kenyan highlanders versus Danes, bottom-up studies are also clearly justified.

Further Reading

The key text in this area is Bouchard et al (1997). Though dating slightly, it should be on the shelves of any serious student of the subject.

References

Beunen G, Thomis M 2004 Gene powered? Where to go from heritability (h^2) in muscle strength and power? Exercise and Sport Sciences Reviews 32:148–154

Bodmer W F, Cavalli-Sforza L L 1976 Genetics, evolution, and man. San Francisco, W H Freeman

Bouchard C, Malina R M 1983 Genetics of physiological fitness and motor performance. Exercise and Sports Sciences Reviews 11:306–339

Bouchard C, Perusse L 1994 Heredity, activity level, fitness and health. In: Bouchard C, Shephard R J, Stephens T (eds) physical activity, fitness and health. Champaign, IL, Human Kinetics p 106–118

Bouchard C, Lesage R, Lortie G et al 1986a Aerobic performance in brothers, dizygotic and monozygotic twins. Medicine and Science in Sports and Exercise 18:639–646

Bouchard C, Simoneau J A, Lortie G et al 1986b Genetic effects in human skeletal muscle fiber type distribution and enzyme activities. Canadian Journal of Physiology and Pharmacology 64:1245–1251

Bouchard C, Perusse L, Leblanc C 1990 Using MZ twins in experimental research to test for the presence of a genotype-environment interaction effect. Acta Geneticae Medicae et Gemmelologiae 39:84–89

Bouchard C, Dionne FT, Simoneau J A, Boulay M R 1992 Genetics of aerobic and anaerobic performances. Exercise and Sport Sciences Reviews 20:27–58

Bouchard C, Malina R M, Perusse L 1997 Genetics of fitness and physical performance. Champaign, IL, Human Kinetics

Bouchard C, Rankinen T, Chagnon Y C et al 2000 Genomic scan for maximal oxygen uptake and its response to training in the heritage family study. Journal of Applied Physiology 88:551–559

Bouchard T J Jr, Propping P 1993 Twins: Nature's twice-told tale. In: Bouchard T J Jr, Propping P (eds) Twins as a tool of behavioural genetics. Chichester, Wiley, p 1–15

Bromfenbrenner U, Ceci S J 1993 Heredity, environment and the question 'how?' – a first approximation. In: Plomin R, McCleary G E (eds) Nature-nurture and psychology. Washington, American Psychological Association, p 313–324

Christian J C, Norton J A, Sorbel J, Williams C J 1995 Comparison of analysis of variance and maximum likelihood based path analysis of twin data: Partitioning genetic and environmental sources of covariance. Genetic Epidemiology 12:27–35

Christian J C, Williams C J 2000 Comparison of analysis of variance and likelihood models of twin data analysis. In: Spector T D, Snieder H., MacGregor A J (eds) Advances in twin and sib-pair analysis. London, Greenwich Medical Media, p 103–118

Clark P J 1956 The heritability of certain anthropometric characters as ascertained from measurements of twins. American Journal of Human Genetics 7:49–54

Fagard R, Bielen E, Amery A 1991 Heritability of aerobic power and anaerobic energy generation during exercise. Journal of Applied Physiology 70:357–362

Falconer D S 1989 Introduction to quantitative genetics. Harlow, Longmans

Frankham R, Ballou J D, Briscoe D A 2002 Conservation genetics. Cambridge, University Press

Galton F 1869 Hereditary genius. London, Macmillan

Galton F 1875 The history of twins as a criterion of the relative powers of nature and nurture. Fraser's Magazine Nov: 566–576

Hagberg J M, Moore G E, Ferrell R E 2001 Specific genetic markers of endurance performance and $\dot{V}O_{2max}$. Exercise and Sport Sciences Reviews 29:15–19

Heath A C, Neale M C, Hewitt J K et al 1989 Testing structural equation models for twin data using LISREL. Behavior Genetics 19:9–35

Howald H 1976 Ultrastructure and biochemical function of skeletal muscle in twins. Annals of Human Biology 3:455–462

Huygens W, Thomis M A, Peeters M W et al 2004 Determinants and upper-limit heritabilities of skeletal muscle mass and strength. Canadian Journal of Applied Physiology 29:186–200

Kang K W, Christian J C, Norton J A 1978 Heritability estimates from twin studies. 1: Formulae of heritability estimates. Acta Geneticae Medicae et Gemmellologiae 27:39–44

Karlsson J, Komi P V, Viitasalo J H 1979 Muscle strength and muscle characteristics in monozygous and dizygous twins. Acta Physiologica Scandinavica 106:319–325

Klissouras V 1971 Heritability of adaptive variation. Journal of Applied Physiology 31:338–344

Klissouras V 1997 Heritability of adaptive variation revisited. Journal of Sports Medicine and Physical Fitness 37:1–6

Klissouras V, Pirnay F, Petit J-M 1973 Adaptation to maximal effort: genetics and age. Journal of Applied Physiology 35:288–293

Komi P V, Viitasalo J H T, Havu M, Thorstenssohn A et al 1977 Skeletal muscle fibres and enzyme activities in monozygous and dizygous twins of both sexes. Acta Physiologica Scandinavica 100:385–392

Lewontin R C 1993 The Doctrine of DNA: Biology as Ideology. London, Penguin

Maes H H M, Beunen G P, Vlietinck R F et al 1996 Inheritance of physical fitness in 10-yr-old twins and their parents. Medicine and Science in Sports and Exercise 28: 479–1491

Nimmo M A, Wilson R H, Snow D H 1985 The inheritance of skeletal muscle fibre composition in mice. Comparative Biochemistry and Physiology 81A: 109–115

Noakes TD, Harley YXR, Bosch AN et al 2004 Physiological function and neuromuscular recruitment in elite South African distance runners. Equine and Comparative Exercise Physiology 1: 261–271

Payne J, Montgomery H 2004 Angiotensin-converting enzyme and human physical performance. Equine and Comparative Exercise Physiology 1:255–260

Perusse L, Lortie G, Leblanc C et al 1987 Genetic and environmental sources of variation in physical fitness. Annals of Human Biology 14:425–434

Perusse L, Tremblay A, Leblanc C, Bouchard C 1989 Genetic and environmental influences on level of habitual physical activity and exercise participation. American Journal of Epidemiology 129:1012–1022

Prud'Homme D, Bouchard C, Leblanc C et al 1984 Sensitivity of maximum aerobic power to training is genotype-dependent. Medicine and Science in Sports and Exercise 16:489–493

Purcell S 2000 Statistical methods in behavioural genetics. In: Plomi R, DeFries J C, McClearn G E, McGuffin P (eds) Behavioural genetics, 4th edn, New York, Worth p 327–371

Rende R D, Plomin R, Vandenber S G 1990 Who discovered the twin method? Behavior Genetics 20:277–285

Saltin B, Larsen H, Terrados N et al 1995 Aerobic exercise capacity at sea level and at altitude in Kenyan boys, junior and senior runners compared with Scandinavian runners. Scandinavian Journal of Medicine & Science in Sports 5: 209–221

Scott R A, Moran C, Wilson R H et al 2004 Genetic influence on East African running success. Equine and Comparative Exercise Physiology 1:273–280

Simoneau J-A, Bouchard C 1995 Genetic determination of fibre type proportion in human skeletal muscle. FASEB Journal 9:1091–1095

Simoneau J-A, Lortie C, Leblanc C, Bouchard C 1986 Anaerobic work capacity in adopted and biological siblings. In: Malina R M, Bouchard C (eds) Sport and Human Genetics. Champaign, Human Kinetics, p 165–171

Spector T D 2000 The history of twin and sibling-pair studies. In: Spector T D, Snieder H., MacGregor A J (eds) Advances in twin and sib-pair analysis. London, Greenwich Medical Media, p 1–10

Spurway N C 1992 Aerobic exercise, anaerobic exercise and the lactate threshold. British Medical Bulletin 48:569–591

Spurway N C 2004 The secret of East African running prowess? Personal reactions to the Glasgow conference of 15 May 2004. Equine and Comparative Exercise Physiology 1:293–294

Sundet J M, Magnus P, Tambs K 1994 The heritability of maximal aerobic power: A study of Norwegian twins. Scandinavian Journal of Medicine and Science in Sports 4:181–185

Tanner J M 1949 The fallacy of per-weight and per-surface area standards and their relation to spurious correlation. Journal of Applied Physiology 2:1–15

Thomis M A I, Beunen G P, Maes H H et al 1998 Strength training: importance of genetic factors. Medicine and Science in Sports and Exercise 30:724–731

Tiainen K, Sipila S, Alen M et al 2004 Heritability of maximal isometric muscle strength in older female twins. Journal of Applied Physiology 96:173–180

Winter E M, Neville A 1996 Scaling: Adjusting for differences in body size. In: Easton R, Reilly T (eds) Procedures and data for kinanthropometry and exercise physiology. London, Chapman & Hall p 321–335

Chapter **3**

Types of skeletal muscle fibre

Neil Spurway

CHAPTER CONTENTS

LEARNING OBJECTIVES:

After studying this chapter, you should be able to . . .

1. Outline the history of our understanding that the fibres making up skeletal muscles are not all the same.
2. Understand the basic procedures of histology, enzyme histochemistry (qualitative and quantitative), biochemistry, electron microscopy, immunocytochemistry and physiological experimentation, as applied to mammalian and human skeletal muscle.
3. Discuss the validity of the concept that stable adult muscle fibres can be classified into definable types.
4. Describe the three major types into which large-mammal (including human) fibres have traditionally been divided since about 1970, giving their alternative names and both biochemical and physiological properties. Indicate two or three exceptions to this basic classification and make one comment on the significance of each.
5. Associate the properties and recruitment-order of the different sizes of motor unit with those of their constitutive fibre types.
6. Present the evidence that nerve activity is the predominant determinant of muscle fibre type, but name at least three competing non-neural influences.
7. Discuss the differences in fibre-type composition between different human muscles and the muscles of different humans – relating the former to function and the latter to sporting aptitude and mode of training.
8. Cite evidence from a range of animal muscles demonstrating the range of possible relationships between the different metabolic and contractile properties of muscle fibres.
9. Discuss the contractile properties of muscle fibres in relation to their chemical and structural features.
10. Comment on the relations of myosin types 2X and 2M to the isoforms you listed under objective 4.

MUSCULAR DIVERSITY

People's muscles differ. Even between 'identical' twins, and between the left and right sides of the same person, there are some differences. Between a 115 kg male rugby forward and a 45 kg desk-bound woman who spends her leisure watching television they are very much greater; and over the life-spans of each of these people, from infancy to very old age, they will be even greater still.

Nevertheless, the differences which are most obvious are differences of size, exact shape, and precise location relative to other body parts – differences of gross anatomy. All of these, insofar as they can be expressed numerically, will take the form of continuous variables: none of them are differences of kind.

Yet there *are* differences of kind, within the make-up of every given muscle in the body. Some are differences at molecular level, such as in the kind of myosin molecules incorporated into the contractile apparatus or the activities of the enzymes constituting a metabolic pathway. Others, although they, too, involve underlying molecular differences, are more evident at the level of ultrastructure; examples are the structure of the M line or the morphology of the sarcoplasmic reticulum. All such properties, molecular or structural, extend throughout the volume of any one muscle fibre, but will as likely as not be different between that fibre and its neighbour. However, an important further generalization, some evidence for which we shall explore below, is that the various properties tend to group, so that one pattern of molecular properties is usually found together with a particular pattern of structural ones and particular ranges of the quantitative ones. Consequently we may speak of different types of fibre – specific *fibre types*. This is only a first-order simplification, and is much more tenable in stable muscles than in a muscle undergoing rapid change through growth, injury, disease or training. Nevertheless, it will be a great help to our study.

There are also different fibre types both within the heart and between the various smooth muscles of the body, but it is on the fibre types of skeletal muscle that we shall focus in this book.

History

The grossest indication of different fibre types occurs where whole muscles or groups of muscles are made up of one type of fibre, and other muscles or groups of muscles in the same individual are made of another type. This does not happen in large mammals such as humans, but there are instances in smaller mammals such as guinea pigs (one of the rodents) and rabbits (one of the lagomorphs), and in many birds. The most striking instances of fibre-grouping, however, are in fish. Primitive humans, as soon as they had tools sufficient to cut across the after-body of a free-swimming fish (Fig. 3.1), must have been aware that in most species the bulk of the cross-section is

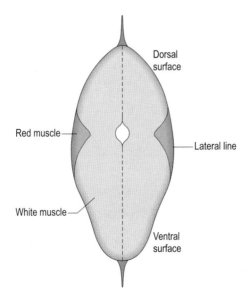

Figure 3.1   Section through the muscular part of a continually-swimming fish such as mackerel. 'Red' (red-brown) muscle lies immediately beneath the skin, about half-way up each side, just deep to the sensory structure called the lateral line. The rest of the musculature is white. Modern electromyography (Johnson et al 1977) shows that the red muscle is all that is used in normal, 'cruising-speed' swimming; white muscle is recruited only for power bursts, in hunting or escape. Often there is a 'pink' band between the red and white regions; in these cases, the pink zone is recruited at intermediate speeds. Obviously such functional differences could not have been known to our pre-scientific ancestors, but they could not have failed to notice the basic colour differentiation.

white, but a band of brown or reddish muscle runs lengthwise down the middle of each side, just deep to the line of structures on the skin where the colour changes from dark above to pale beneath – what we now call the 'lateral line'.

This is the most classical distinction between types of skeletal musculature. The two types are known as *white muscle* and *red muscle*, although the 'white' may often be cream-coloured or very pale pink, and the 'red' is often russet or brown. The first written description of the red/white distinction in mammalian muscle which modern historians of science have recognized was by an Italian, Lorenzini, in the 1670s. His account, which was of rabbit muscles, did not reach down to the microscopic level, however, and the scientist usually accredited with the first description of white versus red *fibres* is Ranvier (1873). However, Figure 3.2, from a paper by Bowman (1840), indicates that the distinction had already been effectively observed by that date: the smaller, more granular fibres are the ones which, grouped together in bulk, look red; the larger, less granular, look white. Bowman does not refer to this difference in his text, and it would be interesting to know whether this was because the distinction was already well-known, or because he did not think it important. But we should note that he (or his draughtsman, if this was not Bowman) saw the two main types in representative vertebrates of every main class – fish (in this case a bony fish), amphibians, reptile, birds and mammals – although the distinction in the mammal he chose, the human, is less clear than in the other species. We shall see later that it is still much clearer in all smaller mammals, and many other large ones, than it is in the human, especially when that human is untrained.

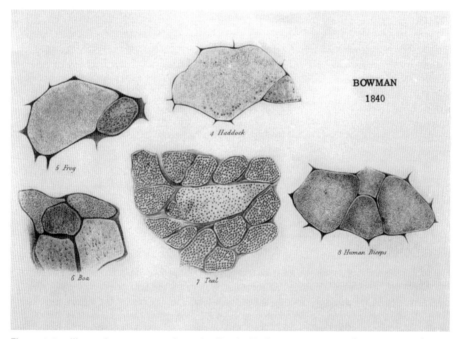

Figure 3.2 Illustration to a paper from the first half of the 19th century (Bowman 1840), showing that the existence of two types of muscle fibre – small, granular and pigmented versus large, agranular and pale – was already recognized in representatives of each of the major vertebrate classes, although less clearly demarcated in humans than the other species.

Ranvier's true innovation was to find that functional differences were associated with the differences of appearance. Stimulating red muscles, he found that their responses to a single electrical shock (their 'twitches') were three to four times longer than those of white muscles. So the generalization, 'red = slow twitch, white = fast twitch', entered the literature. We shall see below that this is not entirely valid, but it was a useful start. What Ranvier was not able to do was to compare the *fatigue resistances* of red and white muscles. He was working just a few years before Ringer described the first true physiological saline, containing appropriate amounts of potassium and calcium salts as well as sodium chloride. In the solutions available to Ranvier, neither white nor red would have gone on contracting very long. If he *could* have stimulated them repeatedly in well oxygenated Ringer's solution, he would have found that red muscles retained the ability to contract long after white ones had fatigued down to almost zero excitability. And *this* generalization would have proved universally valid, because redness is due to the presence of iron-containing pigments – what we would now refer to as myoglobin and the cytochromes – enabling aerobic metabolism to continue as long as oxygen supply is maintained. So, merging modern knowledge with Ranvier's findings, we should really say that red muscles (and their constitutive fibres) are *usually* slow-twitch, but *always* of high fatigue resistance.

(You can get a strong hint of the correct understanding here simply by looking at the muscles of birds in a poulterer's shop. Chickens and turkeys, which scarcely fly at all, have very pale breast [pectoral] muscles, but in ducks and geese, which can fly long distances, the pectorals are rich red-brown. Yet the leg muscles of all these species, at least if they have been allowed to live free-range, are relatively pigmented because the legs are in use for walking or swimming all day.)

In the hundred years following Ranvier's publication, people came increasingly to feel that in most species of vertebrate it was useful to designate a third type of fibre. But what that fibre's properties were would be stated differently according to species, age, fitness status, and technique of study. For instance, with the best techniques available in the middle of the 20th century, conclusions about the domestic fowl, a widely studied species, would differ significantly according to whether a battery-reared or free-range bird was used. In this situation, far-sighted perceptions were often obscured by subsequent misunderstandings, or mistakenly-assumed equivalences. To see the reasons for some of the false trails, as well as following how modern understanding developed, we need to look thoroughly at the techniques employed – particularly those developed since about 1950.

HISTOLOGICAL AND HISTOCHEMICAL TECHNIQUES
Classical Histology

The light microscope has been a crucial tool in the study of muscle fibre types, individual fibres being too narrow to be examined effectively by eye. Until well into the 20th century, microscopical sections could be cut only from blocks of tissue which had been chemically preserved ('fixed'), then dehydrated in alcohols before being embedded in hot wax – the sections being cut when the wax had cooled again. All fixatives destroy enzymic activity: as far as the enzymes involved in post-mortem degradation are concerned, this is part of the very purpose of fixation. With these techniques the main structural components of muscle fibres could be seen – sarcolemma, contractile filaments, mitochondria and (in special silver- or gold-impregnated preparations) sarcoplasmic reticulum and neuromuscular junction. The only chemical features identifiable, however, were bulk accumulations of relatively unreactive substances, essentially the metabolic stores of *lipid* and *glycogen*, plus the oxygen-handling protein, *myoglobin*.

Mitochondria, lipid droplets and myoglobin are all involved in oxidative (aerobic) metabolism, the first two being also the major contributors to the kind of granular appearance predominant in the small fibres of Figure 3.2; thus rough indicators of aerobic capacity were available from an early stage. Glycogen could be assumed to be at high concentration only in fibres with high glycolytic capacity, which would therefore be capable of vigorous anaerobic metabolism, although of course glycolysis could also be aerobic if the fibre had sufficient mitochondria and oxygen was not in short supply. These indicators were, however, indirect and fairly crude, and in any case they gave no information, however indirectly, about the mechanical properties of muscle, such as twitch-duration or shortening velocity.

Histochemistry

For these contractile features, as well as for markers of other aspects of metabolic capacity, *histochemistry* was required. Histochemical preparations are not fixed but simply frozen very rapidly – 'quench frozen'. The best technique involves taking specimens of tissue, measuring only a few mm in at least two if not all three directions, and plunging them into an organic liquid which itself is cooled in liquid nitrogen. (If the specimen is dropped directly into the nitrogen it will instantly boil the liquid nearest to it, and thereafter be enclosed in bubbles of N_2 gas which constitute an insulating layer and retard the tissue's cooling.) The intermediate organic liquid selected will be one which is liquid from tissue temperature down almost, if not quite, to that of liquid nitrogen ($-192°C$); tissue specimens dropped into it produce vigorous convective stirring and thereby cool much of their thickness to below the freezing points of their constituent fluids in less than a second. Ice crystals formed so fast are tiny, even by the standards of a high-resolution light microscope, whereas ones which take longer to form have time to grow large, and leave visible holes ('ice artefact') in the tissue.

Once the block is frozen, sections are cut from it using a microtome enclosed in a refrigerated compartment, a 'cryostat'. These sections are collected on glass cover-slips, air-dried in a few seconds at room temperature, and then subjected to a specific chemical reaction, usually to demonstrate a particular enzyme in the tissue (*enzyme histochemistry*). Although only one reaction can be carried out on any one section, quite broad chemical characterisations of individual fibres can be built up using serial sections, cut transversely through the sample of muscle tissue (Fig. 3.3). Helped by the shapes of the subdivisions ('fasciculi') within the muscle, and local anatomical landmarks such as small blood vessels, it is usually quite easy to identify the same fibres in all the sections, however they have been reacted. The resultant multi-reaction description of an individual muscle fibre is termed its *histochemical profile*.

Metabolic Enzymes

It happens that the first category of enzymes readily demonstrated histochemically were aerobic ones, such as *succinate dehydrogenase* (SDH), a mitochondrial enzyme of the tricarboxylic cycle. Another widely-used reaction was for *NADH-tetrazolium reductase*, an artificial marker of oxidative function which was usually, but not quite always, proportional to the true, biological capacity for aerobic metabolism. Its name, however, is instructive: 'tetrazolium' (four-nitrogen) salts were the reagents used to

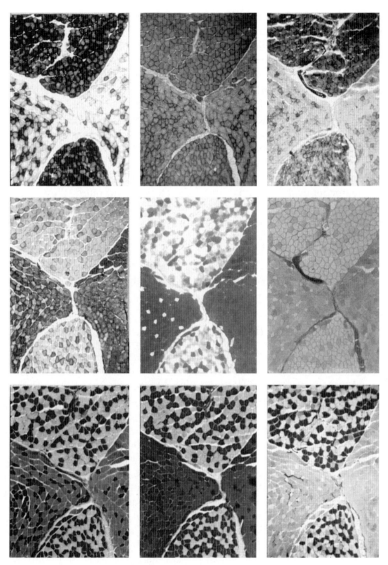

Figure 3.3 Series of nine closely-adjacent transverse cryostat sections from a single block of muscles taken from the rear lower leg ('calf muscles') of a mouse, at the point where two 'slow' muscles (top: soleus; bottom: a specialized region of medial gastrocnemius found only in small rodents) meet two 'fast' ones (right: lateral gastrocnemius; left: plantaris). Top row: three reactions indicative of aerobic capacity (succinate dehydrogenase, NADH-tetrazolium reductase and the Sudan Black stain for stored lipid). Middle row: indicators of anaerobic capacity (α-glycerophosphate dehydrogenase, the active 'a' form of glycogen phosphorylase, and PAS reaction for stored glycogen). Bottom row: myosin ATPase reactions (respectively after alkaline pretreatment, negligible pretreatment following a method of Brooke & Kaiser, and after acid pretreatment). Preparation: Mrs Anne Ferrel. From Figure 2 of Spurway (1981), with permission

capture electrons from the particular substrate which had been introduced into the reaction medium – succinate and NADH in our respective examples. The tetrazolium salts would do this in proportion to the tissue's activity of the enzyme specific for that substrate, and would then precipitate out, at the site of the reaction, to form an insoluble, dark (usually purple) deposit. Because these rather remarkable reagents came early onto the scene, and conveniently also made a bridge with what could be deduced by the older, histological techniques, aerobic capacity was the first property of muscle fibres to be well studied. At that stage (roughly 1940s–1960s), if a third fibre type was identified, in addition to the small, slow, 'red' and the large, fast, 'white' ones of Ranvier, it would invariably be one of intermediate aerobic capacity. Usually it would be assumed to be of intermediate speed as well, but this assumption was entirely unsupported by evidence and often, as we shall see, seriously misleading.

Other histochemical methods were developed, although they were often considerably more complicated than those for oxidative enzymes. Thus it gradually became possible to study the main pathways for both lipid and carbohydrate metabolisms (*lipolysis* and *glycolysis*), along with the enzymes directly involved in handling glycogen. The one responsible for breaking down stored glycogen to feed hexose units into the glycolytic pathway, *glycogen phosphorylase* (GP or PPL, often referred to simply as 'phosphorylase'), was another reaction with reasonably convenient properties, and was widely used.

Myosin ATPase – Basic Reactions

All the foregoing, from SDH to GP, are *metabolic enzymes* – enzymes concerned with the supply of ATP. A balanced picture of muscle fibre chemistry could not be achieved until the systems consuming ATP could also be studied. Necessarily, these are all *ATPases*. Most important for our understanding has been the ATPase of force generation – that by which the acto-myosin cross-bridge hydrolyses ATP to perform a cross-bridge cycle. The activity of this enzyme is a chemical indicator of the velocity at which the intact fibre could shorten. However, there are other ATPases in each muscle fibre. Those responsible for pumping calcium ions back into the sarcoplasmic reticulum (SR) after a contraction are also important, and indicate twitch duration. The surface membrane ATPase driving the sodium/potassium pump, and the ATPases of the mitochondria themselves, are present and active too.

The basic procedure for demonstrating ATPases utilizes the phosphate produced when these enzymes hydrolyse their substrate. Cryostat-cut sections are incubated in a medium containing ATP and a salt whose cation will readily precipitate out when it encounters phosphate ions. The deposit is then made visible by follow-up reactions which replace the precipitated phosphate (white) by a dark substance – usually cobalt sulphide (brown). However, if the initial incubation is done in conditions close to those of living cytoplasm all the ATPases of the cell catalyse similar reactions and the whole cross-section of every fibre finishes up an indiscrimate brown. Selective ATPase reactions therefore depend on finding circumstances in which all other ATPases are more or less completely inhibited, yet the one being investigated still functions. In the 1950s and early 1960s Padykula and her co-workers identified such conditions for the ATPase of the myofibrils. At a pH of 9.4 (more than 2 full units alkaline of normal cytoplasm), in a solution containing 10–20 mmole·L^{-1} calcium (~10^4 times more than in contracting muscle!), an ATPase capacity of the myosin headgroups is activated and precipitates calcium phosphate from ATP, while all other ATPases of the cytoplasm are more or less strongly inhibited. This high-pH, calcium-activated ATPase does not involve the actin filaments, so it is termed the *myosin ATPase* (mATPase), but fortunately its activity correlates fairly closely with that which would have been displayed by the true force-generating *acto-myosin ATPase* (amATPase) at cellular pH, and hence with the speed of contraction (Barany 1967). Consequently, a muscle fibre which stains strongly under the mATPase reaction may be taken to have been a fast-contracting fibre, and one which stains weakly may be classified as slow.

Myosin ATPase Reaction After Pre-treatments

The discrimination achieved by the basic mATPase reaction is not always a bold one, but a number of different pre-treatments ('pre-incubations'), performed before the incubation in ATP-containing medium, enhance the fast–slow distinction. One of the most widely used of these pre-incubating media (Brooke & Kaiser 1970, Guth & Samaha 1969) is a buffer solution of even higher pH than the subsequent ATP-containing medium – typically pH 10.4 – usually preceded by a short fixation in cold, dilute formaldehyde. Such a multi-stage reaction is properly called an 'alkali-pre-incubated mATPase reaction' or, almost universally, *'alkaline ATPase'* for short. It is important to appreciate that the alkaline step referred to is the pre-incubation at ~10.4, *not* the incubation at 9.4. The logic of this becomes evident when an alternative pre-incubation at pH ~4.4 (without the formaldehyde step) is considered. This is the 'acid-pre-incubated mATPase reaction', or *'acid ATPase'*. Incubation with ATP at this pH would produce no deposits, not only because calcium phosphate is soluble at such acidity but also because ATPase enzymes are inactive. So the adjectives 'acid' and 'alkaline' refer to the *pre*-incubations; the not-quite-so-alkaline incubation which follows is the same for both. Note that the effects of the pre-treatments are permanent – selective 'denaturings' of some enzymes while others survive. Contrast this with 'inhibition', a reduction of activity in a particular medium which is reversed if the medium is changed. Figure 3.4 shows the sequence of reactions diagrammatically.

What the acid pre-incubation does is to destroy the ATPase capacity of fast myosin, but maintain or even enhance that of slow; so slow fibres stain dark when the subsequent hydrolytic reaction and its follow-up visualization steps are carried out, while fast fibres remain pale. At least, this is what happens when the acid step has been applied strongly. Slightly less severe treatment, normally achieved by adjusting the pH to 4.65–4.8, but affected also by such factors as the molarity and temperature of the medium and the duration of the treatment, subdivides the fast fibres: the largest are left with a moderate stain, and only the smaller fast fibres are completely pale. The same distinction can be made with the alkaline pre-treatment: the largest fast fibres stain most strongly in most mammalian species, with the smaller ones intermediate between these and the slow fibres. In rodent muscle, however, the small fast fibres are darkest. This is important, because the physiological evidence (described below) is that these smaller 'fast' fibres are not quite as fast, either in terms of twitch duration or of shortening speed, as the larger ones. The alkali-pre-treated reaction in the muscles of most mammals could suggest that the less-fast fibres contain a mixture of fast and slow myosins. However, the rodent picture, and the effects of acid pre-treatment, combine to rule this out. The smaller fibres have a third form of myosin, not a mixture.

Physiological Experiments

As we acknowledged at the beginning of this chapter, a few mammalian muscles do consist of only one type of fibre: soleus in the guinea pig, for instance, is composed entirely of slow, red fibres, and most if not quite all of rabbit psoas entirely of fast,

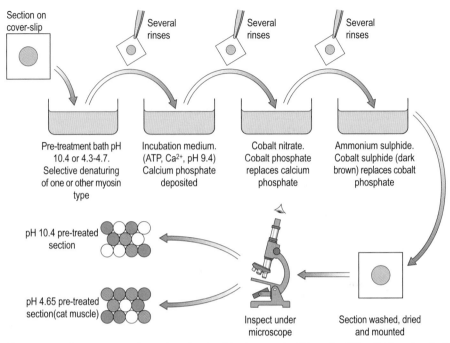

Figure 3.4 The sequence of reactions involved in the myosin ATPase ('mATPase') histochemical reaction, with acid or alkaline pre-treatment.

white ones. Comparisons involving different species, however, are complicated by many factors other than fibre type, only within a species, and better still within a single muscle of that species, can properties which are entirely the consequences of fibre type be convincingly studied.

Work of this kind flourished in the 1970s, immediately after the histochemical methods described above had become established. The biological feature making them possible is that muscle fibres controlled by a single motor nerve fibre – i.e. the fibres comprising a single *motor unit* – have proved to be all of one type. Thus if single motor axons are exposed by experimental surgery, and then electrically stimulated, the fibres which contract in response to the stimulus will all be of one type

Because the fibres of a single motor unit do not lie side-by-side in the muscle, instead being distributed quite widely through it, a further technical development was necessary to identify them. The standard method was to fatigue a motor unit, after establishing its properties, by repeatedly stimulating its nerve axon (normally at the ventral root, Fig. 3.5) while the blood supply to the limb was cut off by a tourniquet, till the unit was almost incapable of producing any force at all. This depleted the glycogen stores of the muscle fibres making up that unit, so that when the part of the muscle which had been active was subsequently either fixed, or rapid-frozen and sectioned in a cryostat, the fibres of the motor unit concerned would be negligibly stained in sections reacted for glycogen. However, their other reactions had no cause to be affected; so, by following the same fibres in neighbouring sections, their overall histochemical profiles could be built up. For accounts of the methods described in this section, as they were developed and applied to the muscles of laboratory animals, see Burke et al (1973), Burke & Edgerton (1975) and Burke (1980).

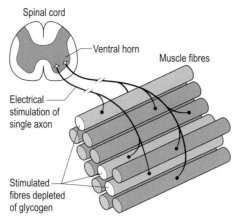

Figure 3.5   Diagrammatic summary of procedure involved in glycogen depletion of muscle fibres belonging to a single motor unit.

Obviously these techniques cannot be applied exactly as described to human muscles, but Garnett et al (1979) came impressively close by stimulating single axons near where they entered the medial gastrocnemius, and taking biopsies for the subsequent histochemistry.

CHEMICAL QUANTIFICATION

Biochemistry

Routine histochemical methods lead to descriptions of fibres in terms of adjectives ('dark', 'light' and 'intermediate') or visual assessment of reaction-intensities on scales from '0' to '+++' or '++++'. Progress beyond such semi-quantification was first achieved biochemically.

However, everyday biochemical methods require quite sizeable samples of tissue. Thus they are again limited by the fact that muscles consisting of only one fibre type are rare in mammals, and there is no laboratory species with two different muscles, respectively consisting 100% of one type of fibre in one and 100% of another type in the other. Early attempts to introduce the quantitative precision of biochemistry into fibre-type comparisons were based on relaxing this condition slightly, by using some muscles in which a given fibre type was only strongly, not 100%, predominant. Guinea pigs and rabbits provided some of the most suitable material (Peter et al 1972).

A further contribution from biochemical studies of multi-fibre muscle samples was the concept of 'constant proportion groups'. Analysing a wide range of muscles, from invertebrates as well as mammals and birds, Pette and colleagues found that any specimen in which, say, succinate dehydrogenase displayed high activity would have all other enzymes of oxidative metabolism (tricarboxylic acid cycle and oxidative phosphorylation) such as malate dehydrogenase, citrate synthase and cytochrome c reductase, high too. Conversely, where one of these activities was low, all would be low. Different muscles could vary as much as two orders of magnitude in their activity, but each member of this oxidative group would vary in close proportion one to another, the maximum range of within-group variation being about two-fold. Other such 'constant proportion groups' were the enzymes of lipolysis, those of glycolysis and those of glycogenolysis. This meant that any one member of such a group could be taken as representative of them all, except where extreme precision was required. To do so had been histochemical practice for some time, but it had not been quantitatively justified before.

The original publications on constant proportion groups were in German, although an English-language review giving them reasonable mention was provided by Pette & Hofer (1980). A further step, however, was presented from early on in English: this was to compare the activity of a representative enzyme from one constant proportion group with that of a different enzyme representing another group (Bass et al 1969). Such *'discriminative ratios'* could exceed 1000 – e.g. the ratio of glycolytic to TCA cycle activities in the fast, wholly white-fibred rabbit muscles psoas major and adductor magnus. The same ratio was ~10 in certain wholly-red muscles such as soleus and masseter, so it varied, within that single species, by two orders of magnitude. Another example was glycogenolytic capacity: although consistently in close proportion to glycolytic, this was ~100 times greater than that of hexokinase (HK) in the fast, white muscles yet of the same order of activity as HK in slow, reds. As HK functions to convey glucose units, just adsorbed from the blood, directly into the glycolytic pathway, this shows that such direct metabolism of glucose is a substantial feature of red muscles whereas, in white, glucose is virtually always routed into the glycogen stores. In the mammalian muscles studied, lipid oxidation was always closely proportionate to the TCA cycle, but it was much less in bee flight muscles whose oxidative metabolism was essentially of carbohydrate. One should note, however, that no rabbit muscle comes near to being homogeneously composed of the third type of fibre which we shall consider extensively below – the fast, red fibre – so Bass et al could not study these, although Peter et al, by using guinea pigs, were able to do so. Histochemical evidence suggests that, in some mammalian species, lipolytic capacity may fall considerably short of oxidative in some if not all fast, red fibres.

The paucity of whole muscles consisting even predominantly, let alone wholly, of one type of fibre gave the impetus to a key technical breakthrough in this field, the introduction of *single fibre biochemistry*. In this technique, muscle specimens are fast-frozen as if for histochemistry, but then vacuum-dried before dissection with sharp needles which cut the fine connective tissue strands holding the muscle fibres together. Complete fibres do not need to be isolated: lengths of about 1 cm, of reasonably large-diameter fibres, suffice to allow qualitative assay for two to four metabolic enzymes – which were usually chosen with constant proportion groups and discriminative ratios in mind. The laboratories of Saltin, Lowry and Pette took the lead in these elegant techniques, their work being reviewed by Pette & Staron (1990). At first, the myosin type was determined in a fragment of each fibre by essentially histochemical, qualitative reactions, leaving the continuous-variable, quantitative assessments to be made only on the metabolic eznzymes. More recent developments, however, utilize electrophoretic and molecular-biological methods (for the latter see Ch. 4) to study the myosin heavy chain (MHC) isoforms and their precursor RNAs, with results that are not only highly discriminative qualitatively but are also quantitative. Pette et al (1999) have reviewed these methods.

Quantitative Histochemistry

Even single-fibre biochemistry has shortcomings: it is biased towards the larger-diameter fibres, narrower ones being harder to dissect and to analyse, and only the crudest information about anatomical location can be retained. A complementary approach, avoiding these problems, was also explored about the same time, namely

(A)   (B)

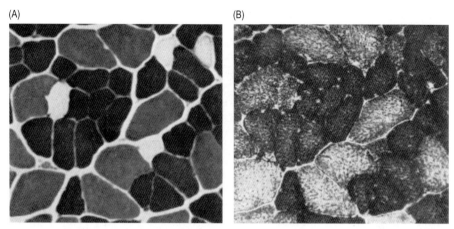

Figure 3.6   Serial transverse cryostat sections of mouse gastrocnemius (deep medial part). (A) mATPase reaction after alkaline pre-treatment: three types of fibre are clearly distinguished. (B) Succinate dehydrogenase reaction giving a wide and continuous distribution of mean densities.

quantitative histochemistry (Spurway 1980). In this technique the narrow light-beam of a microphotometer is passed through the cross section of one fibre at a time, or better still a series of small portions of one fibre at a time, and an assay of the mean density of the reaction product in that fibre is arrived at. The main problems with this are optical: only where the product is uniformly deposited across the area scanned is the light absorbtion strictly proportional to the amount of product. This problem ('distribution error') is approximately, but only approximately, compensated for by averaging the readings from many small areas – sophisticated 'scanning microdensitometers' do this semi-automatically. Despite this compensation being less than perfect, quantitative histochemistry and single-fibre biochemical analysis point to the same general conclusion – that the majority of fibres in stable, mature skeletal muscles can be typed fairly decisively by the kind of *myosin* they contain, but the *metabolic* variables within each myosin-based type vary over wide ranges, often overlapping those of other myosin types. This tallies with the impression given by visual inspection of histochemical preparations (Fig. 3.6).

ELECTRON MICROSCOPY

Electron microscopy (E/M) has been brought to bear intermittently from early in the modern period of fibre-type research. The ultrastructural features which can easily be correlated with light microscope histology and histochemistry are the presence, and locations within fibres, of mitochondria and fat droplets. In the early period, even authors well placed to notice correlations also with mATPase reactions in fact placed their emphases on structures involved in oxidative metabolism. As one would expect, the correlations were almost 1:1: not only the packing densities of mitochondria and lipid droplets but their locations within the fibres tallied extremely closely with descriptions from light microscopy. A widespread feature of highly oxidative fibres, for instance, was that the greatest density of mitochondria was just beneath the sarcolemma ('subsarcolemmal mitochondria': see smaller fibres in Fig. 3.7).

Gradually, however, specific features related to the contractile filaments came to be appreciated. Gauthier (1969) had noticed that the Z lines varied in thickness between

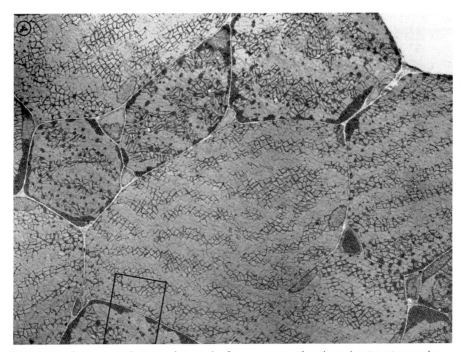

Figure 3.7   Low power electron micrograph of transverse section through rat gastrocnemius muscle. Black profiles (subsarcolemmal clumps, intracytoplasmic spots and fine networks) are aggregates of mitochondria, perhaps in latter case associated with sarcoplasmic reticulum. Large fibres (type 2B) have only the networks, constituting a small fraction of fibre volume. Mitochondrial volume fractions in smaller fibres (probably all type 2A in this specimen) are much higher, and include characteristic subsarcolemmal aggregates. Reproduced from Figure 4 of Schiaffino et al (1970) by copyright permission of The Rockefeller University Press.

different types of fibre. Later the same proved true of the M lines. The sarcoplasmic reticulum and, to less striking extents the T-tubes, also differ, but more sophisticated *'stereological'* (space-studying) methods than simple application of a ruler are required to quantify the comparisons. Stereology involves the laying of various forms of grid over a series of micrographs, and counting the intersections of grid lines with membranes, or the incidence of other components within grid-squares. Most features of the contractile apparatus and membrane systems could be most readily seen in longitudinal sections; by contrast, it is easier to assess mitochondrial density and distribution in sections cut transversely.

Electron microscope studies of different mammalian fibre types, and methods for quantification of observed features, were reviewed by Eisenberg (1983).

IMMUNOCYTOCHEMISTRY (IMMUNOHISTOCHEMISTRY)

This is the most recent microscopical technique we need to consider. First a protein – almost always, in muscle studies, a myofibrillar protein such as troponin or, most commonly of all, myosin (whole molecule or a sizeable component: typically the myosin heavy chain, MHC) – is prepared from the tissues of one animal. Emphasis is placed on getting this protein from a tissue sample containing only one type of fibre: fortunately fish or bird muscle, in which this condition is much more easily met, is as useful for many purposes as mammalian. A series of injections of the protein is then made into a host animal, which usually *is* a mammal, whose immune system is thereby challenged to make antibodies against the original protein. After sufficient time for the antibody titre to build up, serum is taken from the injected animal, and the antibody separated out. The antibody will be named first by the host animal which produced the antibody, then the source and type of protein. An example might be 'goat anti-turbot white-muscle MHC', meaning an antibody raised in a goat by injecting it with myosin heavy chains from the white musculature of a turbot.

After preparation, the antibody molecules are labelled or 'tagged' in a way which makes them visualizable on a microscope section. The labelled antibody is kept refrigerated until, in very dilute solution, it is applied to a section (usually from a cryostat, but in some cases fixed) of a third animal's muscle. The tag may be a fluorescent marker such as fluorescein (*fluorescent antibody technique*) or a non-mammalian enzyme which will catalyze the formation of a visible product. Horse radish peroxidase is a favoured choice; a subsequent reaction with hydrogen peroxide in the presence of di-amino benzene (DAB) creates a stable brown deposit where the selective antibody bound to the tissue (*immunoperoxidase technique*). Since fluorescence fades with use whereas the DAB product does not, this latter method is now more commonly used; fluorescence may enable smaller amounts of labelled material to be detected, but this will not often be a problem in skeletal muscle fibre typing because almost all the proteins studied are present in high concentration.

When the antibody interacts with the sectioned tissue it binds, in the ideal case, only to molecules which have a sequence of amino acids identical or closely similar to a group on the original molecule against which the antibody was raised. This group is termed the 'antibody determinant'. There are generally several sites on a protein capable of eliciting an antibody response, so not even all goat anti-turbot MHC antibodies will have identical properties, and ones which turn out to be really good are treasured. The value of the technique is that large parts of molecules with like functions are identical or closely similar in all vertebrates, their amino acid sequences having been evolutionarily conserved (Ch. 1). So an antibody raised against, say, fish fast-muscle myosin will have high affinity for one or more forms of fast myosin in a sectioned muscle from a mouse or man.

Various techniques exist for improving the selectivity of antibodies raised as described above. But much greater precision can be obtained if the injected protein is not obtained by extraction from a sample of whole tissue but synthesized by cloned bacteria into which a short gene sequence specifying part of the protein of interest has been introduced by molecular biological techniques (cf. Ch. 4). Antibodies produced this way are termed 'monoclonal'. Alternatively, a modern variant of the traditional technique is to inject into a host animal not the whole protein but a short specific amino acid sequence, synthesized in the laboratory – an 'epitope'. Both of these methods may be expected to give rise to antibodies of greater selectivity than the traditional method, but the possibility that some functionally homologous molecules will escape demonstration is increased.

While the sections stained by antibodies look quite similar to, and are often serial with, others reacted histochemically, there is an important distinction between them. With the exception of the few reactions for bulk substances like carbohydrates and lipids, histochemistry demonstrates enzyme activity. Most non-enzymes, such as thin-filament proteins, cannot be demonstrated histochemically – but they *can* be demonstrated immunohistochemically. Conversely, if the same catalytic action is capable of being performed by more than one structure of molecule, all of these different *isoenzymes* ('isozymes') are liable to be demonstrated simultaneously by enzyme histochemistry; such an effect can only be avoided if one of the isoenzymes is active in conditions which inhibit others, such as the high-pH, high-calcium medium for mATPase. Immunohistochemistry, at least when the antibody used is monoclonal or epitopic, is likely to be much more specific because it is not demonstrating the catalytic site but some other region randomly located on the molecule. The chance that an identical *non-catalytic* region occurs on, say, both myosin and the mitochondrial ATPase molecule, is not great. In any case, such an eventuality can be nowadays excluded by a 'blast' search of a computer data base for lengths of identical amino acid sequence in the different proteins – provided their structures are all known.

The intensity of fluorescence or staining which results from antibody binding is rarely proportional to the number of binding sites involved. Instead, quite a low tissue concentration of the detected molecule is often demonstrated almost as strongly as a high concentration. This feature is often noticeable in the case of the molecule of greatest importance to us, myosin; however, this has the rather uncommon but extremely useful property of being demonstrable by both enzymic and antibody methods. If a fibre contains two types of myosin, even in quite disparate proportions like 10% of one, 90% the other, antibodies to both myosins will react significantly with it. There would be no prospect of demonstrating the 10% component histochemically unless the two isoenzymes can be differentially inhibited, and even then that component will react only weakly. Consequently, immunohistochemistry is more sensitive than enzyme histochemistry to minor degrees of such myosin 'hybridity', but it gives a poorer indication of the ratios involved.

In the above outline of antibody techniques, the account of how a bound antibody is made evident to the microscopist ('visualized') was kept basic. A sophistication now widespread is to apply two or more antibodies to the section in series. The second antibody will be one raised against the proteins of the animal from which the first antibody was derived, and it is the second not the first which will be labelled. A third stage may even be employed, as when antibody no 2 is peroxidase-labelled, and antibody 3 is an anti-peroxidase (the 'peroxidase–anti-peroxidase', or PAP method). The advantages of these indirect visualizations are that sensitivity is markedly increased, because many tertiary antibody molecules can be bound to one primary, *and* that non-specific staining (cross-talk) is diminished. This counter-intuitive outcome is due to the fact that the primary antibody can be applied at much greater dilution because its presence is going to be so sensitively detected; when more dilute, it is more selective. Further detail on antibody methods, and other aspects of immunocytochemistry, can be found in Polak & Van Noorden (1997).

OBTAINING SPECIMENS

Before ending our discussion of techniques, we should finally note the various ways in which muscle specimens can be obtained. If a small experimental animal such as rat or mouse is sacrificed, blocks of tissue containing the whole cross-section of a muscle, or from a mouse even a group of muscles, can be dissected out and quench-frozen for histochemistry or immunocytochemistry. (Fig. 3.3, p 67, is an example of this.) From a rabbit, cat or any larger animal, pieces of muscles will have to be used, although it is often useful to freeze small pieces from two or more muscles together as one block, so that their fibres can be compared after absolutely identical reactions. Samples of human muscle taken at autopsy can be treated in the same way as fresh animal material, and will still respond normally for many days, even to most enzyme-histochemical reactions, provided the body has been stored in the cold. (Fig. 3.19, p 98, is from such a specimen.)

However, most studies of human muscle, whether clinical or scientific, make use of a different technique, *needle biopsy*. Biopsy in general is the taking of small samples of tissue from a living animal or subject. This may be done surgically, in which case local anaesthesia will be employed. But a biopsy needle allows samples perhaps 2–3 mm in all dimensions to be taken through the skin, with only a topical anaesthetic or none. The muscle 'kicks' as the fibres are cut, because rupturing their membrane depolarizes them and triggers action potentials, but the small wound left by the needle is readily tolerated by most subjects. The sample of muscle tissue is quench-frozen within about 5 seconds, and thereafter treated like any other specimen for microscopical or biochemical study.

The chief limitation of needle biopsy is that it can provide specimens only from the outer surfaces of a few, large muscles, and even then is restricted to regions where neither significant nerves nor substantial blood vessels lie between the surface and the muscle. Vastus lateralis is the most suitable human muscle and, although in a young-adult male it contains roughly half a million muscle fibres (Lexell et al 1988), only a few thousand occupy the region commonly sampled. Gastrocnemius and deltoid are among the others accessible to skilled hands, but the regions of these muscles which can be sampled are even more circumscribed. Needle biopsy is thus well suited to comparisons between individuals, or in one individual over time. (A skilled biopsist can take about half a dozen samples from one lateral vastus before scar tissue from earlier biopsies interferes with new ones.) But reliance on this technique would give very biased pictures of the overall volume even of the muscles on which it can be used. In small-animal limbs there is a marked preponderance of small, red fibres deep down, near the bones, and large, white ones near the surface. In large animals, including humans, the depth-to-surface gradient is less extreme, but in most muscles still significant. So, even for muscles accessible to biopsy, accounts of the deeper regions, and estimates of the overall percentages of different fibre types, must be based on cadaver studies. One of the most extensive of these was performed by Johnson et al (1973); they gave percentage figures, for fast and slow fibres in 43 human muscles, which are still widely cited. Some examples are given in Table 3.1; an alternative tabulation, culling data from many sources, is Table 8 of Saltin & Gollnick (1983).

Specimens for electron microscopy must be fixed within seconds of removal from a live source, or of the animal's death. Needle biopsy is thus applicable, where more leisurely dissection methods are not.

THE THREE MAIN FIBRE TYPES

We began this chapter with the simple binary description, 'slow, red' versus 'fast, white', derived from Ranvier. By the middle of the 20th century this had become consolidated under the labels *type 1* and *type 2*. Nevertheless, it was widely recognized as inadequate. What was much less clear was how it should be extended. The common assumption was that these were the two extremes, but 'intermediate' fibres should also be acknowledged. Since both traditional histology and early enzyme histochemistry most readily gave information about oxidative capacity (correlating

Table 3.1   Means, rounded to two significant figures, of % type 1 ('slow, red') fibres in selected muscles of human young-adult males, from a study of six cadavers by Johnson et al (1973). 95% confidence intervals for the population means averaged about +/-10% of these sample means, but ranged from +/-6% (36–49%) for deep rectus femoris to +/-15% (46–76%) for superficial deltoid. Note that there is sometimes no surface-depth difference (tibialis anterior, triceps) but, where there is one, the mean counts invariably showed more type 1 fibres in the deeper parts of the muscle. The most predominantly-slow muscle sampled was soleus, with tibialis anterior second; the most predominantly-fast was triceps, with rectus femoris (averaging its deep and superficial samples) second.

Muscle	Mean % type 1
Biceps brachii (surface)	42
Biceps brachii (deep)	51
Biceps femoris	67
Deltoid (surface)	53
Deltoid (deep)	61
Gastrocnemius (lateral: surface)	44
Gastrocnemius (lateral: deep)	50
Gluteus maximus	52
Iliopsoas	49
Latissimus dorsi	51
Pectoralis major	42
Rectus abdomis	46
Rectus femoris (surface)	30
Rectus femoris (deep)	42
Soleus (suface)	86
Soleus (deep)	89
Tibialis anterior (surface)	73
Tibialis anterior (deep)	73
Triceps brachii (surface)	33
Triceps brachii (deep)	33
Vastus lateralis (surface)	38
Vastus lateralis (deep)	49
Vastus medialis (surface)	44
Vastus medialis (deep)	62

closely with redness) the word usually meant fibres seen to be of intermediate oxidative capacity. It would usually be assumed that their other properties – glycolytic capacity, contraction speed, endurance – were intermediate too. By the later 1960s, however, serious efforts were being made to check this. It applied quite well to the sedentary human, and so was acceptable clinically; for many other species, however, it was not true. Most animals and birds in the wild, small ones even if caged, and also athletically trained people, had fibres which were very red in colour yet whose contractile properties were fast, not slow. So the type 2 fibres were divided into two sub-groups: fast, red fibres were labelled *type 2A*, while the traditional fast, whites became *2B* (Brooke & Kaiser 1970).

In this and later papers Brooke & Kaiser also recognized a fourth fibre type, which they termed 2C. It was never common but could be seen in certain animal and human

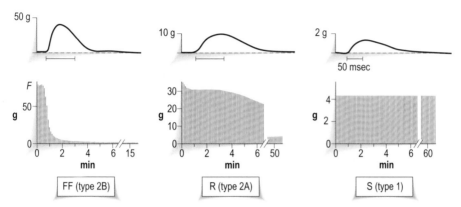

Figure 3.8 Records of twitches on fast time-scale (upper trace) and repeated tetani on slow time-scale (lower trace), from three motor units of cat gastrocnemius. Note different ordinates. Original nomenclature (Fast Fatiguing, Fast fatigue-Resistant, Slow) supplemented by now-accepted designations of fibre types involved. Reproduced from Figures 1, 2 and 3 of Burke et al (1973) by permission of Blackwell Publishing Ltd.

muscles, particularly when either immature, recovering from injury or undergoing a major change of exercise regime. This fibre seemed to have many characteristics which suggested a cross between types 1 and 2A, but its mATPase activity was often found to be even more acid-stable than that of type 1 fibres, and thus quite unlike the 2As. It now seems that 2C fibres, as originally identified, contained substantial quantities of a foetal or neonatal myosin, not stable in adult muscle. The term (sometimes extended to include 1C as well as 2C) has subsequently been applied to fibres containing mixtures of types 1 and 2A, or 2A and 2B myosins (Pierobon-Bormioli et al 1981). We shall examine later whether these are rare or common.

Physiological experiments did not immediately contradict the uncritical assumption that the 2A fibre was intermediate between types 1 and 2B in all respects. Burke et al (1973) found three main classes of motor unit in cat gastrocnemius muscles (Fig. 3.8). The slow-twitch units ('S', in their terminology) consisted of relatively few muscle fibres, and so developed fairly small forces, but resisted fatigue extraordinarily well. Histochemical analysis confirmed that they consisted of highly oxidative fibres with marked capacity to metabolize lipids but usually rather limited capacity for glycolysis, and always type 1 myosin. The largest, most forceful units fatigued very quickly, and were termed fast, fatiguing (FF) by these investigators. Their metabolism was weakly oxidative and entirely non-lipolytic; they always had high glycolytic capacity and 2B myosin. The units containing 2A myosin were of medium size, twitched fairly fast, and resisted fatigue quite well too: Burke and colleagues labelled these fast, resistant (FR) units.

Other combined physiological and histochemical studies were made on rodent limb muscles by such workers as Kugelberg (1973) and Close (1972), with only minor differences in their findings, and on human limb muscles by Garnett et al (1979) and Andreassen & Arendt-Nielsen (1987). (See Fig. 3.9.) On this basis, therefore, it was possible to tabulate a wide range of properties of the three main fibre types found in stable, adult, skeletal muscles of mammalian limbs and trunk, with confidence that the same types of fibre were being characterized, whichever the property described (Table 3.2). But thinking of the 2A fibre as intermediate between the others was not contradicted by these data.

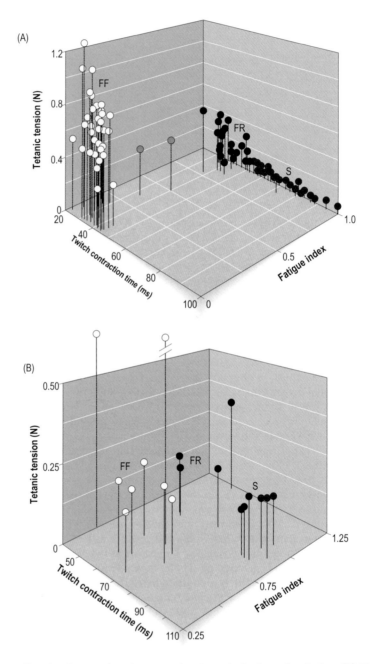

Figure 3.9 Functional properties of motor units, shown in '3-dimensional' plots. (A) 81 cat gastrocnemius units: all but two fall into one of three clusters, labelled as in Figure 3.8, original nomenclature. From Figure 5 of Burke et al (1973) with permission from Blackwell Publishing Ltd. (B) 17 human gastrocnemius units, displaying a tendency to fall into three clusters analogous to those in (A). Reproduced from Figure 4 of Garnett et al (1979) with permission from Blackwell Publishing Ltd.

Table 3.2 Characteristics of the three main types of stable human muscle fibres. Top row (myosin type) is also the name by which the fibre type is nowadays most often designated. The label 2X, for the fastest human fibre type, has been increasingly adopted since the mid-1990s. Hyphenated descriptions ('medium-high', etc.) mean that the property can range from medium to high in fibres of this type, depending on the size of the fibre and the individual's training state. The bottom six rows (*italicized*) are enzyme activities measured in healthy but untrained young males by Essen & Henrikson (cited by Saltin & Gollnick 1983). The units are μmol product $g^{-1} \cdot min^{-1}$ at 25°C. The enzymes represent, from top to bottom, capacities for glycogenolysis, glycolysis, pyruvate reduction, fat metabolism, tricarboxylic acid cycling and oxidative phosphorylation. Note that in most other species, 2B fibres would be listed as consistently larger than types 2A and 1; often 2X would too. However, in sedentary young-adult humans relative sizes differ little, while in highly trained people type 1 fibres may be larger or smaller than the types 2 according to the training mode. Note also that in rodents, but not in larger mammals, myosin ATPase activity after alkaline pre-treatment is highest in 2A fibres.

Myosin type	1	2A	2X (formerly '2B')
Description	Slow, red (oxidative),fatigue resistant	Fast, red (oxidative), fatigue resistant	Fast, white (glycolytic), readily fatigued
Abbreviated description	SO	FOG	FG
Motor neurone size	Small	Medium	Large
Recruitment frquency	Low	Medium	High
Contraction speed	Slow	Fast	Slightly faster still
Endurance	High	Medium-high	Low
Motor unit nomenclature	Slow (S)	Fast, fatigue-resistant (FR)	Fast, fatiguing (FF)
Myosin ATPase activity after pH 10.3 treatment	Low	High	Slightly higher still
Ditto, after pH 4.6 treatment	High	Low	Medium
Ditto, after pH 4.3 treatment	High	Low	Low
Mitochondrial density	High	Medium-very high	Low
Oxidative capacity	High	Medium-very high	Low
Myoglobin content	High	Medium-high	Low
Glycolytic capacity	Low-medium	Medium-very high	High
Phosphorylase	*2.8*	*5.8*	*8.8*
Phosphofructokinase	*7.5*	*13.7*	*17.5*
Lactate dehydrogenase	*59*	*221*	*293*
3-hydroxyacyl dehydrogenase	*14.8*	*11.6*	*7.1*
Succinate dehydrogenase	*7.1*	*4.8*	*2.5*
Citrate synthase	*10.8*	*8.6*	*6.5*

Nor did electron microscopy (Schiaffino et al 1973; Eisenberg 1983) do anything to correct this assumption. Z lines were found to be thickest and M lines thinnest in type 1 fibres; Z thinnest, M thickest in 2B; and both intermediate in 2A.

However, the acid and alkaline pre-treatments used with the mATPase reaction told a different story. The fact that 2A myosin was more acid-labile than 2B in all species studied, and in rodents more alkali-stable too, made clear that these fibres contained a third type of myosin, not a mixture of types 1 and 2B. When sufficiently selective antibodies became available, immunohistochemistry consistently confirmed this.

The final step of understanding came from the finding that, in almost all small animals and birds, fibres with 2A myosin are actually the most oxidative of all (Kugelberg 1973, Peter et al 1972, Spurway 1980). This can also be true in fit larger animals sampled in their natural environments, and in certain highly trained human athletes. In these cases it is the type 1 fibre which is oxidatively intermediate. We shall consider what determines oxidative capacity later. Meanwhile, we can appreciate that this type of 2A fibre, with high or sometimes very high aerobic capacity, usually high or very high anaerobic capacity, fast yet not the fastest contractile properties and high, though probably never the highest fatigue resistance, can profitably be thought of not as a rather ill-defined compromise but as a 'super fibre' (Kugelberg 1973), having the best all-round balance of properties for animals aerobically fit enough to use them.

Table 3.2 collates the structural, chemical and physiological properties of the three main types of fibre whose identity we have now established. For completeness it also includes one important piece of information for which we must look ahead of our historical account – namely that many fibres classified as 2B in the 1970s are now known to have a slightly different myosin, termed 2X. In animals where both occur, 2X myosin is slightly less fast than 2B myosin, and is characteristically found in fibres of slightly higher oxidative capacity. In species having only 2X – which are now known to include the human, at least as far as large limb and trunk muscles are concerned – 2X fibres perform all the functions elsewhere associated with 2B fibres, but must be assumed to do so with rather greater endurance. This in turn may perhaps explain a previously puzzling phenomenon: namel, that the fastest, least oxidative human fibres are not routinely larger than the other types. More will be said about 2X myosin, with references, in the final section of this chapter.

VALIDITY OF THE FIBRE TYPE CONCEPT

Quantitative Histochemistry

The idea that it is possible to classify the majority of muscle fibres into discrete types is not universally accepted. For reasons which will be evident, writers concerned mainly with metabolic enzymes are particularly inclined to question the idea. However, mATPase histochemistry strongly suggests that a very large percentage of the fibres of a stable, adult muscle can be unequivocally classified. Quantitative histochemistry supports this. Figure 3.10 illustrates the point visually.

Cluster Analysis

This approach was pressed to its limit by taking equal account of 10 different indicators (all the nine histochemical reactions illustrated in Fig. 3.3, plus fibre diameter). Graphs cannot be drawn to display more than three reactions quantitatively, but the technique

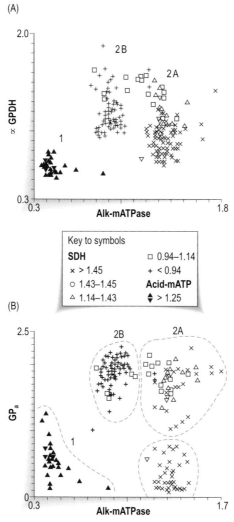

Figure 3.10 Optical absorbance values for 200 mouse muscle fibres, from specimen illustrated in Figure 3.3. All but perhaps 3–4 fall cleanly into three groups in terms of their alkali-pre-treated myosin ATPase reactions (abscissa). (In this species, unlike larger mammals, 2A myosin reacts more strongly than 2B after alkaline pre-incubation.) The two fast myosin types, however, are both associated with a wide range of activities for the metabolic enzymes shown in Figure 3.10A (glycolytic, indicated by α-glycerophosphate dehydrogenase, on the ordinate, oxidative – succinate dehydrogenase – by symbol). If glycogen phosphorylase *a*, the active form of an enzyme associated with glycogenolysis rather than glycolysis is used (Fig. 3.10B), the distinction between high and low capacities for carbohydrate metabolism divides the 2A fibres into two subgroups, all but one of the weakly glycogenolytic fibres being in the highest range of oxidative capacity. Type 1 and 2B groupings are not significantly affected by the change of anaerobic marker. Modified from Figures 11 and 10 respectively of Spurway (1981).

of *cluster analysis* attempts to do the equivalent in as many so-called 'dimensions' as one has measurements for. The chief limitation is that the human observer, looking at a graph, uses a range of criteria simultaneously in deciding what constitutes a cluster of points homogeneous enough to represent – in our case – one type of fibre. The observer takes account of the density of points, separations between groups, spread of the extremes, and many other criteria. Computer programs can utilize only one criterion at a time. So, in practice, the researcher runs a number of separate analyses, each embodying a different criterion, and looks for groupings which are recognized using each of several independent criteria. The basic procedure was described very briefly by Spurway (1980) and exhaustively by Spurway (1981). For a more sophisticated version, see Spurway & Rowlerson (1989).

The relevance of cluster analysis in discussion of the fibre type concept is that three to five closely comparable fibre groupings are indeed recognized in multi-reaction data-sets by several independent clustering criteria, so the contention that the diversity of fibre properties falls into identifiable groups has objective support. Almost equally interesting is that, if one seeks to extract only two-cluster patterns from multi-reaction data, different cluster-defining criteria select different patterns – oxidative capacity ('redness') being picked out by one method, glycolytic by another, and mATPase activities ('contraction speed') by a third. The conclusion indicated is that binary subdivisions (red versus white, fast versus slow, etc.) can be made on several bases, but the different ones will not coincide; however classifications into slightly more types can do so. While these conclusions had already been drawn from subjective assessments of histochemical reactions, to have them confirmed quantitatively and objectively was most encouraging.

Different Muscles

The mouse data of Figure 3.10 and the follow-up cluster analyses showed no marked and consistent differences between fibres classified as of one type, depending on the muscle in which they were found. Nevertheless if we look at other species, and muscles of more widely divergent function, we may see such differences. Figure 3.11, from a rabbit study, illustrates this, and should not be dismissed as academic even by sports scientists, as work with rabbits has contributed extensively to our present understanding of muscle; some important examples will be seen later in this chapter.

The example of Figure 3.11 illustrates the fact that fibres of a given type in one location sometimes differ from those with similar mATPase in another location. The 2B fibres of diaphragm, top right in the plot, are more strongly glycogenolytic than any of those in psoas major or extensor digitorum longus, and at the same time more oxidative than most of them. Another common instance, though not seen in this example, is for type 1 fibres in a predominantly-slow muscle, with a largely postural function, such as soleus, to differ in size and/or metabolic capacities from those in muscles like gastrocnemius or vastus lateralis where such fibres are a minority. However, if we consider the relative roles of a given fibre type within the various muscles in which it is found, these roles are almost always found to be consistent. Type 1 fibres are always the slowest in a given muscle, 2B (or 2X) the fastest, and any 2A fibres as small as or smaller than the type 1s will prove to be the most oxidative of all. Furthermore, while sizes and metabolic capacities may vary considerably, the mATPase reactions, ultrastructure, electrophysiology and contractile characteristics rarely differ much between the various muscles of a given animal or species.

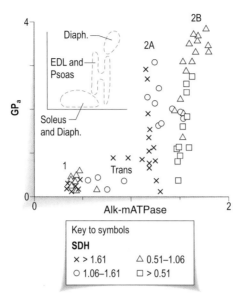

Figure 3.11   Reactions and plotting conventions as in Figure 3.10B, but this time for 65 rabbit fibres from diaphragm, extensor digitorum longus (EDL), psoas major and soleus. In this species, and all larger ones, 2B fibres react more strongly than 2A for myosin ATPase after alkaline pre-treatment. 'Trans' = hybrid fibres, presumed transitional. A major distinction between different muscles displays itself: 2B fibres of diaphragm (see insert) are in a different metabolic group from those of EDL and psoas. Modified from Figure 5 of Spurway (1980).

Different Species

A second version of the same argument can be based on the equivalent fibres in different animals. As argued many decades ago by the great biophysicist A. V. Hill (1950), geometrical and biomechanical limitations must impose massive differences of speed and metabolic capacity upon the muscles of species which differ widely in size. Everyday observation shows that mice and cats, or horses, dogs and hares, run on level ground at speeds which do not greatly differ – if they did, for the larger ones to chase the smaller would either be pointless or trivially easy. This means that the linear speeds of movement of their feet must be similar. However, far more sarcomeres are shortening in series to achieve this in the large species than in the small, so the speed at which individual sarcomeres shorten, and the rate at which cross bridges cycle, are many times greater in the small animals. The frequency of their strides (much greater in small animals) demonstrates the same point, as does that of wing-beats in birds or tail-movements in fish. So the mATPase activity of type 1 mouse fibres is many times greater than that of type 2B cat fibres, and greater still than those of horses.

   This, in turn, implies that the capacity for aerobic metabolism per unit weight of a small animal has to be many times greater than that of a large, if it is to re-synthesize ATP fast enough to power its cross-bridges. This is just as well, because the surface-to-volume ratio of a large animal is much less, so it could not dissipate its metabolic heat at the rate necessary for a small one. The implications of this are summarized as the 'Mouse-elephant law' (Klieber's law), and the overall subject of scaling effects such as these is known as *allometry*. An excellent introduction is a little book by Schmidt-Neilsen (1973).

The implication for muscle fibre properties is that contraction-speed markers like mATPase, as well as markers of aerobic activity such as SDH, will be found many times more active in a given fibre type of a small animal than of a large one. (It is less safe to generalize about glycolytic capacity, presumably because this system functions near its limits only for short periods, in which heat accumulation is not limiting.) However, slow fibres serving predominantly postural functions and having acid-stable mATPases, and faster ones with alkali-stable mATPases, together with the relative metabolic profiles which are by now familiar, have been found in every species studied. As cell-types adapted to equivalent functions in an immense range of species, the concept of fibre types is not eroded but strongly supported by the modifications imposed by body scale. In the limb and trunk muscles of almost all large mammals (Fig. 3.12) the picture is in fact simpler than in smaller species, although their smallest muscles (extra-ocular, laryngeal, middle ear, etc), together with some specialist larger muscles such as those involved in mastication, may be considerably more complicated than the limb and trunk muscles.

Hybrid Fibres

In the data-sets of Figures 3.10 and 3.12, only 1–2% of fibres do not fit readily into one or other of the three to four clusters. In Figure 3.11, the figure is ~6%. The mATPase reactions of the ambiguous fibres were not clear-cut, suggesting that they might contain more than one type of myosin – 'hybrid' fibres. It is important to note that the muscles incorporated in all of these analyses were in stable states. In preparations taken from muscles which were in the course of adapting to changed circumstances, such as an altered exercise regime or, conversely, splinting of the limb concerned, hybrid fibres may be up to 10× more common; overlap of metabolic profiles is even greater too. Accordingly, myosin hybridity detectable by traditional mATPase reactions is widely interpreted as indicating that the fibre concerned was in transition from one condition to another, perhaps even one type to another. The fibre-type concept is not usually considered to be invalidated by such instances. Instead it facilitates description of the particular transition which appears to be taking place.

However, studies using monoclonal antibodies have found much higher percentages of fibres with some degree of hybridity. This is true even of the myosin heavy chains (MHCs) which carry the enzymatic capacity. When other proteins of the contractile system – myosin light chains, troponin, Z-line protein (α-actinin) and proteins of the sarcoplasmic reticulum – are added to the picture, the situation becomes extremely complex. Each of these proteins occurs in at least two forms ('fast' and 'slow'), and several of them in three or more (in which case at least one will most commonly occur in association with 2A MHCs). A simplistic anticipation would be that the fastest MHC would normally be found with the fastest SR and matching light chains, troponin, etc – and equivalently for the other MHCs. There need be no surprise when the matches are imperfect during the period of response to any change of regime or circumstance; only if the turnover rates of all the proteins were identical could this form of transient hybridity be avoided. However, Stephenson (2001), reviewing this topic, cites one instance where ~20% of fibres in a large limb muscle of apparently-stable adult rats were hybrids even in respect of their MHCs, although there were also instances in which no such hybrids were seen. If the concept of hybridity is extended to embrace the other proteins, it must be considered a common phenomenon, not a rare one, even in stable adult muscles.

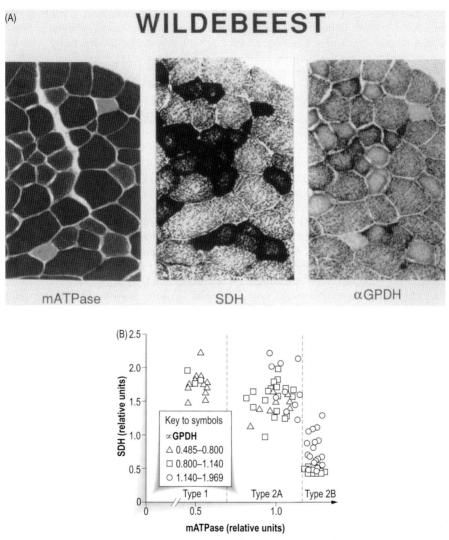

Figure 3.12   Biopsy studies of semimembranosus (a hamstring muscle) of a typical large mammal, the wildebeest. (A) Histochemical reactions in serial cryostat sections: left, actomyosin ATPase (Mabuchi/Sreter reaction, considered to relate particularly closely to contraction speed); centre, succinate dehydrogenase; right, α-glycerophsphate dehydrogenase. (B) Optical absorbance values for 100 fibres from this specimen, plotted on relative scales: note that ordinate here is SDH, with αGPDH indicated by symbols. This figure illustrates the fact that the classification of most large-animal fibres in stable conditions is clear-cut, but the anaerobic capacity of 2A fibres ranges widely; **a** shows that the smallest 2As are very high in both aerobic and anaerobic capacities, while many larger ones are slightly less aerobic but only moderately anaerobic, giving a weakly positive correlation between the two metabolic pathways within this fibre type. Figure 3.12A from Spurway et al (1998), with permission; Figure 3.12B modified from same source.

Some researchers take such instances as further indications that the fibre-type concept is invalid. Others, including the present authors, consider that even in these extreme cases it provides reference-criteria by which to define the hybridity – i.e. by saying which types the hybrids fall between. Either view is permissible; which is preferred will be principally a matter of temperament.

THE SIZE PRINCIPLE

We must now consider two important ideas which emerged from the work of Henneman and colleagues during the 1950s and 1960s (Henneman 1957, Henneman et al 1965, Henneman & Mendel 1981). The first idea was that the ease with which it is possible to excite the neurones controlling skeletal muscles ('α-motor neurones' in English writing, 'α-motoneurons' in American) depends on their size: small diameter neurones are stimulated easily, large-diameter ones only with difficulty. This is true whether the stimulation is by an experimenter's electrode or is natural. Reflex responses which are elicited by only mild stimuli, or voluntary actions which take place very regularly, involve only the smallest motor neurones. By contrast, actions elicited only by strong stimuli, or occuring voluntarily only when great effort is consciously involved, recruit all neurones, including the largest. Notice, though, that they do not recruit *only* the large ones; neurones sensitive to weak activation cannot avoid being stimulated also by strong activation unless they are subject to powerful selective inhibition – and of this there is little convincing indication. Such evidence as there is refers to special circumstances, such as high-force ballistic and eccentric efforts, and the involvement of certain muscles in actions different from their main ones (Enoka & Stuart 1984). These circumstances are unlikely to affect the adaptation of the muscle fibres to their main pattern of activities.

Henneman and colleagues published two more papers in 1965, consecutive with the one referenced above. In the last one, they showed that the neurones which were hardest to excite were also easiest to inhibit. In the same group of papers they pointed out that the mechanism for the size-dependence of neuronal excitability might be based upon simple biophysics. If their membrane properties per unit area are the same, small neurones will be more easily depolarized than large ones: specifically counteractive features of the synaptic inputs would be required if this were not to happen. In fact the membrane properties are not identical, but several of the other factors operating reinforce, rather than oppose, this basic aspect (Kernell 1992).

It has not been universally accepted that the size principle applies generally to human muscle actions, consciously controlled. A complication is that it is much harder to make effective studies of the large, limb muscles than of small muscles, easily accessible from the surface of the body, such as those of the hand and face. These are all specialized, with functions markedly different from those of the limb muscles which are usually the concern of the sport and exercise scientist, and whose animal equivalents were originally studied. Sometimes, in addition, these small muscles have a range of different uses: extensor digitorum communis (EDC), for instance, is involved in the extension of each of the four fingers, and its motor units have been found to be recruited in different sequences for different fingers (Schmidt & Thomas 1981). Yet almost certainly those preferred for a given finger have the best biomechanical location for action on that finger, so it seems permissible to wonder whether EDC should be thought of as one muscle or, rather, a fusion of four. There are certainly other hand muscles which behave entirely in accord with Henneman's model (Fig. 3.13).

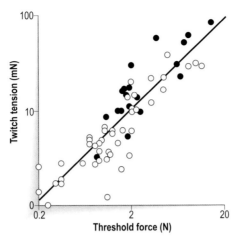

Figure 3.13 Proportional relationship between thresholds of recruitment of human thumb adductor motor units and the forces they develop. Reproduced from Figure 3 of Milner-Brown et al (1973) with permission from Blackwell Publishing Ltd.

Match of Motor Unit Properties to Demand

The second idea to emerge from Henneman's work was that the properties of the motor units fitted the requirements of their recruitment patterns. Units activated every time the muscle of which they are part produces force will be used often, so must have high fatigue resistance. Not surprisingly, they are found to be composed of fatigue-resistant, oxidative fibres. Conversely, the most rarely-recruited units consist of fibres with little oxidative capacity but high glycolytic. Units in the middle of the recruitment order are likely, other things being equal, to have intermediate metabolic profiles. However, more than the resistance of motor units to fatigue can be deduced by thinking about their tasks. Forces which are low, relative to the weight of the limb, are likely to be required for slow movements, or static posture, so it seems reasonable that the motor units lowest in the recruitment order should consist of slow-contracting, type 1 fibres. When maximal force is called upon, an attempt (successful or not) to achieve high speeds is frequently in hand, so we may predict that the fibres will contain 2B or 2X myosin. In between, type 2A is obviously appropriate. As one of the papers in the 1965 series put it: 'The size of the cell determines its excitability, its excitability determines the degree of use of the motor unit, and its usage in turn specifies or influences the type of muscle fibre required'.

So much for the properties of the muscle fibres. What of their number – i.e. how many will make up a motor unit? When the existing force is small, upward or downward adjustments in large steps would produce disconcertingly jerky behaviour; it is appropriate therefore for readily-recruited motor units to be small. The individual fibres do not need to be small on this basis – if they are, it will be for other reasons – but the number of fibres in the unit must be modest. At the other end of the scale, when near-maximal forces, and perhaps speeds, are required, tiny adjustments in either direction are pointless: large motor units, recruitment or de-recruitment of which makes a worthwhile difference, are appropriate. (There is a close analogy here to the operation of sensory systems, traditionally summarized under the

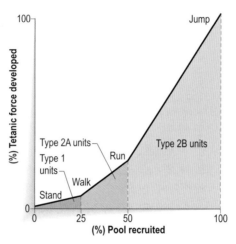

Figure 3.14 Recruitment model for the cat medial gastrocnemius motor unit pool. The solid line represents the force developed by full tetanic recruitment of every motor unit up to the percentage indicated on the abscissa. Modified from Burke (1980).

'Weber–Fechner law'. For instance, if only one light is illuminated in a large hall, turning on one more will be very noticeable. But if 100 were already burning one more would scarcely be noticed; indeed, something like another 100 would be needed to give the same apparent increment as when the second bulb was added to the first.) Given the extent to which evolution has responded to selective pressures, it is hardly a surprise to find that the mechanical equivalent of this relationship is exactly the situation which prevails: the most-often recruited units are small, slow and fatigue resistant (S units, in Burke's terminology, with type 1 myosin and highly aerobic metabolism); the most rarely-recruited units are large, fast and easily fatigued (FF units, with type 2B myosin and essentially glycolytic metabolism); and the units of intermediate excitability have largely intermediate properties (medium sized, FR units, with type 2A fibres and oxidative capacity which is at least moderately high). Figure 3.14 summarizes this picture, and adds indications of the activities for which the various units are typically recruited in the large, leg muscles of a cat. The human situation is considered to be comparable.

There is, of course, another way in which force production can be modified, namely, by 'rate coding' – adjusting the frequency of action potentials (APs) in the motor axons. This mechanism operates much more in small muscles of the head and extremities than in large limb muscles, presumably adding an even finer level of control, but the sequence of recruitment continues to fit with motor unit size. For further discussion, see Chapters 12 and 13 of McComas (1996).

WHAT DETERMINES MOTOR UNIT PROPERTIES?

Perhaps even more interesting than the mere fact of this elegant match of properties to requirements, is how it comes about. An important initial sign is the basic fact that the muscle fibres of a given unit are closely similar to one another, which strongly suggests that the motor nerve controlling them powerfully influences their properties.

Unit Size

Considering unit size first, it may be that this is mainly a direct, mechanistic consequence of neurone size. The overall process of foetal and neonatal muscle growth is complex and we need not consider it in detail. (McComas 1996, Chapter 5, provides a clear account.) For our purpose it suffices to note that growth starts without the influence of nerves: multi-nucleate muscle fibres are formed by the fusion of mononucleate precursors, and motor axons only grow when the multi-nucleate cells already exist – probably much the same number of them as in the mature muscle. At first, the axons branch vigorously, and innervate many muscle fibres. It is believed that all fibres thus become innervated by at least two and often several motor nerves, with rudimentary 'synaptic' (end-plate) connections. Gradually, however, one nerve fibre becomes dominant over a given muscle fibre, and the others regress from it, though themselves often becoming dominant over other fibres. Now the transmitter substance used by such nerves, acetylcholine, and almost certainly other substances with trophic rather than transmitter functions, are synthesized in the cell body, immediately adjacent to the nucleus from which mRNA emerges to control the biosynthesis – usually indirectly, its direct role being in the production of the enzymes which will in their turn control the biosynthesis of the smaller molecules we are discussing. Inevitably, small neurones can synthesize less of these substances than large ones, and it could be simply for this reason that they end up dominating far fewer muscle fibres than their large competitors. Even if other factors are at work too, it seems inevitable that this mechanism plays a part.

Nerve Cross–Union Experiments

When we turn from the number of muscle fibres in a unit to their individual properties, the evidence about the main mechanism is strong, for these properties can be changed not only in early life but in the adult. The first observations which led to current understanding were made by Buller et al (1960). These investigators cut the motor nerves to two similar-sized muscles in the lower hind limbs of young cats, and cross-united ('cross-sutured') them (Fig. 3.15). The muscles they used were soleus

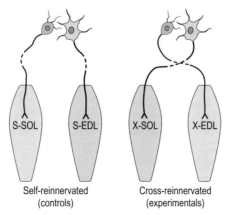

Figure 3.15   Diagrammatic representation of the procedure adopted in nerve cross–union experiments.

(SOL) and extensor digitorum longus (EDL). These muscles function respectively to flex and extend the paw, and the question the experiments were designed to answer was whether the cat's nervous system would re-learn the functions of the muscles to which the nerves had been surgically redirected. In the event, re-learning did not happen: over periods of at least nine months, cross-reinnervated soleus muscles (X-SOL) continued to contract at the points in the gait-cycle appropriate to EDL contraction, and *vice-versa*. However, being very good experimenters (J. C. Eccles would shortly be awarded a Nobel prize for another aspect of his work), Buller et al noticed that something very significant *had* changed: the respective muscles had almost completely inverted their individual contractile properties.

The point was that, choosing on the basis of opposite actions yet similar sizes, the investigators had been led by chance to select one muscle (SOL) in which almost all fibres were slow in this species and another (EDL) in which they were all fast. What *was* different, after nine months or more, was that X-SOL now contracted fast, and X-EDL contracted slowly. Later experimenters (reviewed by Close 1972), following up this observation on several species of laboratory mammal (Fig. 3.16), found that all the properties associated with speed in Table 3.2 had changed as well: X-SOL had high glycolytic capacity and, in most of its fibres, type 2B myosin; only a few of its fibres had 2A myosin and high oxidative capacity as well as glycolytic. Conversely, X-EDL's fibres now predominantly had type 1 myosin, medium-to-high oxidative capacity and low glycolytic.

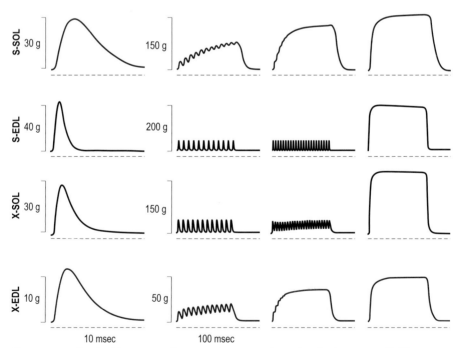

Figure 3.16 Tension/time curves for isometric contractions of self-reinnervated (S-EDL, S-SOL) and cross reinnervated (X-EDL, X-SOL) extensor digitorum longus and soleus rat muscles. Records for each muscle are, from L to R, single twitches and responses to stimulation at 10, 20 and 200 Hz. Reproduced from Figure 1 of Close (1969) with permission from Blackwell Publishing Ltd.

It had thus become evident that the innervating motor nerve was responsible not only for the short-term instructions eliciting contractions but for much longer-term influences determining the speed of those contractions and the metabolic provision for supplying them with ATP. *Nerve tells muscle not only what to do but what to be.*

Effects of Electrical Activation

But how does the nerve do this? Buller et al explicitly stated two alternative hypotheses:

(i)   that active nerve fibres emitted some trophic (growth-stimulating) substance or substances, which diffused across the synaptic gap and influenced the underlying muscle fibre, *or*

(ii) that activation itself had the trophic effects.

Evidence pointing toward the second mechanism came from a young electrical engineer, Salmons, working with an established nerve–muscle physiologist, Vrbova (Salmons & Vrbova 1969). They began with a technique at which Vrbova was already expert, the cutting of SOL's distal tendon ('tenotomy'). This removes the stretch stimulus on the muscles spindles of SOL, so that they cease to fire; the efferent impulse traffic in the α-motorneurones to SOL (a feature of all anti-gravity muscles) therefore also ceases, and the muscle stays flaccid. After some weeks, it proves to have lost its normal resistance to fatigue, and its contractile characteristics have speeded up. (The same happens in any other circumstance where muscle stimulation ceases, including the weightlessness of space travel – a subject on which we know a lot more now than in 1969!) By implanting wire electrodes through the skin of their animals, Salmons & Vrbova could stimulate the SOL nerve electrically, in a way that simulated the sustained low-frequency (LF) firing normally triggered by the stretch reflex. They found that when they did this it slowed again, and recovered its fatigue resistance. They then implanted miniature electrical stimulators under the skin of other rabbits' legs, so as to elicit APs in the normal anatomical nerve to EDL with a pattern of impulses similar to that naturally found in the nerve to SOL, namely steady LF (5-10Hz) firing for many hours per day. The upshot was that EDL became a slow muscle, with all its fibres converted fairly completely to type 1 myosin and highly oxidative, weakly glycolytic metabolism. Carrying this further, Salmons & Sreter (1976) showed that X-SOL could be made even slower than normal SOL by artificial stimulation sustained 24 hours a day, seven days a week – an intensity more extreme than occurs naturally, because even rabbits sleep!

The converse transformation, of SOL fibres to a normal EDL profile was harder to achieve, because the natural excitation of EDL involved only brief high-frequency (HF: typically 40 Hz) bursts of action potentials (APs) at wide intervals. The regular, LF firing, naturally propagating along the axons from the spinal cord, proved dominant over the superimposed but widely spaced HF bursts. However, in later experiments (reviewed by Gunderson 1998) cuffs soaked in local anaesthetic were wrapped around the nerve nearer the cord than ('proximal to') the stimulator, blocking impulse traffic from the CNS. In these situations, only the widely separated HF bursts of artificial stimulation reached the muscle and, sure enough, the anatomical SOL fibres became fast.

It took longest to establish what pattern of firing would promote the formation of 2A fibres. It seems there is more than one. One is the use of rather more numerous HF bursts each day than for 2B fibres; another, however, is sustained stimulation at 2.5 Hz (Mayne et al 1996). Evidently the aggregate number of impulses over an extended

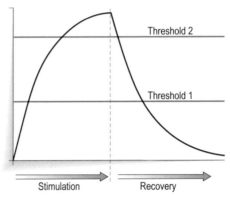

Figure 3.17 Threshold model for changes in skeletal muscle during increased activity ('stimulation') and reduced activity ('recovery'). Ordinate: strength of a notional intracellular signal (e.g. concentration of some signalling substance) responsive to the level of activity. Abscissa: time (several weeks in an experimental animal, perhaps years in human training). Properties which have a high threshold to change are slow to respond to stimulation and quick to return to previous condition when it ceases. For many fibres, natural exercise, however intensive, may involve insufficient activity for the higher threshold(s) to be reached. Diagram reproduced from Figure 1 of Salmons (1994), with permission from Georg Thieme Verlag.

time period is what matters, rather than their frequency within bursts. Sustained 10 Hz stimulation can convert all fibres, however fast they were previously, into type 1; sustained 2.5 Hz stimulation, however, does not cross the necessary 'threshold', but stops short at type 2A. Salmons (1994) developed this concept of thresholds, which also accords with the switch back of properties if stimulation ceases (Fig. 3.17).

Chemotrophism or Impulse–Dependent Mechanisms?

This whole body of results ruled out any suggestion that there was what Salmons & Sreter described as 'a fundamental difference in the chemotrophic character of the motor nerves' – such as different trophic substances being released by small and large nerve fibres, respectively. Instead, they concluded, 'We may confine our attention to impulse-dependent mechanisms'. However, the possibility always remained that some trophic substance, released similarly from the endplates of any motor nerve by each AP, was having the effects observed: the amount of it would depend on the number of APs, so leaving the outcome impulse-dependent. What had to be checked was whether direct electrical stimulation of muscles, perhaps even denervated muscles, could have the same effects. Lomo, in particular, has shown in a long series of papers that it can. After 2 weeks of continuous stimulation, the fastest fibres in a denervated muscle transform into 2As, but it takes at least 2 months more for these 2As to convert into type 1 (Windisch et al 1998). The mechanism within the muscle fibres by which these changes happen will be considered further in Chapter 5, but we can now say confidently that it must be one dependent only on the muscle's activity; chemotrophic influences from the nerves are not involved at all, either as different substances from different nerves or different amounts of one substance depending on their AP frequency. We can also note already that the Lomo group's finding is important clinically as well as theoretically. Traumatically denervated muscles can be maintained in a reasonably normal state by percutaneous or implanted stimulators – an effect which is particularly useful while a severed motor nerve is regrowing.

It might seem that this discovery, of the profound influence of activation-pattern on the properties of muscle fibres, conflicts with the evidence presented in Chapter 2 that the percentages of fibres of one type or another in a given muscle are influenced by genetic factors. (Recall that the extent of the influence found varied rather widely between studies, but there was no dispute that a significant influence occurs.) However, the two standpoints are compatible if it is considered that the direct genetic effect could be on the CNS, with the muscle fibres' properties adjusting in consequence.

Other Influences on Fibre Type

Although the effects of activity-pattern are thus extremely strong, we must acknowledge that other factors can also influence fibre type. The muscle precursor cells in the embryo, 'myoblasts', come in fast and slow lineages. In birds, these types are retained even if the cells are transferred to a new embryo (DiMario et al 1993), although it is less clear whether this is true in mammals. But it certainly is the case in mammals (Condon et al 1990) as well as birds that if the nervous system is prevented from developing, embryonic muscle fibre types can nonetheless differentiate.

Hormonal influences also have relevance. In particular, while anabolic steroids (natural or synthetic) and growth hormone mainly enhance fibre size (Kraemer 1992; although see also Daugaard et al 1998), thyroid hormone has a powerful influence on fibre type: higher levels of the hormone favour the change from slower to faster forms (1→2A, 2A→2X or 2B, etc.) (Caiozzo & Haddad 1996).

Finally, and not only associated with electrical activity but also more like it in being a physical stimulus not a chemical one, *stretch* has long been known to have a powerful trophic influence. Among the more recent investigators of this phenomenon have been the brothers Goldspink, and their respective collaborators. Stretching a normal muscle, with intact innervation, promotes both growth and fast-slow transformation (G. Goldspink et al 1992). At first sight this could be supposed not to involve a separate mechanism at all: it might act solely by eliciting the stretch reflex, and thereby increasing the rate of firing of the α-motor neurones. However, three pieces of evidence oppose this argument. First, muscles stimulated electrically without stretch get smaller – they partially atrophy – whereas the above team showed that muscles subjected to LF electrical stimulation together with stretch became not only slower but larger than under stretch alone. Second, D. F. Goldspink (1977) had shown some time before that stretch stimulates growth of *denervated* muscle; sadly, though, he did not look at fibre types. However, a subsequent experiment in which he participated provides our third strand of evidence. Hnik et al (1985) showed that sustained stretch did *not* elicit enhanced motor nerve activity; over hours and days the chronic electrical activity (indicative of motor nerve firing rate) of muscles stretched with intact innervation is in fact similar to or less than at 'neutral' length. Although the details were very different for the slow, postural soleus from the fast anterior tibial muscles (c.f. the next section of this chapter), it appears that the stretch reflexes in both adapted their sensitivity in the face of sustained extension. Thus all the indications are that the effects of stretch on muscle fibres are direct, and not mediated by changed nerve firing rates.

Of the three non-neural influences just discussed, embryonic cell lineages and stretch must act at particular sites, but hormones have access in principle to all muscles. However, there are indications that the most-used muscles are the most susceptible to hormones. This topic will be taken up again in Chapter 5.

Several of the influences outlined in this subsection will be discussed again, in greater detail, when the effects of particular training patterns are considered later in the chapter. Our question here is how to reconcile the evidence just sketched with the preceding account of neural activation as an apparently sufficient determining factor. One aspect to bear in mind is that activation of a muscle develops tension in it, as does stretch of an inactive one. Nor is it impossible that chronic electrical stimulation provokes some endocrine response – this point does not seem to have been investigated empirically. Many experimenters have also felt that neural stimulation could never entirely over-ride the 'memory' each fibre had of its lineage and other history, but it is doubtful whether that belief can be maintained in the face of the most radical stimulation experiments we described earlier (Salmons & Sreter 1976, Windisch et al 1998). It seems more probable that extreme stimulation regimes, perhaps assisted by concomitant endocrine and stretch effects, can fully over-ride conflicting influences. But such regimes are highly artificial – as is nerve cross-union. In normal physiological circumstances, the various influences must surely be synergistic.

ADAPTATION OF LOCOMOTOR AND POSTURAL MUSCLES TO PARTICULAR FUNCTIONS

Differences Between Muscles

If the properties of motor units fit their patterns of use, it follows that properties of whole muscles must do so too. Even among the large limb and trunk muscles, there are substantial differences in fibre composition within a single individual. We have already referred to some extreme instances in non-human animals, because of their value in the study of fibre type properties. To cite a pair of contrasting muscles from the human, in the group of six young male cadavers autopsied by Johnson et al (1973 and Table 3.1) the surface of the soleus, accessible for sampling by biopsy needles, contained 75–98% type 1 fibres but that of vastus lateralis consisted only of 20–46% type 1 fibres. Soleus is an example of an anti-gravity muscle, steady tension in which is necessary for the maintenance of posture; all such muscles have high percentages of type 1 fibres, which can maintain tone economically. By contrast, muscles such as vastus, used for running and jumping, have higher percentages of type 2 fibres, adapted for contractions which are brief and more or less infrequent.

It is easy to see how these properties could emerge largely, if not solely, from the firing patterns of the innervating motor axons.

Sportspeople's Special Aptitudes

The figures just quoted were from healthy, but relatively sedentary individuals. Among sportspeople, however, the range of variation is greater than in that sample. From quite early in the modern study of skeletal muscle fibre types, it has been known that the locomotor muscles of sprinters have lower and those of long-distance performers substantially higher percentages of type 1 fibres than the population mean (e.g. Costill et al 1976, Gollnick et al 1972). The Costill team sampled gastrocnemius in tack and field athletes and the deltoid in swimmers, but the majority of other results in the literature refer to the particularly accessible vastus lateralis. Despite the fact that

Johnson's data for vastus indicate an average composition of well under 50% slow fibres in sedentary people, figures over 90% have been reported in elite marathon and ultra-marathon runners. At the other extreme, in elite sprinters barely 20% of vastus lateralis fibres may be slow. This inter-individual variation contributes to talents for either endurance or speed/power sports. Nevertheless, in every individual, soleus has more slow fibres than the same individual's vastus.

Figure 3.18 illustrates how other sports relate to the sprint-adapted and endurance-adapted extremes. Probably the most surprising of these, at first sight, is weight lifting. Thinking of the lifter holding the weight aloft, one might assume this was the pre-eminent slow-fibre sport. In fact, skilled technique for many lifts requires that the weight be rapidly accelerated, to carry itself past unfavourable joint-angles of the lifter's body with a considerable contribution from momentum. This alone is a reason why fast fibres may be advantageous. But there is another reason: fast fibres can hypertrophy further than slow ones. In all small species and in large ones which have

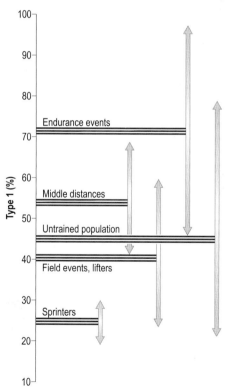

Figure 3.18   Relative percentages of type 1 (slow) fibres in different athletes and in untrained people. Horizontal lines = means, vertical lines = ranges. Summary of biopsy data from several sources including Gollnick et al (1972), Costill et al (1976) and Tesch et al (1984). The muscles sampled were vastus lateralis and gastrocnemius; there is an apparent trend, as predictable from Table 3.1, for the lowest type 1 %s to be found in lateral vastus and the highest in gastrocnemius, but it does not reach statistical significance. Note carefully that this plot is concerned only with fibre numbers, not their sizes. In highly trained people, the most numerous fibres tend also to be larger, amplifying the performance differences suggested by the figures here.

true 2B fibres these are always larger than type 1s, though 2As vary with location and function. In humans, as in horses and some other large herbivores, types 1 and 2 (which are probably in all these instances 2A and 2X, not 2B) are typically of similar sizes from infancy through middle age, and in old age the type 2s commonly atrophy (Lexell et al 1988). However, if a sustained strength-training programme is followed through by human beings at any age, the type 2X fibres increase their diameter most. Thus we may simplify by saying that type 2s are more adjustable in either direction – more 'labile' – than type 1s.

(In people trained solely for endurance the type 1 fibres may become larger than either of the type 2s. This is especially marked if the person is also of advancing years: Figure 3.19. Such large slow fibres are sometimes referred to as 'giant fibres', but their

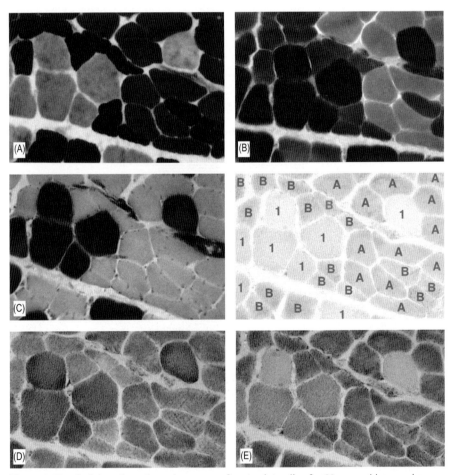

Figure 3.19 Serial sections through an area of vastus lateralis of a 63-year-old man who was a very regular mountain walker. Autopsy specimen, taken several days post mortem. (A) mATPase, alkali pre-treated. (B) mATPase, pre-treated pH 4.7. (C) mATPase, pre-treated pH 4.3. (D) Succinate dehydrogenase. (E) α-Glycerophosphate dehydrogenase. Centre right panel indicates fibre types 1, (2)A, (2)B (i.e. 2X). Note that type 1 fibres are largest, 2B(X) smallest. Preparation: Dr Ian Montgomery.

diameters are not often significantly above the normal range – usually the comparison being made is with adjacent type 2 fibres which have atrophied. Yet, even if it *is* possible truly to hypertrophy type 1 fibres to some extent, this requires a regime lasting many years; it does not contradict the assertion that type 2 are more readily adaptable.)

The existence of the percentage differences sketched in Figure 3.18 depends partly on inheritance, partly on exercise and partly on other environmental factors. Insofar as it is genetic, it suggests inherited predispositions for particular sports. A pointer to this can be found in Figure 3.18 itself, if we look at the ranges, rather than the means, of slow-fibre incidence. The range of the sedentary population extends below the mean for sprinters and above that for endurance performers. This suggests that, had the low % group trained, it would have been at sprints that they would have been good, while the high % people would have been good at endurance events.

Effects of Training

By contrast, the effects of different training regimes clearly recall those of different experimental stimuli. The endurance athlete's training for several hours a day – but with no one movement coming close to maximum speed or power – recalls the chronic LF stimulation which induced transitions from type 2B first to type 2A and ultimately to type 1 in Salmons' experimental animals. However, though conversion of almost all 2B/2X fibres to 2A can be induced by intensive and protracted endurance training (Jansson & Kaijser 1977 and Fig. 3.20; Saltin & Gollnick 1983), most commentators have insisted that there was little firm evidence of the number of type 1 fibres being increased. Even stimulation for 24 hours a day takes many weeks to cross this threshold in rabbits; human muscles would be expected to take longer even if they could be stimulated in that way, and it seems improbable that a person who must eat, sleep, and even do some other things in the waking day than train, could ever achieve this outcome. Cross-sectional data (Thayer et al 2000) do raise the possibility that

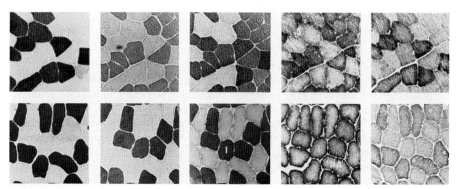

Figure 3.20   Serial sections from gastrocnemius of a control subject (upper row) and vastus lateralis of a highly-trained orienteer (lower row). Reactions, L–R: mATPase after pre-incubation at 10.3, 4.3, 4.6, NADH-tetrazolium reductase (aerobic marker) and α-glycerophosphate dehydrogenase (anaerobic marker). In orienteer specimen note absence of 2B (2X) fibres (reacting positively at pH 4.6 but not at 4.3), plus intense reaction for NADH-tetrazolium reductase and weak one for α-glycerophosphate dehydrogenase in all fibres. Reproduced from Figure 1 of Jansson & Kaisjer (1977), with permission from Blackwell Publishing Ltd.

endurance training sustained over a decade or more can have some effect in this direction, but the problem is that the differences observed may well be due to age, not training. Trappe et al (1995) made a follow-up study of changes in human gastrocnemius muscles over a period of 20 years, and found significant increases in the type 1 fibre percentage in untrained as well as trained subjects. This age-related reduction in the number of type 2 fibres in both sedentary people and endurance athletes parallels that in their size, mentioned above with reference to Lexell et al (1988).

However, the effects of endurance training are not only on the contractile system of the muscle fibres. Adaptations which start much earlier (detectable as little as 2 weeks after commencement of an exercise programme), are universally achieved and quantitatively more important, are not of the myosin using ATP but of the oxidative systems supplying it. Mitochondrial volume and aerobic capacity increase greatly, especially in type 2 fibres, and anaerobic capacity decreases, as Figure 3.20 shows (Holloszy 1975, Jansson & Kaisjer 1977; and, for review, Saltin & Gollnick 1983). Supply of oxygen to the muscle fibres is enhanced by increased capillarization and also, according to normal interpretations, by increased myoglobin content. The net effect is that the ADP produced by ATP hydrolysis is much more efficiently swept up into the mitochondria, so that a higher percentage of the muscle creatine remains phosphorylated, while glycolysis (consuming glycogen) and the myokinase reaction (producing AMP) are both less activated. Even if there were no shift at all toward less prodigal ATP consumption by the myosins, these adaptations would improve endurance many-fold. For a review of early work see Saltin & Gollnick (1983). Sketches of the current states of research are provided by Essig (1996) and Hood et al (2000) for mitochondria, by Mathieu-Costello & Hepple (2002) for capillarization and by Booth et al (1998) for other adaptations not involving myosin type. Mitochondrial biogenesis will also be considered further in Chapter 5.

By contrast, the sprint or power athlete sends a relatively modest number of HF vollies to his/her muscles, then rests for some time before another short burst of intense activity; this pattern is clearly closer to that which induces the formation of fast fibres in experimental animals. The analogies between training and experimental stimulation were explored in a widely-quoted review by Salmons & Henriksson (1981), and more recently, with emphasis on mechanisms determining myosin type, by Booth et al (1998) and Pette (1998). In sprint and power training there is some shift towards types 1 and 2A from 2B/2X attributable to the increased activity, but also the increase in type 2 fibre size mentioned above and illustrated in Figure 3.21.

This occurs especially in resistance training (Howald 1982, Putman et al 2004), so we must look for effects of load as well as stimulation pattern. Goldspink's evidence that stretch is a stimulus to growth, even of denervated muscle, is probably an important clue to the mechanism here: stretch requires load, but in support of the implied hint that the act of elongation itself is also functional not incidental, we may recall that eccentric exercise is widely held to be more effective in developing muscle bulk than isometric exercise (Komi & Buskirk 1972).

There is evidence that another factor in the hypertrophic effect of strength training is the endocrine response. Growth hormone and testosterone (a potent natural anabolic steroid – cf. p 95) both enhance muscle growth, and these hormones are particularly elevated after resistance training. Growth hormone also enhances oxidative metabolism, but probably not as powerfully as thyroxine – also often found to be elevated – which in addition, as we saw earlier, enhances contraction speeds. By contrast with these effects of resistance training, prolonged regimes of *endurance* training somewhat raise thyroxine and growth hormone but *reduce* the circulating

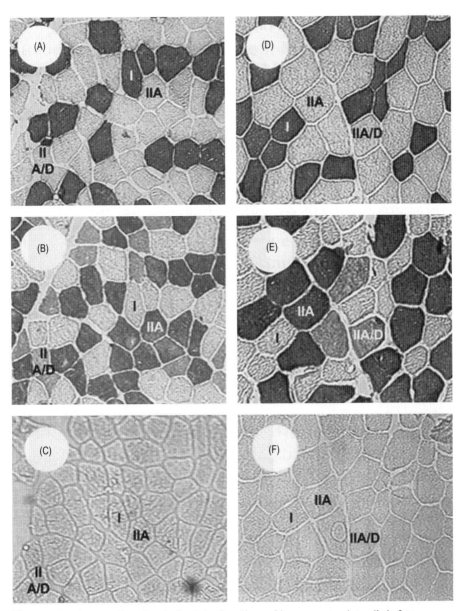

Figure 3.21 Immunohistochemically stained sections of human vastus lateralis before training (A–C) and after 12 weeks of resistance training (D–F). Primary reactions used monoclonal antibodies against human type 1 MHCs (A, D), human type 2A MHCs (B, E), and mouse immunoglobulin as negative control (C, F). The authors employ nomenclature 'D' for the myosin more commonly designated 'X', and Roman numerals for 1 and 2. No pure 2D(X) fibres were present in these sections, but 2A/D hybrids were common. Note significant enlargement of types 2A and 2A/D fibres, but not type 1, after this form of training. Reproduced from Figure 3 of Putnam et al (2004) with kind permission of Springer Science and Business Media.

level of testosterone. They also raise the level of cortisol, the 'stress hormone'. By contrast with all the other hormones named, cortisol has catabolic (tissue eroding) actions, which may well contribute to the fact that endurance training tends to reduce muscle bulk. On the other hand its resting levels are lowered during resistance training. Thus all these factors point to fibre changes in the directions which are in fact observed. For more detail see Kraemer (1992).

INTRACELLULAR SYSTEMS

Two Puzzles

Up to this point all the fibre-type differences and all the changes in response to training we have described should have seemed logical – such that they do not need to be remembered, but can be deduced by simply thinking what is needed. However, two aspects of aerobic metabolism fail to fit this pattern. The first is the distribution of mitochondria, and the second the function of myoglobin.

Early in this chapter, while sketching the contribution of electron microscopy, we noted that the mitochondria of oxidative fibres are markedly more concentrated immediately deep to the sarcolemma than in the main cytoplasm, and if anything tend to be least concentrated of all near the centre. But diffusional constraints point the other way. Oxygen enters the fibre through the sarcolemma and, as a small molecule of reasonable solubility, has a good chance of penetrating several μm into the fibre in a few tens of msec. By contrast, the organic molecules required for and produced by oxidative phophorylation – molecules ranging from pyruvate to ATP – are all quite large and must diffuse relatively slowly. On this logic it ought to be the oxygen which is required to diffuse over the longer intracellular distances, and we should expect to see mitochondria as close to every myofibril as possible and therefore uniformly distributed through the fibre cross-section. Where so much makes sense, this apparent failure of evolution to come up with the optimum distribution indicates that there is some factor operating which we have not yet understood.

The other anomaly is conflicting evidence about the function of myoglobin (Mb). This oxygen-binding pigment may be thought of molecularly as a simple version of haemoglobin (Hb) – it has a high affinity for oxygen (O_2) at lower pressure than Hb itself. This gives it three potential functions: storing O_2, reducing the O_2 partial pressure on the cytoplasmic side of the cell membrane, and facilitating O_2 diffusion through the cytoplasm (Wittenberg & Wittenberg 1989). The storage function is only significant where the time between breaths is exceptionally high, which it normally is only in diving mammals (whose almost-black flesh is due to extremely high Mb concentrations) and to a lesser extent in diving birds. The other two functions, however, have been universally considered to contribute to aerobic metabolism in terrestrial mammals and in birds, and the Wittenbergs and their co-workers have shown experimentally that chemical blockade of Mb's O_2 affinity impairs muscle function. This tallies with the fact that Mb concentrations almost double with endurance training in many species – though admittedly much less so in humans. It was therefore a shock when Garry et al reported (1998) that mice which had been manipulated genetically so that they could not synthesize Mb ('Mb knock-out mice') showed no statistically significant impairment of aerobic performance. It is extremely hard to square this finding with either molecular understanding or prior observation, but it has been suggested that compensatory adaptations may occur during the development of a genetically-modified animal for which there is not time during an acute intervention.

Independent Variation of the Several Systems

So far we have been able to think in terms of three stable types of fibre, recognizably similar in all adult mammals including humans. Does this imply that some genetic or developmental interaction dictates, say, that the fastest myosin in an animal must be coupled to high glycolytic and glycogenolytic activity, and low oxidative and lipolytic? Or that the slowest myosin must be coupled to the converse metabolic pattern? And that the slightly less fast myosin must have high oxidative capacity, but is more tolerant in its glycolytic requirements?

If we confined ourselves to mammals, we might reasonably feel that these general rules were approximately true – at any rate representing powerful trends, from which only second-order departures were feasible. It is instructive, therefore, to look briefly at some examples from animals in other zoological orders which show that no such rigid couplings operate. We shall do this by positing three possible generalizations, which might seem valid if we considered only mammals, and then refuting them by looking more widely.

(1) Is lipolytic capacity necessarily high, where oxidative capacity is?

Compare the flight muscles of two insects: locusts and honey bees. Both are very active, and accordingly highly aerobic. Locust flight muscle also has very high lipolytic capacity. Bees, however, metabolize the carbohydrate they collect almost solely, and their flight muscles have negligible lipolytic capacity (Bass et al 1969). Thus it need be no surprise that although, in mammals, all type 1 fibres have high lipolytic capacity, that of 2A fibres may be moderate or variable (Burke et al 1973).

The opposite generalization, however, *has* to be true: lipolytic capacity cannot be high where oxidative is low. This is because the products of fatty acid oxidation would provide no energy if they could not feed into the TCA cycle and thence to oxidative phosphorylation.

(2) Is glycolytic capacity always high when oxidative is low?

The broad trend in mammals and birds – the warm-blooded species – is for fibres to have high capacity for *either* glycolytic *or* oxidative metabolism. If only fibre types 1 and 2B were present, the negative correlation coefficients (r values) between glycolytic and oxidative markers would be at least 0.8. type 2A, the 'superfibres', many of which in small animals and all of which in large ones are high in both capacities, weaken this relationship to give $r \sim -0.6$ (Spurway 1981), but this is still a strongly negative overall correlation. Nevertheless, one sometimes observes, within a given muscle or even a single fasciculus, that fibres of a given fast type (2B or 2A) show a positive oxidative/glycolytic correlation, those better endowed for one type of metabolism being better endowed for the other too.

This, however, is only a very mild expression of the possibility for positive correlation. In cold-blooded vertebrates ('poikilotherms') of every kind, but most strongly in amphibians (frogs and toads), fibres are either well equipped for both streams of metabolism or poorly equipped for both (Figs 3.22, 3.23) – diametrically converse to the general mammalian situation. Speculating on the reason for this in terms of evolutionary advantage, one might suppose that animals solely breathing air climbed high mountains sufficiently rarely in evolutionary history that a shortfall in oxygen supply need not be provided for. On the other hand they carried their whole weight and could not afford sufficient cardio-respiratory capacity to supply all muscle

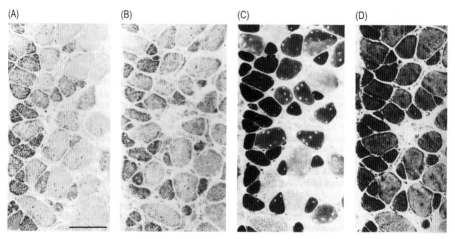

Figure 3.22 Serial sections from frog rectus abdominis reacted histochemically for (A) succinate dehydrogenase, (B) β-hydroxybutyrate dehydrogenase (a marker of fat metabolism), (C) PAS (indicating glycogen) and (D) α-glycerophosphate dehydrogenase. Note the very large extent to which fibres stained strongly in A and B (aspects of aerobic metabolism) are also stained strongly in C and D (aspects of anaerobic metabolism). Reproduced from Figure 1 of Rowlerson & Spurway (1988), with kind permission of Springer Science and Business Media.

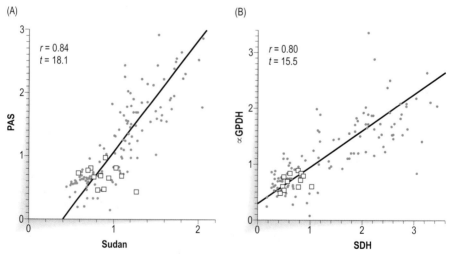

Figure 3.23 Plots of data from microphotometric assays of reaction intensities in frog sartorius muscle fibres. (A) Glycogen (PAS stain) versus fat stores (Sudan black). (B) Glycolysis (α-glycerophosphate dehydrogenase) versus oxidative metabolism (succinate dehydrogenase). Statistics of the strongly positive correlations are indicated. Squares = tonic fibres. From Figures 1a, b of Spurway & Rowlerson (1989), with the publisher's permission.

fibres with oxygen fast enough to meet maximum demand (cf. Chap 1, 97); the fibres least likely to be recruited were thus equipped with the alternative, glycolytic system. By contrast, animals liable to systemic hypoxia, under water or during confined air-breathing, might equip the most-used fibres generously for both means of metabolism, and the least-used sparsely for both.

Whatever the truth of that suggestion, the possibility of finding such a positive correlation between the two main ATP-supply systems, at least within subgroups of mammalian fibres, should not be discounted: Figure 3.12A provides an example.

(3) Are slow fibres always highly oxidative?

Birds, reptiles and amphibians have classes of fibre radically slower than mammalian type 1 fibres. They are not activated by APs, but simply by 'electrotonic' spread of depolarization from their motor endplates. To make this more feasible, however, each such fibre has several endplates spread along its length. These fibres contract and relax many times more slowly even than type 1 mammalian fibres. They are called 'tonic fibres' (Hess 1970). Now tonic fibres have greater resistance to fatigue even than the type 1 fibres of an elite endurance athlete, yet they are not significantly aerobic. Indeed, so free are they of both mitochondria and lipid droplets that early experimenters called them 'clear fibres', and identified them by this criterion when dissecting them under dark ground illumination. Thus, in total reversal of Ranvier's dictum described at the start of this chapter, we find that the slowest, most enduring fibres are among the least 'red' ever found. Yet, in keeping with our discussion of point 2 (above), they have very low glycolytic capacity too (Fig. 3.24).

To see how this can be, consider what is essential for very high endurance. The criterion is that ATP shall be suppliable at least as fast as it can possibly be used. Stating this requirement mathematically, it is that:

Maximum rate of oxidative ATP supply/Maximum rate of ATP consumption ≥ 1

When cross-bridges are cycling at high speed, they need very high aerobic capacity to supply their ATP needs – consider the very strong oxidative staining of 2A fibres in small-medium mammals. type 1 fibres can have the same endurance with ~1/3 as much aerobic capacity, because their cross-bridges cycle at ~1/3 the rate of those in 2A fibres. Pressing the same thinking to its extreme, we see that avian and amphibian tonic fibres can be less oxidative than any others if their XB cycling rates are also lower than the others – which they are.

A convincing mammalian demonstration of this 'demand and supply' model can be found in the results of chronic 10 Hz stimulation of rabbit muscles which were initially of largely 2B fibre composition. Oxidative enzymes and mitochondrial volumes (Fig. 3.25) initially rise steeply, but peak at 2–3 weeks and then fall off again, although settling to levels higher than before the experiment. When they are highest the myosin present is still fast (2B and some 2A); their decline coincides with the beginning of its transition to type 1. The final levels, after 12 or more weeks, are those required to maintain ATP supply in continually-active type 1 fibres (Henriksson et al 1986).

Significance of Non-Mammalian Situations for this Book

The observations from non-mammalian species quoted in this sub-section should be interesting in themselves. However, the purpose of introducing them in a book for human exercise physiologists is to underline the fundamental independence of the

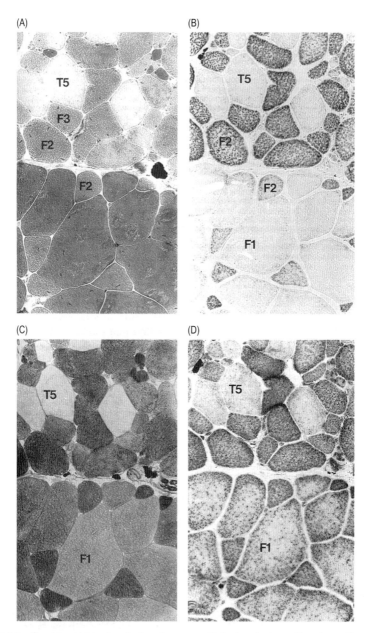

Figure 3.24 Combined histochemical and immuno-histochemical reactions in sections of frog iliofibularis muscle, showing tonic fibres (T5) compared with three fast types (F1-3). (A) Acto-myosin ATPase reaction (Mabuchi-Sreter method: considered to represent contraction speed particularly closely), (B) succinate dehydrogenase, (C) rabbit anti-chick tonic myosin polyclonal antibody, (D) α-glycerophosphate dehydrogenase. The tonic fibres are as low in oxidative and lower in glycolytic activities than the largest, fastest 'white' fibres (F1). Reproduced from parts of Figure 2 of Rowlerson & Spurway (1988), with kind permission of Springer Science and Business Media.

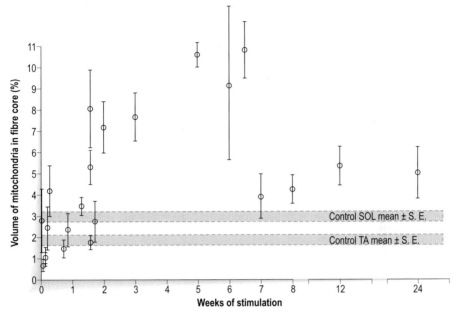

Figure 3.25   Effects of long-term stimulation on mitochondrial volume fraction in electron micrographs of rabbit tibialis anterior muscle fibres. Shaded areas represent mean ± standard error for control fast and slow muscles. Note very high volumes between 1 1/2 and 6 1/2 weeks' stimulation, decreasing from 7 weeks onwards. Reproduced from Figure **N** of Eisenberg & Salmons (1981), with permission.

several metabolic systems, each adapting to meet the particular requirements of a individual fibre. The strong tendencies for fibres in any species to group into types, and for essentially the same types to be identifiable in all species of any given taxonomic family, results from common clusters of demands, not automatically-linked gene expression. In Chapter 4 onwards these common clusters of demands will be seen to be expressed through the parallel activation of the respective signal transduction pathways.

FACTORS AFFECTING FIBRE SIZE

Skeletal muscle fibres are the second longest cell type in the body, only large neurones being longer. It is intriguing that the neurones never have more than one nucleus, whereas the biggest muscle fibres may have several thousand nuclei. The explanation usually offered is that this massive number of nuclei is necessary to control the growth and maintenance of the large volume of cytoplasm in the muscle fibre, and relative to most other cell types this looks reasonable: the ratio of fibre volume to number or nuclei, which must give a rough indication of the domain of cytoplasm under the control of any one nucleus, is greater than the volume of a typical epithelial of connective tissue cell. Yet the volume of cytoplasm in a large neurone can be at least two orders of magnitude greater still, so there must be factors here which we do not yet understand.

In small muscles, such as those moving the eye (extra-ocular muscles) and those within the hands and feet, all fibres run most of the muscle's length. In large pennate muscles, such as soleus, they occupy the full diagonal from muscle surface to the central aponeurosis or tendon. By contrast, in the largest human limb and trunk muscles, such as quadriceps or latissimus dorsi, it is usually considered that no one fibre is much more than half the length of the muscle – typically perhaps 15 cm. Yet it should be noted that this is not an easy figure to arrive at. The usual method has been to tease apart a whole muscle after treatment to hydrolyse or digest its collagen; but in this process the longest fibres can readily be broken. The alternative, trying to trace fibres throughout the volume of such a muscle by conventional histology, would require an almost astronomical number of serial sections, taken from a great many abutting tissue blocks, and an anatomist with the patience of Job! So the possibility that 15 cm is an underestimate should probably be borne in mind.

In the face of these difficulties, probably only the more prominent correlations between fibre length and cytoplasmic properties have been noticed, but it seems safe to say that the longest fibres are ones of large diameter, containing one or other of the fast myosins. Slow myosin is usually found in fibres which are not among the very longest, and more often lie deep in a muscle rather than near its surface; however, as noted earlier, this tendency is much more marked in small animals than large ones such as humans.

What is usually meant by the 'size' of a fibre is, in fact, its mean diameter – or, more accurately, its cross-sectional area. The previous paragraph indicates that this broadly correlates with the whole fibre's volume, but an exact relationship must not be assumed. We can be more confident, however, about the main factor influencing size in this cross-sectional sense: it is oxygen diffusion. It seems likely that no fibre relying on oxidative metabolism can be of greater diameter than allows the partial pressure of oxygen to be maintained above the limiting value for successful respiratory chain function in its deepest-lying mitochondria. Where that constraint is absent, fibres can grow bigger. That is why the adjectives 'large' and 'white' are almost always found together. If there is a puzzle here, it is why in some but not all large animals, humans included, the white fibres are *not* generally larger than the red. Perhaps it is related to the fact (of which we shall see more below) that no human fibres are as purely glycolytic as those of many other species.

Turning to the red fibres, we can make immediate sense of the diameters we see. Not only are none of these fibres big, in species which have very big white fibres. It is also the case that the most highly oxidative – staining darkest in reactions for succinate dehydrogenase, for instance – are smaller than those of intermediate oxidative capacity. We have already noted that the most oxidative in these species are invariably 2A fibres (though not all 2As are so extreme). As this myosin is in the fast group, to find their diameter lowest of all would otherwise seem paradoxical.

Such ultra-aerobic 2A fibres are only common in species which have rather low percentages of type 1 fibres: the figure is about 10% in mice, by contrast with a mean of ~50% in humans. In such instances, it appears that the most often-recruited 2A motor units share endurance functions performed exclusively by type 1 fibres in humans. Their exceptional aerobic capacity makes this possible.

TWITCHES, TETANI AND SHORTENING VELOCITY

So far this chapter has referred to the 'speed' of a muscle or fibre, without clearly distinguishing the different properties which might be implied. Usually it has meant twitch speed (more exactly, twitch *duration*), the simplest property, and one which every investigator from Ranvier to Burke could measure. A property directly associated with twitch duration, and also studied by Burke et al (1973), is the stimulation frequency needed to produce a smooth tetanus. The requirement for a smooth tetanus is that the second stimulus of a train reaches the muscle while the tension elicited by the first one is still rising at its maximum rate; then the third stimulus while the tension is still rising at maximum rate following the second one .... and so on. It follows that, if the twitches of muscle S take four times longer than those of muscle F, yet are of essentially similar shape, S will be able to respond with a smooth tetanus to stimulation at a quarter the frequency required by F: i.e. the 'tetanic fusion frequency' (TFF) of S is 1/4 that of F.

Thus TFF is causally, and therefore inescapably, linked to twitch duration. Another property which is, as a matter of fact, almost equally closely correlated with twitch duration is shortening speed (more precisely, shortening *velocity*). Muscles whose twitches take 3–4 times longer than other muscles almost always shorten roughly 3–4 times more slowly, under equivalent conditions of stimulation and load. However, shortening velocity is a function of the rate at which the cross-bridges (XBs) between myosin and actin cycle, while the concentration of calcium ions ($[Ca^{2+}]$) in the cytoplasm bathing them stays supra-maximal for force-generation. But twitch duration probably depends primarily on how long that $[Ca^{2+}]$-elevation lasts, which is determined by the membrane systems of the sarcoplasmic reticulum (SR): if muscle S's SR lets $[Ca^{2+}]$ stay supra-maximal around the contractile filaments for 3× longer than does the SR of muscle F, then S's twitch will last 3× longer. Insofar as this is correct, twitch duration and shortening velocity chiefly depend on unrelated systems, with no causal link between them. The fact that they are actually closely correlated is a consequence of evolutionary adaptation, not shared mechanism. If a twitch takes a long time, it can afford a slow contraction; if it is short-lived, it must elicit a fast response. But fast response is costly (hydrolysing a lot of ATP per unit time) so providing it will only be advantgeous where the reasons just stated mean that there is no useful alternative.

That account of twitch duration implicitly assumes that the period of force production coincides exactly with the period of elevated $[Ca^{2+}]$. In fact, there is some lag at the beginning, because the XBs take finite times to attach and generate force, and probably greater lag at the end while they complete their cycles and detach. Both these processes *do* depend, absolutely, on the cycling rate. So there are two aspects of twitch duration, one of which – probably normally the major one – is only evolutionarily related to shortening velocity, but the other is directly related to it because it stems from the same cause.

It is because of this close relation between twitch duration and shortening velocity that we have been able loosely to speak of them both as indicators of 'speed'. In all consideration of large, limb muscles it is only when precise, quantitative measures are under discussion that it is necessary to be explicit about which is meant. Some anomalies have, however, been reported in small muscles, notably of the hands and feet. For example, the ball-of-the-thumb muscle, adductor pollicis, has 80% type 1 fibres, so that its shortening velocity (though difficult to measure with any precision in a muscle of that shape) must be presumed to be low. Yet its twitches are unexpectedly brief (Round et al 1983). Presumably the period for which $[Ca^{2+}]$ is high enough to activate force generation is atypically short after a single AP in this muscle, but this has not been proved.

In a final return to general principles, note that shortening velocity falls off with load at different rates in different types of fibre. Only when there is no load does shortening velocity provide a simple indication of XB cycling rate. Unless otherwise specified, therefore, 'unloaded shortening velocity' will always be meant, both here and in other scientific literature.

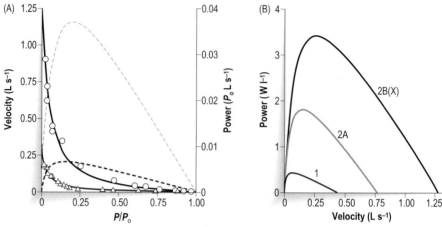

Figure 3.26 Curves relating force, velocity and power in skinned human muscle fibres. (A) Force–velocity and force–power curves (full and broken lines respectively) for representative type 1 and 2B(X) fibres at 12°C. Force ('pull') at each finite shortening velocity is expressed as a fraction of that at zero velocity, P_o; curves for type 1 fibres are the lower ones, for both force and power. (B) Velocity–power curves for representative fibres of each main type, indirectly deduced from the data. Reproduced from Figures 5a, b of Bottinelli et al (1996), with permission from Blackwell Publishing Ltd.

An important series of papers by Bottinelli et al reported unloaded shortening velocities, measured directly and by extrapolation from the lowest of a series of finite loads, in preparations first of rat and then of human single fibres (Bottinelli et al 1996). The preparations were dissected fibres from which the plasmalemma and SR had been removed by detergent so that the properties of the myofibrils could be directly studied. Shortening velocities, and a number of properties related to force and power production (Fig. 3.26), were found to follow an elegantly logical order in accord with the MHC composition of the fibres, type 1 being slowest, then in sequence 1+2A hybrids, 2As, 2A+2B hybrids and finally what Bottinelli et al still called 2B being fastest (Fig. 3.27). Maximum isometric force per unit cross-section was also somewhat lower in type 1 fibres, supporting a widespread but not universal finding on whole muscles. Whether this is due to less force-production by the cross-bridges of type 1 myosin is not yet clear; it might simply result because a greater percentage of the cross-section of such fibres than of 2Bs and all but exceptionally-trained 2As is occupied by mitochondria (or, in detergent-treated fibres, the spaces left by mitochondria). Either way, it provides yet another reason why strength athletes normally have more type 2 than type 1 fibres.

THE VARIETY OF MYOSINS

Identification of Type 2X

Much earlier in this chapter we saw that the initial division into just slow and fast fibres, powered by either slow or fast myosins, had been extended by about 1970, on the basis of acid- and alkali-pre-treated mATPase reactions, into three types: 1, 2A and 2B. Papers as recent as that of Bottinelli et al (1996), just cited, were expressed in such

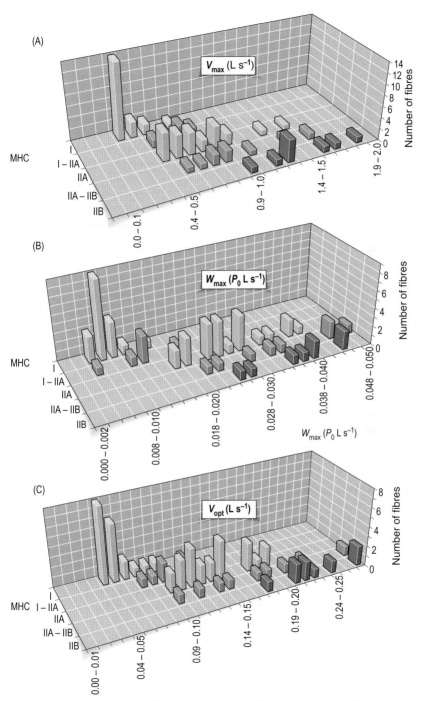

Figure 3.27   Properties of 151 skinned human muscle fibres, grouped according to their myosin heavy chain (MHC) content. (A) Maximum shortening velocity, (B) maximum power, (C) velocity at which maximum power is produced. Reproduced from Figures 6a–c of Bottinelli et al (1996), with permission from Blackwell Publishing Ltd.

terms. However, from the mid-1980s, a third fast MHC, and fibres containing it, were identified first in rat, then in other laboratory animals, in the laboratories of both Schiaffino (Schiaffino et al 1985, 1989, Schiaffino & Reggiani 1996) and Pette (Bar & Pette 1988, Pette & Staron 1990). The former group called it 2X, the latter one 2D (they had recognized it first in diaphragm fibres). The descriptions from the two labs were not identical, but the divergences could be attributed to differences of technique, species and even individual muscle: gradually it became accepted that the two descriptions were of the same entity, and the designation 2X slowly emerged as the more widely-accepted label.

2X myosin was definitively identified by monoclonal antibodies, but could also be distinguished by enzyme histochemistry if one was prepared to bring to bear a sufficient gamut of techniques, and to apply different criteria for every separate species (Hamalainen & Pette 1993). Finally, in the mid-1990s, 2X myosin was shown, not merely to exist in human muscle, but in fact to be the form which had until then always been known as 2B (Sant'ana Pereira et al 1997, Smerdu et al 1994). True 2B myosin is faster than 2X, and probably occurs only in small animals. Thus all earlier work on human fibres can be instantly translated by reading '2X' wherever it referred to '2B' (as in Table 3.2, p 81). Findings for smaller animals require more care, but can usually be sufficiently deduced with the knowledge that 2X fibres contract at speeds intermediate between those of 2A and true 2B, and are on average more oxidative than the latter but less so than the former. Therefore what were previously thought of as the more oxidative 2B fibres were more than likely in fact 2X.

The main properties of human motor units are summarized, in these terms, in Figure 3.28.

2M

About 1980, Rowlerson made a number of observations indicating that the masseter muscles of cats had fibres whose myosin was faster than that of 2B fibres and histochemically distinguished by being not only alkali stable but also more acid stable even than type 1 or '2C' myosins. In a series of papers she and colleagues showed that this 'superfast' or 2M (masseteric) myosin occurred in the jaw-closer muscles of almost all carnivores and all primates except humans – the rule seeming to be that it was present wherever the animal regularly used its bite aggressively, whether in attack or defence. It seems to be confined to the region embryologically originating in the first branchial arch (Rowlerson et al 1983). In addition to the jaw closers these include muscles of the middle ear, where very fast adjustments to sound levels are required. According to Hoh & Hughes (1988), 2M myosin continues to form in jaw muscles transplanted to limbs and innervated by limb-muscle nerves. Overall, it is thus a very interesting adaptation. However, never having been found in limb muscles, it is unlikely to be of direct concern in exercise science.

Others

Currently, about ten MHCs have been identified in adult vertebrate muscle fibres. Embryonic and neonatal myosins can be found in such fibres during regeneration after injury. Although the common type 1 MHC appears to be identical to the major large-animal cardiac form, MHCβ, both heart and slow skeletal muscle can express other forms, including the one commoner in small animal hearts, MHCα. A variety different from and faster than both 2B and 2M is found in extra-ocular muscles. And

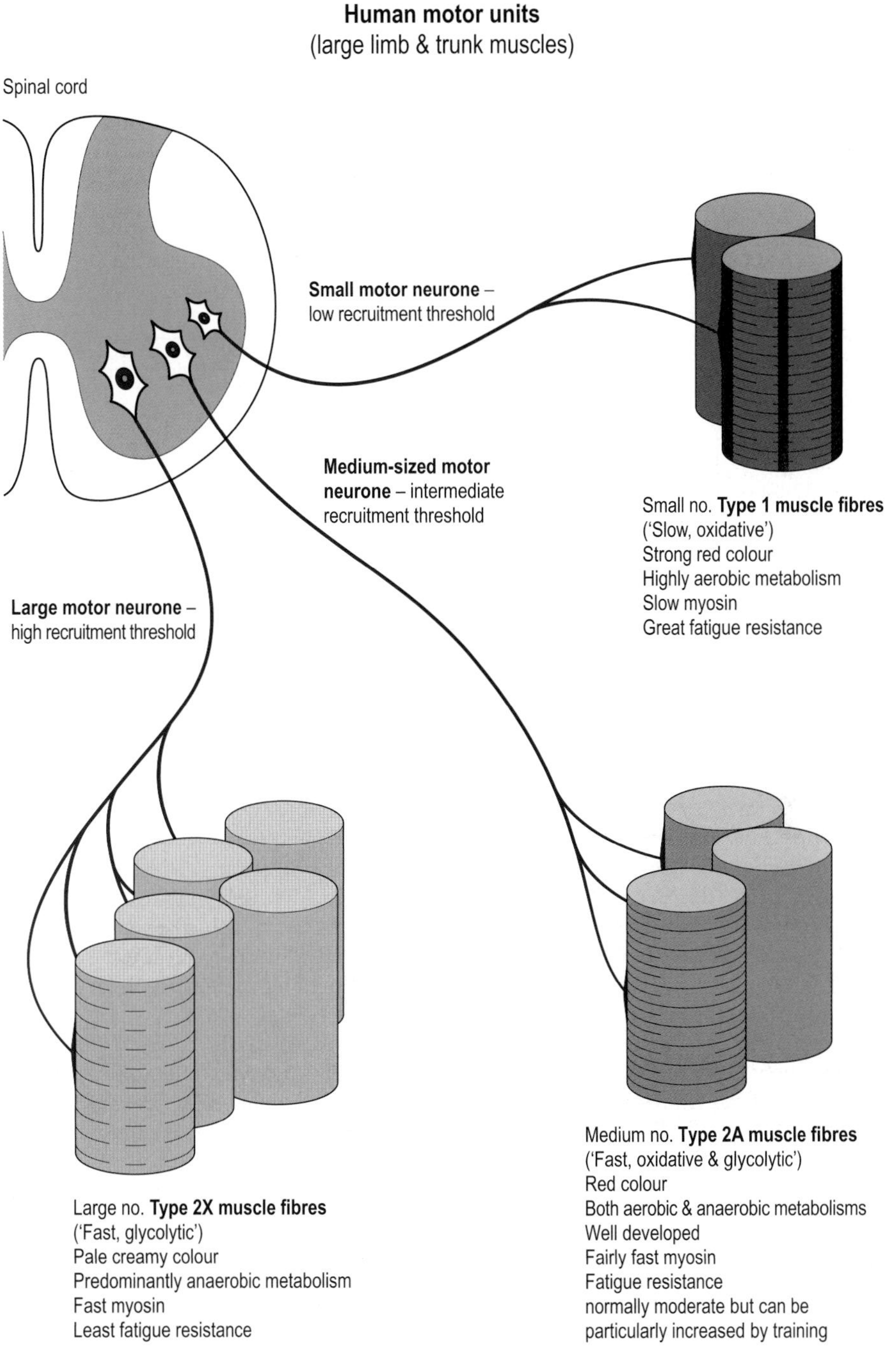

Human motor units
(large limb & trunk muscles)

Spinal cord

Small motor neurone –
low recruitment threshold

**Medium-sized motor
neurone –** intermediate
recruitment threshold

Large motor neurone –
high recruitment threshold

Small no. **Type 1 muscle fibres**
('Slow, oxidative')
Strong red colour
Highly aerobic metabolism
Slow myosin
Great fatigue resistance

Large no. **Type 2X muscle fibres**
('Fast, glycolytic')
Pale creamy colour
Predominantly anaerobic metabolism
Fast myosin
Least fatigue resistance

Medium no. **Type 2A muscle fibres**
('Fast, oxidative & glycolytic')
Red colour
Both aerobic & anaerobic metabolisms
Well developed
Fairly fast myosin
Fatigue resistance
normally moderate but can be
particularly increased by training

Figure 3.28   Diagram summarizing the properties of the three principle types of motor unit found in large human muscles, and their component muscle fibres, as indicated by the accumulated evidence of this chapter.

so on! Quite possibly more will be reported before this book reaches print. But it seems fairly unlikely that forms not yet identified will be of direct concern to the sport and exercise scientist.

It is therefore appropriate to turn to the techniques by which it is now possible to investigate the *formation* of the myosins and other molecules in skeletal muscle fibres, and hence of the intracellular structures in which they are incorporated. These, and the resultant findings, will be the subject of the rest of this book.

KEY POINTS

1. In many species of fish and birds, the naked eye can readily see that parts of the musculature are red-brown and other parts pale. Behavioural or electro-myographic observations show that the red-brown regions are utilized sustainedly, the pale ones only occasionally.

2. From roughly 1840 to 1970, microscopists came to recognize that the colour differences resided in the individual muscle fibres, and that 'red' and 'white' extremes (although often accompanied by various intermediate forms) were mixed together in the majority of mammalian muscles – including all human ones involved in posture and propulsion.

3. Histochemical, ultrastructural and biochemical techniques demonstrated that the redness was due to myoglobin and the respiratory molecules of mitochondria, which gave these fibres aerobic endurance lacked by the white fibres. In many species, but not generally in humans, the red fibres are substantially smaller than the white, presumably to facilitate oxygen diffusion.

4. Different contractile proteins, especially the myosins, were also involved. White fibres of fish, birds and mammals always contained fast (type 2B) myosin, and red fibres with postural or slow-speed functions contained slow (type 1). However, where repeated fast contractions were required, the fibres were also red (sometimes redder than the slow fibres) and contained a third type of myosin (type 2A) only marginally less fast than 2B. More recently, a myosin with properties intermediate between 2A and 2B, usually designated 2X, has been identified, and found to be the fast myosin of human limb and trunk muscle fibres, previously classified as 2B. In species which have both, 2X myosin is found in fibres slightly more aerobic and less large than 2B – tallying with the fact that human fibres differ less than those of many other animals.

5. 2X myosin was revealed by immunohistochemistry; its difference from 2B is extremely hard, though possible, to detect histochemicaly. Much the same is true of 'hybrid' fibres (fibres having more than one isoform of a particular protein, notably myosin). A few of these may be present in mature muscles in stable states; far more occur during growth, injury and recovery, and during adaptation to a changed activity or training regime. Nonetheless, most researchers into human/mammalian muscle find the concept of three main fibre types useful; at a minimum it is a basis for nomenclature and the classification of hybridity.

6. Overwhelmingly the most powerful determinant of muscle fibre type is contractile activity, which is physiologically a result of neural activity. Consequently, each normal motor unit is essentially homogeneous in its muscle fibre type.

7. Neurone size, recruitment threshold and motor unit size (number of muscle fibres, not *their* sizes) correlate strongly (the 'size principle'). The smallest motor neurones control the smallest, and therefore weakest, units and are the most easily recruited; this requires their muscle fibres to have the highest resistance to fatigue, so they

are red (highly oxidative) fibres with the slow, and therefore economical, type 1 myosin. The largest neurones control the largest, strongest units, but are hardest to recruit; being thus used only rarely, they develop the least fatigue resistance, but have the fastest (and least economical) myosin in the species – type 2B or 2X. Units intermediate in all respects have type 2A fibres.

8. Enzymes within a given metabolic pathway vary in near-constant proportions. However, comparative studies, especially of non-mammalian vertebrates (whose enzymes, both contractile and metabolic, are molecularly closely similar to those of mammals) show that there are few obligatory relationships, either positive or negative, between different pathways. High lipolytic activity *must* be associated with high oxidative, but aerobic and anaerobic activities can be positively correlated, though always overall negative in mammals; and the condition for high endurance is that the ratio of ATP consumption rate to aerobic ATP production rate does not exceed 1: where the former is very low, so may the latter be.

Further Reading

The review by Saltin & Gollnick (1983) covers a wide range of the subject matter of this chapter lucidly, and with greater emphasis than we have placed on the human. Although inevitably unaware of 2X myosin, it is otherwise remarkably little dated.

More recent reviews of fibre types are those of Schiaffino & Reggiani (1996) and Booth et al (1998). The earlier of these links particularly closely to our subsequent chapters, but a newcomer to the field is likely to find it heavier going. By contrast, the papers of Gunderson (1998) and Pette (1998), in the same symposium as that of Booth et al, together provide lucid coverage of much of our field.

For general background on skeletal muscle function, in the context of fibre types and physical performance, see Spurway (1999), and the chapters by Greenhaff & Hultman, Hamilton et al, and Sharpe & Koutedakis in the same volume.

For more details on motor unit properties, see McComas (1996), and on muscle biochemistry Maughan et al (1997). Finally, on muscle in general see also Jones et al (2004)

References

Andreassen S, Arendt-Nielsen L 1987 Muscle fibre conduction velocity in motor units of the human anterior tibial muscle: a new size principle parameter. Journal of Physiology 391: 561–571

Bar A, Pette D 1988 Three fast myosin heavy chains in adult rat skeletal muscle. FEBS letters 235: 153–155

Barany M 1967 ATPase activity of myosin correlated with speed of muscle shortening. Journal of General Physiology 50: 197–218

Bass A, Brdiczka D, Eyer P et al 1969 Metabolic differentiation of distinct muscle types at the level of enzymatic organisation. European Journal of Biochemistry 10: 198–206

Booth F W, Teng J S, Fluck M, Carson J A 1998 Molecular and cellular adaptation of muscle in response to physical training. Acta Physiologica Scandinavica 162: 343–350

Bottinelli R, Canepai M, Pellgrino M A, Reggiani C 1996 Force-velocity properties of human skeletal muscle fibres: myosin heavy chain isoform and temperature dependence. Journal of Physiology 495: 573–586

Bowman W 1840 On the minute structure and movements of voluntary muscle. Philosophical Transactions of the Royal Society of London 130 Part II: 457

Brooke M H, Kaiser K K 1970 Muscle fibre types: how many and what kind? Archives of Neurology 23: 369–379

Buller A J, Eccles J C, Eccles R M 1960 Interactions between motor neurones and muscles in respect of the characteristic speeds of their responses. Journal of Physiology 150: 417–439

Burke R E 1980 Motor unit types: Functional specializations in motor control. Trends in Neurological Sciences 3: 255–260.

Burke R E, Edgerton V R 1975 Motor unit properties and selective involvement in movement. Exercise and Sport Science Reviews 3: 31–81

Burke R E, Levine D N, Tsairis P, Zajac F E 1973 Physiological types and histological profiles in motor units of cat gastrocnemius. Journal of Physiology 234: 723–748

Caiozzo C, Haddad F 1996 Thyroid hormone: modulation of muscle structure, function and adaptive responses to mechanical loading. Exercise and Sport Science Reviews 24: 321–361

Close R I 1969 Dynamic properties of fast and slow skeletal muscles of the rat after nerve cross-union. Journal of Physiology 204: 331–346

Close R I 1972 Dynamic properties of mammalian skeletal muscles. Physiological Reviews 52: 129–197

Condon K, Silberstein L, Blau H M, Thompson W J 1990 Differentiation of fibre types in aneural musculature of the prenatal rat hindlimb. Developmental Biology 138: 275–295

Costill D L, Daniels J, Evans W et al 1976 Skeletal muscle enzymes and fibre composition in male and female athletes. Journal of Applied Physiology 40: 149–154

Daugaard J R, Lausten J L , Hansen B S, Richter E A 1998 Growth hormone induces muscle fibre type transformation in growth-hormone deficient rats. Acta Physiologica Scandinavica 164: 119–126

DiMario J X, Fernyak S E, Stockdale F E 1993 Myoblasts transferred to the limbs of embryos are committed to specific fibre types. Nature 362: 165–167

Eisenberg B R, Salmons S 1981 The reorganization of subcellular structure in muscle undergoing fast-to-slow type transformation. A stereological study. Cell and Tissue Research 220: 449–471

Eisenberg B R 1983 Quantitative ultrastructure of mammalian skeletal muscle. In: Peachey LD, Adrian RH, Geiger SR (eds) Skeletal muscle. Handbook of physiology, sect. 10. Bethesda, American Phyiological Society: p 73–112

Enoka R M, Stuart D G 1984 Henneman's 'size principle': Current issues. Trends in Neuroscience 7: 226–228

Essig D A 1996 Contractile activity-induced mitochondrial biogenesis in skeletal muscle. Exercise and Sport Science Reviews 24: 289–319

Garnett R A F, O'Donovan M J, Stephens J A, Taylor A 1979 Motor unit organization of human medial gastrocnemius. Journal of Physiology 287: 33–43

Garry D J, Ordway G A, Lorenz J N et al 1998 Mice without myoglobin. Nature 395: 905–908

Gauthier G F 1969 On the relationship of ultrastructural and cytochemical features to color in mammalian skeltal muscle. Zeitschrift fur Zellforschung und mikroscopische Anatomie 95: 162

Goldspink D F 1978 The influence of passive stretch on the growth and protein turnover of denervated extensor digitorum longus muscle. Biochemical Journal 171: 585–602

Goldspink G, Scutt A, Loughna P T et al 1992 Gene expression in skeletal muscle in response to stretch and force generation. American Journal of Physiology 262: R356–R363

Gollnick P D, Armstrong R B, Saubert C W et al 1972 Enzyme activity and fibre composition in skeletal muscle of untrained and trained men. Journal of Applied Physiology 33: 312–319

Gundersen K 1998 Determination of muscle contractile proprerties: the importance of the nerve. Acta Physiologica Scandinavica 162: 333–341

Guth L, Samaha F J 1969 Qualitative differences between the actomyosin ATPase of slow and fast mammalian muscle. Experimental Neurology 25: 138–163

Hamalainen N, Pette D 1993 The histochemical profiles of fast fibre types IIb, IId and IIa in skeletal muscles of mouse, rat and rabbit. Journal of Histochemistry and Cytochemistry 41: 733–743

Henneman E 1957 Relation between size of neurons and their susceptibility to discharge. Science 126: 1345–1346

Henneman E, Mendell L M 1981 Functional organization of motoneuron pool and its inputs. In: Burke RE (ed) The nervous system. Handbook of physiology, vol II, part 1. Bethesda, MD, American Physiological Society: p 423–507

Henneman E, Somjen G, Carpenter DO 1965 Functional significance of cell size in spinal motoneurones. Journal of Neurophysiology 28: 560–580

Henriksson J, Chi M M-Y, Hintz C S et al 1986 Chronic stimulation of mammalian muscle: Changes in enzymes of six metabolic pathways. American Journal of Physiology 251: C614–C632

Hess A 1970 Vertebrate slow muscle fibres. Physiological Reviews 50: 40–62

Hill A V 1950 The dimensions of animals and their muscular dynamics. Science Progress 38: 209–230

Hnik P, Vejsada R, Goldspink D et al 1985 Quantitative evaluation of EMG activity in rat extensor and flexor muscles immobilized at different lengths. Experimental Neurology 88: 515–528

Hoh J F Y, Hughes S 1988 Myogenic and neurogenic regulation of myosin gene expression in cat jaw-closing muscles regenerating in fast and slow limb muscle beds. Journal of Muscle Research and Cell Motility 9: 59–72

Holloszy J O 1975 Adaptation of skeletal muscle to endurance exercise. Medicine and Science in Sports and Exercise 7: 155–164

Hood D A, Takahashi M, Connor M K, Freyssenet D 2000 Assembly of the cellular powerhouse: Current issues in muscle mitochondrial biogenesis. Exercise and Sport Science Reviews 28: 68–73

Hoppeler H, Luthi P, Claasen H et al 1973 The ultrastructure of the normal human skeletal muscle. A morphometric analysis on untrained men, women, and well-trained orienteers. Pflugers Archiv – European Journal of Physiology 344: 217–232

Howald H 1982 Training-induced morphological and functional changes in skeletal muscle. International Journal of Sports Medicine 3: 1–12

Jansson E, Kaijser L 1977 Muscle adaptation to extreme endurance training in man. Acta Physiologica Scandinavica 100: 315–324

Johnston I A, Davison W, Goldspink G 1977 Energy metabolism of carp swimming muscles. Journal of Comparative Physiology 114: 203–216

Johnson M A, Polgar J, Weightman D, Appleton D 1973 Data on the distribution of fibre types in thirty-six human muscles. Journal of the Neurological Sciences 18: 111–129

Jones D, Round J, Haan A 2004 Skeletal muscle from molecules to movement. Edinburgh, Churchill Livingstone

Kernell D 1992 Organizational variability in the neuromuscular system: a survey of task-related adaptations. Archives Italiennes de Biologie 130: 19–66

Komi P V, Buskirk E R 1972 Effects of eccentric and concentric muscle conditioning on tension and electrical activity of human muscle. Ergonomics 15: 417–434

Kraemer W J 1992 Hormonal mechanisms related to the expression of muscular strength and power. In: Komi PV (ed) Strength and power in sport. Oxford, Blackwell, p 64–76

Kugelberg E 1973 Histochemical composition, contraction speed and fatiguability of rat soleus motor units. Journal of the Neurological Sciences 20: 177–198

Lexell J, Taylor C C, Sjostrom M 1988 What is the cause of the ageing atrophy? Total number, size and proportion of different fibre types studied in the whole vastus lateralis muscle from 15- to 83-year-old men. Journal of the Neurological Sciences 84: 275–294

Mathieu-Costello O, Hepple R T 2002 Muscle structural capacity for oxygen flux from capillary to fiber mitochondria. Exercise and Sport Science Reviews 30: 80–84

Mauhan R, Gleeson M, Greenhaff P L 1997 Biochemistry of exercise and training. Oxford, Oxford University Press

Mayne C N, Sutherland H, Jarvis J C et al 1996 Induction of a fast-oxidative phenotype by chronic muscle stimulation: Histochemical and metabolic studies. American Journal of Physiology 270: C313–C320

McComas A J 1996 Skeletal muscle form and function. Champaign, IL, Human Kinetics

Milner-Brown H S, Stein R B, Yemm R 1973 The orderly recruitment of human motor units during voluntary isometric contractions. Journal of Physiology 230: 359–370

Peter J B, Barnard R J, Edegerton V R et al 1972 Metabolic profiles of three fibre types of skeletal muscles in guinea pigs and rabbits. Biochemistry 11: 2672–2683

Pette D 1998 Training effects on the contractile apparatus. Acta Physiologica Scandinavica 162: 367–376

Pette D, Hofer H W 1980 The constant proportion enzyme group concept in the selection of reference enzymes in metabolism. In: Evered D, O'Connor M (eds) Trends in enzyme histochemistry and cytochemistry. Ciba Foundation Symposium 73 (new series). Amsterdam, Excerpta Medica, p 231–144

Pette D, Peuker H, Staron R S 1999 The impact of biochemical methods for single fibre analysis. Acta Physiologica Scandinavica 166: 261–277

Pette D, Staron R S 1990 Cellular and molecular diversities of mammalian skeletal muscle fibres. Reviews of Physiology, Biochemistry and Pharmacology 116: 1–76

Pierobon-Bormioli S, Sartori S, Libera L D et al 1981 'Fast' isomyosins and fibre types in mammalian skeletal muscle. Journal of Histochemistry and Cytochemistry 29: 1179–1188

Polak J M, Van Noorden S 1997 Introduction to immunocytochemistry. Oxford, BIOS

Putnam C T, Xu X, Gillies E et al 2004 Effects of strength, endurance and combined training on myosin heavy chain content and fibre-type distribution in humans. European Journal of Applied Physiology 92: 376–384

Ranvier M L 1873 Propriétés et structures différentes des muscles rouges et des muscles blancs, chez les lapins et chez les raies. Comptes Rendue des Académie de Sciences 77: 1030–1034

Round J M, Jones D A, Chapman S J et al 1983 The anatomy and fibre type composition of the human adductor pollicis in relation to its contractile properties. Journal of the Neurological Sciences 66: 263–292

Rowlerson A M, Mascarello F, Veggetti A, Carpene E 1983 The fibre type composition of the first branchial arch muscles in carnivora and primates. Journal of Muscle Research and Cell Motility 4: 443–472

Rowlerson A M, Spurway N C 1988 Histochemical and immunohistochemical properties of skeletal muscle fibres from *Rana* and *Xenopus*. Histochemical Journal 20: 657–673

Salmons S 1994 Exercise, stimulation and type transformation of skeletal muscle. International Journal of Sports Medicine 15: 136–141

Salmons S, Henriksson K 1981 The adaptive response of skeletal muscle to increased use. Muscle and Nerve 4: 94–105

Salmons S, Sreter FA 1976 Significance of impulse activity in the transformation of skeletal muscle type. Nature 263: 30–34

Salmons S, Vrbova G 1969 The influence of activity on some contractile characteristics of mammalian fast and slow muscles. Journal of Physiology 201: 535–549.

Saltin B, Gollnick P D 1983 Skeletal muscle adaptability: significance for metabolism and performance. In: Peachey L D, Adrian R H, Geiger S R (eds) Skeletal muscle. Handbook of physiology, sect. 10. Bethesda, American Physiological Society, p 555–631

Sant'Ana-Pereira J A A, Ennion S, Sargeant A J et al 1997 Comparison of the molecular, antigenic and ATPase determinants of fast myosin heavy chains in rat and human: a single fibre study. Pflugers Archiv – Euroopean Journal of Physiology 435: 151–163

Schiaffino S, Reggiani C 1996 Molecular diversity of myofibrillar proteins: gene regulation and functional significance. Physiological Reviews 76: 371–423

Schiaffino S, Hanzlikova V, Pierobon S 1970 Relations between structure and function in rat skeletal muscle fibers. Journal of Cell Biology 47: 107–119

Schiaffino S, Sagin I, Viela A, Gorza I 1985 Differentiation of fibre types in rat skeletal muscle visualized with monoclonal antimyosin antibodies. Journal of Muscle Research and Cell Motility 6: 60–61

Schiaffino S, Gorza L, Sartore S et al 1989 Three myosin heavy chain isoforms in type 2 skeletal muscle fibres. Journal of Muscle Research and Cell Motility 10: 197–205

Schmidt E M, Thomas S J 1981 Motor unit recruitment order: Modification under volitional control. In: Desmedt J E (ed) Progress in neurophysiology 9. Basel, Karger, p 145–148

Schmidt-Nielsen K 1973 Scaling: why is animal size so important? Cambridge, Cambridge University Press

Smerdu V, Karsch-Mizrachi I, Campione M et al 1994 Type IIX myosin heavy chain transcripts are expressed in type IIB fibres of human skeletal muscle. American Journal of Physiology 267: C1723–C1728

Spurway N C, Murray M J, Montgomery I, Gilmour W H 1996 Quantitative skeletal muscle histochemistry of four east African ruminants. Journal of Anatomy 188: 455–472

Spurway N C 1980 Histochemical typing of muscle fibres by microphotometry. In: Pette D (ed) Plasticity of muscle. Berlin, de Gruyter, p 31–44

Spurway N C 1981 Objective characterization of cells in terms of microscopical parameters: An example from muscle histochemistry. Histochemical Journal 13: 269–317

Spurway N C 1999 Muscle. In: Maughan R J (ed) Basic and applied sciences for sports medicine. Oxford, Butterworth-Heinemann, p 1–47

Spurway N C, Rowlerson A M 1989 Quantitative analysis of histochemical and immunohistochemical reactions in skeletal muscle fibres of *Rana* and *Xenopus*. Histochemical Journal 21: 461–474

Stephenson G M M 2001 Hybrid skeletal muscle fibres: a rare or common phenomenon? Clinical and Experimental Pharmacology and Physiology 28: 692–702

Tesch P, Thorsson A, Kaiser P 1984 Muscle capillary supply and fibre type characteristics in weight and power lifters. Journal of Applied Physiology 56: 35–38

Thayer R, Collins J, Noble E G et al 2000 A decade of aerobic endurance training: histological evidence for fibre type transformation. Journal of Sports Medicine and Physical Fitness 40: 284–289

Trappe S W, Costill D L, Fink W J et al 1995 Skeletal muscle characteristics among distance runners: a 20-yr follow-up study. Journal of Applied Physiology 78: 823–829

Windisch A, Gundersen K, Sjaboles M J et al 1998 Fast to slow transformation of denervated and electrically stimulated rat muscle. Journal of Physiology 510: 623–632

Wittenberg B A, Wittenberg J B 1989 Transport of oxygen in muscle. Annual Reviews of Physiology 51: 857–878

Chapter **4**

Introduction to molecular exercise physiology

Henning Wackerhage

CHAPTER CONTENTS

LEARNING OBJECTIVES:

After studying this chapter, you should be able to . . .

1. Explain the nature of DNA, transcription of DNA to mRNA and translation of mRNA to protein.
2. Explain how signal transduction pathways may sense exercise-related signals, integrate this information and regulate the resultant adaptation to exercise.
3. Describe models and methods used in molecular exercise physiology research.

INTRODUCTION

Judged by the activities of the world's leading institutions and by publication impact, exercise physiology research is currently changing one of its major foci towards investigating the cellular and molecular basis of phenomena such as the adaptation to exercise. As a result, a lot of exercise science is currently published in journals like *Nature*, *Science* and *Cell* and findings such as 'marathon mice' and 'super toddlers' are reported by mass media. Unfortunately, much of this research has not yet entered mainstream sports science teaching, with the possible exception of some North American and Scandinavian institutions.

In this chapter we focus on molecular exercise physiology related to skeletal muscle – which is a field in which a lot of progress has been made. Molecular exercise physiology usually is a continuation of classical exercise physiology and provides explanations for older observations. Important classical exercise physiology findings are the changes in capillarization, muscle enzyme activities, fibre phenotypes and size, that occur as adaptations to exercise. Such skeletal muscle adaptations explain the development of fatigue resistance by endurance training and the greater strength and size that results from a period of resistance training. Classical exercise physiologists consciously or unconsciously used the following research model: *exercise → 'black box' → adaptation*. As a result of applying muscle biopsies and biochemical and histochemical analyses to exercise problems, many of the important skeletal muscle adaptations to exercise were already known at the beginning of the 1980s (Gollnick et al 1983, Holloszy & Booth 1976). Molecular exercise physiology started in the late 80s when exercise physiologists first applied cellular and molecular-biological techniques to physiological problems (Booth 1988). Researchers at that time had to learn and apply tricky molecular and cellular techniques. There were only a few kits or easy protocols for assays. Many cellular and molecular techniques must have been daunting for people trained in measuring oxygen uptake or blood lactate concentration and in staining capillaries. However, the new approach has allowed researchers to open up the black box in the classical exercise physiologist's research model. The new model is: *exercise → signal transduction and gene regulation → adaptation*. The aim is to identify an uninterrupted chain of events which starts with the signals associated with exercise and ends in a specific adaptive response.

Research in this field has now entered its golden era: Signal transduction pathways that regulate adaptations to endurance training such as the expression of 'fast' or 'slow' motor proteins and mitochondrial biogenesis have been discovered and will be discussed in Chapter 5. In contrast to endurance training, the specific adaptation of muscle to resistance training is growth. Recent research has led to the discovery of the major signal transduction pathways that upregulate protein synthesis and satellite cell proliferation after high-intensity exercise and this will be discussed in Chapter 6. Comprehensive overviews of the regulation of thousands of genes by exercise or other interventions affecting skeletal muscle have been obtained by carrying out 'transcriptional' (cDNA microarray) and 'translational' profiling experiments (if the terms in quotes are unfamiliar, they will be explained shortly). The research carried out in this area, especially in the few years of the present century, has given us a much deeper insight into the regulation of adaptation to exercise.

The regulatory events mediating the specific adaptation to various forms of exercise in several organs are just an example of the problems studied by molecular exercise physiologists. Another challenge is to identify the links between genetic variation and athletic ability. Research questions in this field are: 'What determines muscle mass?', 'What determines sprint performance?' or 'What determines a high percentage of slow muscle fibres?'. The research in this field is in its infancy: genes such as those for ACE and actinin-3 have been linked to specific types of athletic performance and trainability. However, as we saw in Chapter 2, it is rare that a single gene variant is a major regulator of a complex trait such as endurance exercise performance. It is probably more like a lottery draw: a combination of several beneficial gene variants is needed in order to have the chance to become an Olympic champion. An elite marathon runner is likely not to be only an individual with a high percentage of slow muscle fibres but one with high running economy, low body weight [there are some very tall marathoners, but they're always very thin; I'm sure body weight is the key], high mitochondrial content, vigorous fat metabolism, excellent glycogen saving, high percentage slow fibres, large heart and high haematocrit. In turn, the majority if not all of these features are influenced by several feature-specific genetic variations.

The recent advent of so-called 'single nucleotide polymorphism' (SNP) or genotyping chips (i.e. a method to scan for thousands of gene variations in an overnight experiment) means that we now have a tool that can be applied to carry out large-scale analyses of genetic variation. These chips will allow us to correlate thousands of genetic variations with specific forms of athletic performance or with the likelihoods of particular diseases. It will be a great challenge for today's exercise physiologists to use such techniques in larger populations in order to obtain sufficient statistical power to be able to discover the combinations of gene variants necessary for particular types of elite performance. At the same time, it will be important to consider ethical issues regarding the use of large-scale genotyping data in sports science.

The preceding paragraphs of this chapter have given an overview of the field of molecular exercise physiology. We define the field thus:

Molecular exercise physiology is the study of genetics and signal transduction in relation to exercise. Molecular exercise physiologists aim to identify the genetic determinants of human performance on a molecular level and characterize the mechanisms responsible for the adaptation of cells and organs to exercise.

The above definition is narrow but we shall use it as a starting point. The aim of this chapter is to introduce the reader not trained in molecular or cellular biology to the basic knowledge on signal transduction and gene regulation that is necessary for understanding molecular exercise physiology findings. We will then discuss the models and the research techniques that are used by molecular exercise physiologists with special reference to skeletal muscle.

DNA

In this section we will cover DNA, its transcription to mRNA and the translation of mRNA into protein. Deoxyribonucleic acid (DNA) is the molecule that carries our genetic information. Its basic units are nucleotides, each consisting of a sugar and a base joined by phosphodiester bonds. There are four nucleotides in DNA, namely adenine (A), guanine (G), cytosine (C) and thymine (T). The nucleotides are linked together as a DNA strand and two *complementary DNA strands* form the double-helix or double-stranded DNA (Watson & Crick 1953). In the complementary strands, A is linked to T via *two* hydrogen bonds and C to G via *three* hydrogen bonds. The complementary strand for ATCG would be TAGC.

Human DNA consists of 3 201 762 515 nucleotide or base pairs according to the *Ensembl* database. Prefixes such as kilo, mega and giga are also used to denote thousands, millions and billions of base pairs and thus we may say that the human genome contains 3.2 giga base pairs or 6.4 giga bases. Only a small part of the DNA,

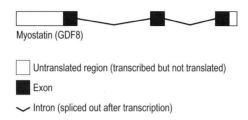

Myostatin (GDF8)

☐ Untranslated region (transcribed but not translated)

■ Exon

⌣ Intron (spliced out after transcription)

Figure 4.1

about 5%, encodes genes. Nearly all genes are blueprints for proteins (some code for ribosomal RNA or for pseudogenes which are genes that are not translated). The use of the gene blueprint to build a protein involves two steps: genes are first *transcribed* (i.e. a copy of the DNA is made) into messenger ribonucleic acid (mRNA) which is then *translated* into a protein. This is known as the 'central dogma' of molecular biology: *DNA → mRNA → polypeptide or protein*. The human genome, i.e. the whole of our DNA, encodes roughly 25 000 genes, which is a surprisingly low number – earlier counts were higher. The number is the same as in some of the higher plants, and there are ~6000 genes in the genome of such a simple, unicellular organism as yeast. The complexity of the human being is therefore not due to a larger number of genes but rather due to a more sophisticated use of the gene products in the building process. The ~95% of the DNA that does not code genes serves regulatory or unknown non-coding functions. Even genes contain non-coding parts: genes consist of so-called *exons* ('expressed DNA', i.e. DNA which is the template for producing a protein) and *introns* (intervening, non-expressed sequences). Introns are *spliced* or cut out of the pre-mRNA before mRNA is translated. Figure 4.1 shows the gene structure for myostatin (GDF8) which is a powerful inhibitor of muscle growth. The picture is redrawn from the information present in the Ensembl database. Three exons are visible in red and the thin, kinked lines in between indicate two introns. The open boxes at the beginning and end show parts of the protein that are cleaved during its processing from the precursor to the mature form.

TRANSCRIPTION, RNA CAPPING AND SPLICING

Exercise regulates the expression of hundreds or even thousands of genes in skeletal muscle and many other tissues. During the first phase, transcription, DNA is transcribed into messenger ribonucleic acid (mRNA) by RNA polymerase II. RNA polymerase is an enzyme that can 'read' DNA and synthesize a complementary RNA copy of the DNA. RNA polymerases I and III exist as well but their function is restricted to synthesizing RNA needed for the synthesis of ribosomes, the factories which build proteins on the bases of the mRNA blueprints.

RNA polymerase II first binds to the so-called *promoter* of a gene. The basal promoter is a ~100 base pair DNA sequence located upstream (or 'to the left' or in the 5' direction) of the gene. Many genes have a so-called TATA box in their basal promoter region but this TATA sequence is not found in all genes. Once RNA polymerase II is positioned on the basal promoter it will scan over the DNA and start transcribing the gene into mRNA. Each base in DNA has an 'opposite number' in RNA. For cysteine this is guanine and for guanine it is cysteine; for thymine it is adenine but for adenine it is *not* thymine. The equivalent of thymine in DNA is uracil in RNA. To give an example, the DNA sequence (DNA is given in upper-case letters) in the following upper line will be transcribed into the lower-line mRNA (RNA is given in lower-case letters) as follows:

DNA	CTC	TTT	AAG	GGT	CAC	CCA	GAG
mRNA	gag	aaa	uuc	cca	gug	ggu	cuc

Several online programmes can be used to 'transcribe' DNA into mRNA *in silico*, as we say (i.e. by computer) or to 'translate' mRNA into the resultant amino acid sequence (protein).

An instance of such a programme can be found at www.nitrogenorder.org/cgi-bin/nucleo.cgi. Enter a DNA or mRNA sequence and the programme will either 'transcribe' the DNA into its mRNA sequence or 'translate' the mRNA into a peptide sequence.

The arrival of so-called *DNA microarrays* (or 'gene chips' (the method will be explained on page 153) has allowed us to investigate the effects of exercise on the expression of nearly all of the ~25 000 human genes. A DNA microarray is produced by using computer chip-printing equipment to print thousands of probes for different DNA molecules on a surface. DNA microarrays are used in conjunction with fluorescent dyes to estimate the concentration of tens of thousands of mRNAs. Such DNA microarray studies have shown that the expression of hundreds or even thousands of genes is changed in response to exercise in skeletal muscle. Good DNA microarray results are often a rich source for research ideas. Molecular exercise physiologists can use published information on these genes in order to develop hypotheses regarding their function. DNA microarray research is thus sometimes described as 'hypothesis-generating' research.

How does exercise affect the expression of genes? Gene expression is a tightly regulated process. It ensures that the specific muscle and heart genes are only expressed in muscle or heart, respectively. In contrast, common 'housekeeping' genes are switched on in nearly all tissues. Many genes are induced at specific time points in the development of the organism; others are only switched on or off in response to environmental stimuli such as exercise. Exercise activates so-called *signal transduction pathways* (discussed in detail below) and some of these pathways activate *transcription factors* which will then direct RNA polymerase II to genes that are upregulated by exercise.

DNA is normally tightly wrapped around so-called histones and in this state it is not accessible for RNA polymerase II. The first step in gene regulation is thus the opening and unravelling of the DNA and the recruitment of RNA polymerase II to the start *codon* (a codon consists of three nucleotides and encodes one amino acid). RNA polymerase II will then copy the DNA into RNA from the start to the stop codon of a gene. RNA polymerase II is directed to the transcription start site of a gene by transcription factors which bind to specific, short stretches of DNA lying in the vicinity of the gene. Binding of a specific set of transcription factors to the promoter region of a gene will lead to the recruitment of RNA polymerase II to the basal promoter of the gene, followed by transcription of the gene (Fig. 4.2).

Transcription factors are only one mechanism by which transcription is regulated. Another class of gene regulation is called epigenetic regulation. Epigenetic regulatory events are associated with regulated changes of the DNA molecule or DNA packaging. One epigenetic mechanism is DNA methylation (methylation means adding a CH_3 group to a base in DNA). This is achieved by the methylation of cytosines in so-called CpG-rich islands (stretches with a high C-G content), a process which leads to inactivation of the gene. Many 'housekeeping' genes (genes that are stably expressed in all cells) possess unmethylated CpG-rich islands at the promoter

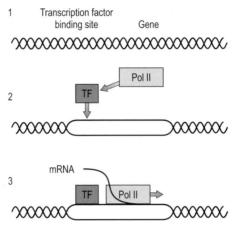

Figure 4.2   Schematic drawing showing the transcription of a gene. (1) DNA is usually densely packed as chromatin. The first step involves the unravelling of the DNA by chromatin remodelling machines (not shown). (2) Transcription factors (TF; only one is shown for simplicity) then bind to transcription factor binding sites and recruit RNA polymerase II (Pol II) to the promoter site which lies just left of the gene. (3) Pol II then scans the DNA from the start to the stop codon and transcribes the DNA sequence into mRNA. mRNA is subsequently spliced and translated into protein (not shown).

region. In contrast, certain CpG-rich islands in the promoter region of tissue-specific genes are methylated in all tissues other than the one where the gene is expressed.

A second class of epigenetic mechanisms involves the packing or unpacking of DNA. The packing can vary from a tightly packed chromosome to dispersed, lose DNA. For example, the packaging of DNA can be regulated by the deacetylation (i.e. removal of a $COCH_3$ group) from histones (DNA packing proteins) by so-called 'histone deacetylases'. Some histone deacetylases are responsive to calcium in muscle (McKinsey et al 2001) and thus might possibly be involved in the regulation of the response to exercise because, of course, cytoplasmic calcium is high during muscle contraction.

Newly synthesized mRNA is modified later ('post-transcriptionally'). This involves the chemical modification of both ends of the mRNA and the splicing of introns. The start (or so-called 5' end) of the mRNA is 'capped' whereas the tail (or 3' end) is polyadenylated (i.e. a tail of up to 200 adenines is added). The cap is important for the recognition of the mRNA by the ribosome – the cellular machine that can translate the mRNA into protein.

A second post-transcriptional event is termed *splicing*. The newly-synthesized mRNA contained introns which are now cut out so that only the exons are translated into a protein. Splicing is facilitated by a protein complex termed a *spliceosome*. In the splicing reaction, the splice sites at both ends of an intron are recognized, the intron is cut out and the resulting mRNA only consists of exons. Splicing seems a wasteful process but it is often a mechanism of producing protein variants from one gene by *alternative splicing*. Alternative splicing refers to a process where different parts of a gene are spliced out. For example, alternative splicing leads to the production of several isoforms of the insulin-like growth factor-1 (IGF-1) as shown in Figure 4.3. For example, in the IGF-1Ea variants, exons 2 and 5 are cut out. The groups led by Goldspink and Harridge work in this area (Hameed et al 2003).

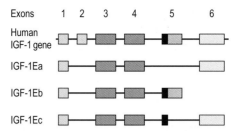

Figure 4.3 Splice variants of the human IGF-1 gene. The function of IGF-1 splice variants is discussed in Chapter 6. Units 3, 4 = the exon, 1 = a universal intron, 2, 5 and 6 = introns which may or may not be present. In IGF-1Ec only the black part of exon 5 is translated. Reproduced from Hameed M et al Journal of Physiology 2003 547:247–254, with permission from Blackwell Publishing Ltd.

Table 4.1   Amino acids and their one- and three-letter symbols as recommended by the IUPAC-IUB Joint Commission on Biochemical Nomenclature (JCBN).

Amino acid	One-letter symbol	Three-letter symbol
Alanine	A	Ala
Aspartic acid or asparagines	B	Asx
Cysteine	C	Cys
Aspartic acid	D	Asp
Glutamic acid	E	Glu
Phenylalanine	F	Phe
Glycine	G	Gly
Histidine	H	His
Isoleucine	I	Ile
Kysine	K	Lys
Leucine	L	Leu
Methionine	M	Met
Asparagine	N	Asn
Proline	P	Pro
Glutamine	Q	Gln
Arginine	R	Arg
Serine	S	Ser
Threonine	T	Thr
Valine	V	Val
Tryptophan	W	Trp
Tyrosine	Y	Tyr
Unknown or 'other' amino acid	X	Xaa

TRANSLATION

Transcription, capping and splicing results in mature mRNA which can then be *translated* into a peptide or protein. Proteins are made from 20 amino acids (Table 4.1), and a one- or three-letter symbol is often used to abbreviate amino acids.

Before explaining how translation works, we must clarify some vocabulary: An amino acid is a small molecule with an amino (NH_2) group at one end and a carboxyl group (COOH) at the other end. Amino acids can be bound together by *peptide bonds* (the NH_2 and COOH groups bind together) producing a peptide. A protein is a large peptide made out of many amino acids. Several proteins often form protein complexes.

Back to translation. Translation is the reaction in which the processed mRNA (the finalized blueprint) is used to synthesize a protein. Thus translation is simply protein synthesis. The 'translation machine' is the *ribosome,* an organelle made out of RNA. Ribosomes are located in the cytosol or on the endoplasmic reticulum and therefore the mRNA needs first to be exported from the nucleus (the site of transcription) into the cytosol. The 'capped' 5' end of the mRNA is then directed into the core of the ribosome. The first three coding nucleotides of the mRNA (i.e. the first codon) are then paired with a so-called 'anticodon' of a *transfer RNA* (tRNA). Each tRNA is bound to one of the 20 amino acids (see Table 4.1). When the reaction proceeds and the next codon is read, another tRNA-bound amino acid is recruited to the mRNA and a peptide bond is formed between the first and second amino acids. An example of the translation of mRNA into a peptide is shown below.

mRNA   gag aaa uuc cca gug ggu cuc is translated into
Protein   Glu Lys Phe Pro Val Gly Leu
See Table 4.1 for an explanation of the three-letter amino acid code.

There are three major steps during translation:

(a) initiation
(b) elongation of the peptide chain
(c) termination.

Factors involved in initiation are termed eukaryotic initiation factors (eIF) and those involved in elongation are termed eukaryotic elongation factors (eEF). Translation starts with the assembly of a ribosome complex that includes mRNA, initiator tRNA, various eIFs and the 60S and 40S subunits of the ribosome and about 80 ribosomal proteins. These components are needed for the 'ready-to-translate' complex.

The capped 5' end of the mRNA is directed with the aid of eIFs to its specific binding site deep inside the ribosome. aug is the start codon of mRNA and it is paired with a tRNA that has an uac anticodon (this start tRNA binds to methionine). This is then followed by the second tRNA whose anticodon will pair with the second codon in the mRNA. A peptidyl transferase (which is an enzyme located inside the ribosome) will then catalyse a peptide bond between the amino acid attached to the first tRNA and the amino acid attached to the second RNA. During translation elongation, this cycle proceeds and the peptide chain will grow, amino acid by amino acid. This process is fuelled by energy derived from hydolysis of guanosine triphosphate, GTP (GTP is similar to ATP) and thus protein synthesis is an energy-consuming process. Translation stops when a uaa, uag or uga 'stop codon' is reached on the mRNA. These codons are recognized by an appropriate tRNA and translation terminates (Fig. 4.4).

ADAPTATION AND SIGNAL TRANSDUCTION

Transcription and translation are the endpoints of a muscle's adaptation to exercise. Both processes are highly regulated and in the following text we will explain the regulatory system that links exercise to adaptive regulation of transcription,

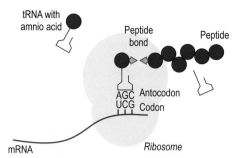

Figure 4.4 Schematic drawing of translation elongation. After initiation of translation the mRNA is read by the ribosome. During elongation each mRNA codon pairs in turn with a tRNA anticodon. tRNA with a specific anticodon can only bind a particular amino acid. For example, tRNA with the anticodon agc only binds serine (Ser). The amino acid bound to the tRNA then forms a peptide bond to the growing peptide. In this reaction, the N-terminal end (the NH_2 group) of one amino acid pairs with the C-terminal end (the COOH group) of another amino acid: amino acid-NH_2 + amino acid-COOH $\rightarrow$ amino acid–amino acid + H_2O.

translation and other cellular processes. Adaptation of a human or other animal not only to exercise but to many other environmental stimuli is essential for the survival of the individuals and species. Evolution is the major long-term adaptive mechanism allowing creatures to pass on life. Short-term adaptation to environmental change such as exercise, however, occurs within the individual and is regulated on two levels: First, whole-body responses are regulated by the nervous and endocrine systems; such adjustments are the stuff of traditional physiology and are not discussed here. Second, all cells contain regulatory systems that respond to hormones and other signalling molecules within the circulation or changes in the immediate surroundings and internal environment of the cell. These regulatory systems lie inside the cell and are termed *signal transduction pathways;* they sense a cell's environment and regulate its adaptation to an environmental change by controlling transcription, translation, cell growth, content, division, breakdown and death.

Most Muscle Adaptation to Exercise is Regulated Locally

Adaptation of skeletal muscle to both resistance and endurance training are mainly regulated at the cellular level and not at the level of the whole organism. For example, myofibrillar protein synthesis increases ~five-fold in an isolated skeletal muscle that is electrically stimulated with a protocol mimicking resistance excersize (Atherton et al 2005). There are obviously no hormonal changes in this model because the rest of the organism is absent. The local nature of the growth response can also be demonstrated by, say, resistance training just the right biceps. If we do that then only the right biceps and not the left biceps (or any other muscles in our body) will hypertrophy. Endocrine changes may now play some role but resistance training predominantly stimulates muscle growth via signalling processes within the trained muscle – although it cannot be excluded that some of the internal mechanisms may enhance the exercised muscle's responses to the hormones.

Similarly, adaptations to endurance training or chronic electrical low-frequency stimulation are regulated mainly locally. For example, chronic electrical low-frequency stimulation of the left tibialis anterior muscle will trigger fast-to-slow fibre phenotype transformation and mitochondrial biogenesis (Chs 3 and 5) only in the left but not the right tibialis anterior muscle of a rabbit or rat (Pette et al 1992, Salmons et al 1981). Similarly, if we endurance-train one leg on a specific one-legged ergometer then only the trained leg will have a higher mitochondrial content and a higher capillary density after the training period (Saltin et al 1976).

The localized nature of both strength and endurance responses underlies the 'specificity' which is a crucial feature of training programmes.

Regulation of Cellular Adaptation

Until the last two or three paragraphs the text so far has probably seemed a bit dry and not very much related to exercise. We shall now look further at how the intracellular molecular processes are connected to physical activity. The specific adaptations of skeletal muscle to endurance or resistance exercise are regulated by a cellular network of signal transduction pathways. There are three major classes of proteins in this regulatory network (Fig. 4.5):

1. Sensor proteins
2. Signal transduction proteins
3. Effector proteins.

Sensor Proteins

Sensor proteins in muscle can be broken down into three classes: (1) membrane and nuclear receptors; (2) small-molecule sensors, and (3) mechanosensors. The first class of sensory proteins are membrane or nuclear receptors which are activated by protein–protein interaction. They are an interface for the endocrine and immune systems. The insulin receptor is an example of a membrane-located hormone receptor. Such receptors can be a link to the endocrine system but several receptors are activated by peptides such as IGF-1 which is produced in part centrally but in part also by the exercised muscle. This type of signalling is termed *autocrine* or *paracrine*. The tumour necrosis factor-α (TNF-α) receptor is a membrane-located receptor activated by TNF-α, which is a signalling molecule within the immune system. By contrast, the receptors to which testosterone and growth hormone bind are nuclear receptors that bind DNA and regulate transcription.

The second class of sensory proteins are small-molecule sensors. Three examples are calmodulin, which has four binding sites for Ca^{2+}, AMP-dependent kinase (AMPK), which is activated by AMP and inhibited by glycogen (not itself a small molecule), and hypoxia-induced factor-1 (HIF-1) which is activated by low oxygen tension. These small molecules (Ca^{2+}, AMP and O_2 in our examples) are sensitive indicators of the internal cellular environment and many of the sensor proteins detecting them are evolutionarily conserved from yeast to humans. Many small-molecule sensors act via *allosteric* mechanisms where the binding of the small molecule to one site on the protein affects the conformation and function of another site which is 'allosteric' – meaning 'at another place'. For example, the binding of Ca^{2+} to calmodulin affects the affinity of another site on calmodulin for other proteins. Ca^{2+}-calmodulin-binding to these proteins, which often have enzymatic functions, then causes their activation or deactivation.

Finally, mechanosensors sense variables such as force and length changes. They are likely to be important in skeletal muscle but little is known about their identity. A class of proteins termed integrins are putative mechanosensors. They are receptor proteins

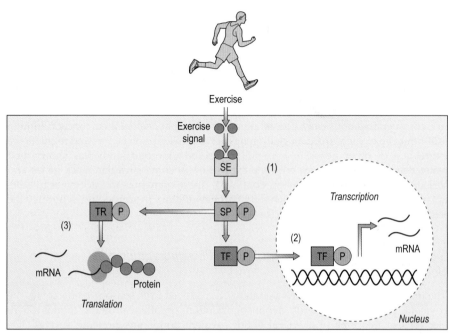

Figure 4.5 Schematic drawing showing the regulation of both transcription and translation by an exercise-activated signal transduction pathway. (1) Exercise signals (e.g. calcium, tension, hypoxia or hormone) are induced by the activity and sensed by sensor proteins (SE – these can be membrane receptors). The sensor proteins activate (or inhibit) signal transduction proteins (SP), often by changing the latter's phosphorylation states. In turn, many signal transduction proteins are kinases which themselves phosphorylate further proteins. (2) In this example, SP phosphorylates and activates a transcription factor (TF; one type of effector protein) which enters the nucleus and binds to specific transcription factor binding sites. This increases the expression of genes regulated by the particular TF. (3) SP can also phosphorylate and activate translational regulators (TR; another type of effector protein). Such translational regulators control the rate of translation (i.e. the rate at which existing mRNAs are translated into protein). Other biological responses such as cell division or changes of cell shape may also be regulated by signal transduction pathways.

that bind to the extracellular matrix (i.e. the mesh of collagen and other fibrillar proteins that surrounds muscle fibres), span the cell membrane from outside to inside and are capable of activating signal transduction proteins in the cytoplasm (Carson & Wei 2000). Mechanosensing is discussed further in Chapter 6.

Hopefully the above discussion of sensor proteins has developed the idea that exercise does not go 'unnoticed' in a skeletal muscle. The changes associated with exercise will be sensed by various sensor proteins which is a necessary first step for regulating adaptation to it. The detection of many signals activates transduction pathways which then regulate effectors of muscle growth or phenotype change. Signal transduction pathways convey the information, amplify it and act as biological 'microchips' that integrate different signals. For example, protein synthesis is regulated by insulin, resistance training, amino acids and myostatin, among other factors. These signals will activate several interconnected signal transduction pathways (one can speak of a signal transduction network) which regulate muscle protein synthesis as an output.

Circadian Clock Genes in Skeletal Muscle

A distinct class of 'input' proteins (different from sensor proteins) are encoded by circadian (from Latin: *circa* = about; *dies* = day) clock genes, which thus give skeletal muscle an endogenous clock consisting of proteins that change their concentration in a 24-hour cycle. Such circadian clock genes act as transcription factors and regulate the expression of other genes in a circadian fashion. A recent study has shown that resistance exercise interferes with the expression of some circadian clock genes and 'resets' the muscle clock (Zambon et al 2003). Developmental and ageing regulators are other time-related genes which modify the regulatory processes and determine the response of the organism to exercise.

Signal Transduction by Covalent Protein Phosphorylation and Dephosphorylation

The major mechanism by which signals are transduced from sensors to effectors is the covalent phosphorylation or dephosphorylation of other proteins (atoms share electrons in this type of chemical bond; covalent bonds are therefore strong). The major breakthrough in protein phosphorylation was made by Fischer and Krebs who demonstrated that the inactive b form of phosphorylase could be converted to the more active a form when ATP and phosphorylase kinase were present (Cohen 2002). Phosphorylase kinase transfers the γ-phosphoryl group of ATP (i.e. the terminal phosphoryl or phosphate groups of an ATP molecule) to a serine residue in the phosphorylase molecule. Protein phosphorylation by protein kinases turned out to be the major signal transduction mechanism and Fisher and Krebs were awarded the Nobel prize for Physiology/Medicine in 1992. About a third of all proteins contain covalently bound phosphate (Cohen 2002) and genes for 518 protein kinases have been identified in the human genome (Manning et al 2002). They may not all be expressed together but several hundred probably are. Generally, serine (Ser), threonine (Thr) and tyrosine (Tyr) residues are the only amino acids of a protein that can be phosphorylated and dephosphorylated by protein kinases. A common feature of these amino acids is that each has a hydroxyl group.

Most protein kinases can phosphorylate either Ser and Thr or only Tyr residues. The position of the phosphorylated amino acid in the protein should always be stated because many proteins are phosphorylated at different sites. The amino acid at the so-called N-terminus of a protein has a free amino (NH_2) group and is amino acid 1. The amino acid at the C-terminus has a free carboxyl (COOH) group and is the last amino acid of a protein. If, for example, Ser388 is phosphorylated then this will be amino acid 388 from the N-terminal end of the protein: 'N-terminus-. . .-Glu386-Ala387-**Ser388**-Lys389-Phe390-. . .-C-terminus'. Some proteins, such as tuberin (TSC2, see Ch. 6) are activated by phosphorylation of one amino acid residue and deactivated by the phosphorylation of a different residue. The statement of the specific phosphorylation site is therefore essential for interpreting a phosphorylation event. Listings of published protein phosphorylation sites on proteins can be found on the Phosphosite website (www.phosphosite.org). Protein kinases phosphorylate specific phosphorylation motifs which are amino acid sequences containing the phosphorylated residue. Scansite (www.scansite.mit.edu) is a programme that allows a search for proteins with a specific phosphorylation motif. For example, one could search for proteins that contain a site which may possibly be phosphorylated by the p38 mitogen activated protein kinase (p38 MAPK).

Most protein kinases contain a eukaryotic protein kinase (ePK) catalytic domain: this is a specific amino acid sequence within the kinase and is the active enzymic region which transfers the phosphoryl group of an ATP to the protein substrate. The structure of the first eukaryotic protein kinase domain was solved in 1991 for cAMP-dependent protein kinase (Knighton et al 1991). The key feature of the ePK domain is a stretch of ~250 amino acids that constitutes the catalytic domain. Of the 518 protein kinases in the human genome, 478 are ePKs (i.e kinases with the ePK domain) and 40 have atypical protein kinase domains (Manning et al 2002). The protein kinase activity of protein kinases is regulated by changing their concentration via transcriptional or translational regulation, their subcellular localization (cytosolic, nuclear) or frequently by phosphorylation of key residues in the ePK catalytic domain by other ePKs upstream (many sensor proteins are ePKs themselves).

The counterparts of protein kinases are protein phosphatases which remove the phosphoryl groups of proteins. The product of the reaction is the unphosphorylated protein and one inorganic phosphate ion. The inorganic phosphate and ADP are then used to resynthesize ATP. There are three categories of protein phosphatases: serine/threonine protein phosphatases (PSTP), dual specificity protein phosphatases (PSTYP) and tyrosine phosphatases (PYP). Protein phosphatase research lags behind protein kinase research but it is becoming clear that the number of phosphatases specified in the human genome is not much different from the number of kinases. A recent human genome search resulted in the identification of 107 protein tyrosine phosphatases which is more than the 90 protein tyrosine kinases (Alonso et al 2004). The number of serine/threonine protein phosphatases and dual specificity protein phosphatases in the human genome is currently unknown.

The facts that a third of all proteins are phosphorylated, that we have ~500 protein kinases and probably a similar number of protein phosphatases, indicate that protein phosphorylation and dephosphorylation is a very common cellular event. What is the effect of protein phosphorylation? Each phosphate group carries two negative charges and phosphate groups can form three or more hydrogen bonds which can substantially change the conformation (i.e. the shape) and activity of the phosphorylated protein. Many phosphoproteins are enzymes and their activity depends on the phosphorylation. Protein phosphorylation can also affect protein binding and the localization of a protein. The phosphorylation of transcription factors often causes their import into the nucleus.

Other Signal Transduction Mechanisms

G-proteins   A less common signal transduction mechanism is the binding of GTP to so-called G-proteins, resulting in their activation. GTP hydrolysis to GDP (which remains bound) and inorganic phosphate is stimulated by so-called 'GTPase-activating proteins' (GAPs) which bind to the G-protein and activate its hydrolysis by the GTP. GDP-bound G-proteins are usually inactive. Guanine exchange factors (GEFs) then bind to the GDP-bound G-proteins and cause the release of GDP from the protein. A fresh GTP molecule then binds rapidly to the empty nucleotide binding site. An example of a G-protein and a GAP that are involved in the adaptation to exercise are the G-protein Rheb whose activity is regulated by the GAP protein tuberin (TSC2). TSC2 is involved in the regulation of protein synthesis in response to resistance exercise (Atherton et al 2005).

Covalent acetylation and deacetylation   An acetyl (COCH$_3$) group is found in acetyl-Coenzyme A, the substrate for the Krebs cycle. However, numerous proteins are also regulated by acetylation and deacetylation, especially on lysine residues. Histones, transcription factors and several other proteins have all been shown to be regulated by acetylation and deacetylation (Kouzarides 2000). For example, muscle development is partially regulated by histone acetylases (HATs) and histone deacetylases (HDACs) (McKinsey et al 2001).

Signal Transduction Networks

We have seen above that human beings have 518 protein kinases, hundreds of protein phosphatases and several other signalling proteins and transcription factors. Not all of these proteins are expressed in skeletal muscle but there must still be hundreds of proteins that are involved in signal transduction. The next question is: how does the system of signalling proteins work as a whole? Does it work as a set of linear signal transduction pathways where each signal independently activates a sensor protein and hence a signal transduction pathway and where each activated signal transduction pathway mediates one or a few adaptations? Or does it work more like a computer, i.e. as an interconnected, information-processing signal transduction network?

Over recent years it has become clear that the signal transduction system functions in the latter way (Wackerhage & Woods 2002). One feature is interconnectivity or cross-talk. This means that many signal transduction proteins are regulated by more than one signal transduction protein upstream of them and that they in turn regulate several downstream signal transduction proteins rather than just one. For example, the 'Kinasource' protein kinase substrate website (www.kinasource.co.uk/database/substrates) currently lists 30 substrates that are phosphorylated by protein kinase B (PKB). Therefore, the activation of protein kinase B by insulin or insulin-like growth factor-1 (IGF-1) could potentially phosphorylate 30 different signal transduction proteins, although not all of these will be expressed in muscle.

Many proteins are also phosphorylated by several upstream protein kinases. To give an example, tuberin (TSC2) is phosphorylated on various sites by different kinases. AMP-activated protein kinase (which is activated by [AMP] or energy stress) phosphorylates TSC2 on Thr1271, Ser1379, Ser1383 and Ser 1387 which will activate TSC2. In contrast, PKB (which is activated by insulin or the muscle-originated insulin-like growth factor (IGF-1)) inhibits TSC2 by phosphorylating its Ser939 and Thr1462 residues.

Several signal transduction proteins work like transistors or microchips in a computer and *integrate* several signals. A good exercise-related example is the signalling unit that consists of TSC2 and the mammalian target of rapamycin (mTOR). Together, these proteins integrate (a) energy stress sensed by AMP-dependent protein kinase (negative effect on output), (b) insulin and insulin-like growth factor (IGF-1) sensed by the insulin/IGF-1 receptor and PKB (positive effect on output), and (c) amino acids sensed by proteins related to mTOR (positive effect on output). Hypoxia is another factor; its mechanism is discussed later. The likely effects of these inputs on the outputs 'mTOR activity and protein synthesis' is shown in Table 4.2.

Effector Proteins

So far, we have discussed the sensing of exercise-related signals by sensor proteins and the ways by which these signals can be transduced and integrated by a signal

Table 4.2   Simplified overview of the input and estimated, relative protein synthesis output resulting from TSC2-mTOR signalling.

Situation	Inputs			Output
	Energy stress	Insulin, IGF–1	Amino acids	mTOR activity and protein synthesis
Resting, before breakfast	0	0	0	0
Resting, after breakfast	0	+	+	+
Endurance training, no meal	++	0	0	0
Endurance training, meal	++	+	++	+
Resistance training, no meal	0/+	++	0	++
Resistance training, meal	0/+	++	++	+++

0 = low/minimal; + = increased; ++ = high; +++ = maximal.

transduction network. The outcome or cellular adaptation to exercise is then regulated by effector proteins. The major classes of effector proteins are:

1. Transcription factors and other transcriptional regulators
2. Translational regulators
3. Other regulatory proteins.

Many examples of these proteins will be given in Chapters 5 and 6. Here, we discuss the basic mechanisms.

Transcription Factors and Other Transcriptional Regulators

The specific expression of many genes is regulated transcriptionally as is evident from DNA microarray experiments which consistently show that the levels of many mRNAs are changed by exercise. The basic mechanism of transcription has been discussed above; here we focus on the function of transcription factors and transcriptional co-factors. Human beings encode nearly 2000 transcription factors in their genome (Messina et al 2004) which once again demonstrates the complexity of the cellular signal transduction network.

(Regulatory) transcription factors are proteins that bind to DNA and thereby enhance or inhibit the expression of a gene. Transcription factors must have a *DNA-binding domain* so that the transcription factor can bind to a specific, short stretch of DNA that usually lies upstream (i.e. in 5′ direction) of the gene that is regulated by the transcription factor. Important DNA-binding domains are the so-called helix-turn-helix, hoemodomain, zinc finger, steroid receptor, leucine zipper, helix-loop-helix and β-sheet motifs. One way or another they all bind to specific short stretches of DNA when given the opportunity.

After DNA binding, transcription factors usually interact with other proteins and recruit RNA polymerase II to the promoter (i.e. the start site) of the gene. *Protein–protein domains* are therefore part of many transcription factors because they facilitate the interaction between the transcription factor and other proteins. Other proteins, such as the peroxisome proliferator-activated receptor-gamma coactivator-1 (PGC-1) are so-called 'transcriptional co-factors': (these do not bind DNA directly but bind and *transactivate* several transcription factors). Finally, the activity of transcription factors is regulated either (a) via an activation domain or (b) by changing the concentration of the transcription factor.

Activation Domains of Transcription Factors

Many signal transduction pathways activated by exercise affect the transcription of genes by modifying the activity of transcription factors. Signal transduction takes place in the cytosol whereas transcription occurs in the nucleus. There is usually a mechanism that causes translocation into the nucleus either of a signal transduction protein, which activates transcription factors there, or of an activated transcription factor. The extracellular signal regulated kinase 1/2 (ERK1/2) is a signal transduction protein that is phosphorylated on Thr202 and Tyr204 by upstream kinases in response to currently unknown exercise signals. Phosphorylation of cytosolic ERK1/2 results not only in its kinase activation but its translocation into the nucleus. Inside the nucleus, ERK1/2 can phosphorylate many substrates among which are a number of transcription factors (see www.kinasource.co.uk/database/substrates for references on ERK1/2 substrates). It seems likely that phosphorylation by ERK1/2 or other signal transduction proteins regulates the DNA binding activities or protein–protein interactions of these transcription factors.

The phosphorylation or dephosphorylation of transcription factors can also directly affect their localization. NFAT is a transcription factor that is dephosphorylated by the exercise-activated protein phosphatase, 'calcineurin'. NFAT contains both a nuclear localization sequence (NLS) and nuclear export sequence (NES). NFAT phosphorylation on serine residues exposes the NES resulting in an export from the nucleus into the cytosol. NFAT dephosphorylation, however, exposes the NLS, resulting in an import of NFAT into the nucleus. Nuclear NFAT binds to DNA resulting in the activation of numerous genes that are involved in the adaptation to exercise (Chin et al 1998).

Regulation of the Concentration of a Transcription Factor

The regulation of the concentration of a transcription factor and any other signal transduction protein can occur via three different mechanisms:

1. Transcriptional regulation
2. Translational regulation
3. Regulated protein breakdown.

Transcription factors can themselves be regulated by transcriptional regulation of the rate at which they are produced. Examples of transcriptionally regulated transcription factors are the so-called myogenic regulatory factors Myf5, MyoD, myogenin and Mrf4, which are expressed at different time points and then drive the differentiation of a myogenic precursor cell into a mature muscle fibre (Buckingham et al 2003).

A second mechanism by which the concentration of a transcription factor can be regulated operates at the translation stage. An example for the translational regulation of a transcription factor is the activating transcription factor 4 (ATF4) (Vattem et al 2004). A unique translational mechanism that involves so-called 'upstream open reading frames' (i.e. DNA or RNA sequences that encode protein) upregulates ATF4 translationally. This mechanism increases the production rate of ATF4 when total translation has decreased, and *vice-versa*. This mechanism might regulate the cellular response to a decrease in protein synthesis.

Finally, the concentration of a signal transduction protein can also be controlled by its rate of breakdown. The response of our organs to reduced oxygen concentrations (as at high altitude) is regulated via such a mechanism. Under normal oxygen concentrations the 'von Hippel-Lindau' (VHL) factor is activated. VHL is a so-called 'E3-ubiquitin ligase'; E3-ubiquitin ligases are involved in attaching a ubiquitin to proteins and ubiquitinated proteins are then recognized by the protein breakdown machinery and degraded (Maxwell et al 1999). A specific substrate of VHL is hypoxia-induced factor 1. Due to the activity of VHL, HIF-1 is ubiquitinated and constantly degraded when oxygen is normal. However, the VHL activity decreases during hypoxia which reduces the ubiquitination and breakdown of HIF-1. The reduction in protein breakdown results in a higher HIF-1 concentration when oxygen is low. HIF-1 itself is a transcription factor upregulating many genes during hypoxia.

Transcription Factor Binding Sites

Do transcription factors bind DNA at random? No, they bind to specific sites in the vicinity of a gene which regulates the recruitment of the RNA polymerase II complex to the basal promoter. Transcription factor binding sites are usually 5–8 base pairs long (a typical example is the TGAGTCA binding site for the jun/fos transcription factor). However, these transcription factor binding sites are often variable, their function depending on the location. For example, there are many TGAGTCA sites in the human genome but jun/fos transcription factors will only bind to some of these in the right DNA context (Wasserman & Sandelin 2004). It has been estimated that 10–50 binding sites for 5–15 different transcription factors are not unusual for the regulation of one single gene (Wray et al 2003). The transcription factor binding sites can lie any distance, from a few hundred base pairs to >100 kilo base pairs, away from the transcription start site. Many transcription factor binding sites are 'clustered' – i.e. several transcription factor binding sites occur close together. If the occurrence of transcription factor binding sites could be successfully predicted then this could be used to explain the gene expression changes that take place in response to exercise. However, the computational prediction of these sites is difficult (Wasserman & Sandelin 2004).

Signal Integration at the Level of the Promoter

There are two different types of gene expression patterns (Louis & Becskei 2002): binary or graded. A binary or on/off expression pattern means that the gene is expressed either fully or not at all. For example, skeletal muscle housekeeping genes are fully expressed in muscle but only slightly or not at all in brain. Another example is the expression of type IIb/IIx myosin heavy chain in fast muscles. It is expressed in an unstimulated muscle but several weeks of chronic 10 Hz stimulation of that muscle will shut down the expression of these myosin heavy chain isoforms (Jarvis et al 1996). In contrast, mitochondria and their genes are always expressed in muscle but the expression pattern is graded as opposed to binary. More exercise increases the expression of mitochondrial genes in skeletal muscle in a dose-dependent manner but no exercise ever leads to a complete cessation of mitochondrial gene expression.

Earlier we described how TSC2 and mTOR signalling was a mechanism that integrated energy stress, IGF-1/insulin and amino acid signals. The outcome of this TSC2-mTOR regulatory module was the regulation of protein synthesis. Signal integration also occurs at the level of the promoter. First, developmental and other transcriptional mechanisms regulate the expression of many genes both spatially (e.g. expression of muscle genes in the leg but not the brain) and temporally (expression of muscle genes at the appropriate time during development). These events turn undifferentiated somatic cells into muscle fibres. A second set of transcription factors regulates the adaptive responses to environmental stimuli such as exercise, feeding and so on. Therefore a lot of developmental and environmental signal information is integrated by the transcription factors which bind to the appropriate sites in the promoter region of a gene.

Some transcription factors integrate several signals similar to the TSC2-mTOR complex. For example, the transcription factor 'forkhead' in rhabdomyosarcoma (FKHR) is phosphorylated by several upstream protein kinases (Woods & Rena 2002). Therefore, the phosphorylation of these sites by each upstream kinase (every one activated by a different signal) will modify the activity and localization of FKHR and the transcription rate of genes which it regulates. If one looks at all steps where the integration (or computing) of signals occurs then it becomes clear that the cellular signal transduction network must work like a cellular brain. Most exercise-related signals probably activate 10 or so signal transduction pathways. These pathways will cross-talk and affect in some cases the activity, localization and expression of a plethora of transcription factors. Again, it seems likely that some genes are regulated by 5–15 different transcription factors binding to 10–50 transcription factor binding sites. Some of these transcription factors will depend on exercise signals whereas others may be necessary for the muscle-specific expression of this gene.

Translational Regulation

Translation initiation, elongation and termination were discussed above. Several eIFs, eEFs and ribosomal proteins are regulated by translational regulators. Translational regulation is the major mechanism by which muscle protein synthesis is upregulated after resistance training. We will discuss these regulators in detail in Chapter 6.

Regulation of Gene Expression by Small Interfering RNA (siRNA) and microRNA (miRNA)

Transcription can also be affected by siRNA and miRNA, which are two classes of small RNA. Both are short, single-stranded RNA molecules, 21–22 nucleotides long. An miRNA termed miR-1 was found to occur preferentially in heart and skeletal muscle and to down-regulate 96 mRNAs that are less expressed in muscle than other tissue. This suggests that miR-1 reduces the mRNA of non-muscle genes in muscle tissue (Lim et al 2005). A recent study suggests that gene regulation via miRNAs is widespread (Xie et al 2005) and regulation of some exercise responses by miRNA is a possibility.

EXPERIMENTAL MODELS USED IN MOLECULAR EXERCISE PHYSIOLOGY OF MUSCLE

Muscle Cell Culture

Primary, secondary and satellite cell cultures (defined below) can be grown first as mononucleated cells and then differentiated into multinucleated myotubes. The main advantages are that these cultures are genetically homogenous and relatively easy to manipulate with pharmacological agents or molecular biology techniques; also there are few ethical concerns especially if secondary cell cultures are used. The disadvantages are that cultured muscle cells are not fully developed fibres and that the survival of many of these cells in the differentiated stage is limited to 1 or 2 days in the L6 model (below) and up to a few weeks in models such as the suspended muscle cell culture (Kubis et al 2002). In addition, 'exercising' these cells is difficult, although this has been achieved in some sophisticated models (Kubis et al 2002). Finally, muscle cell culture is expensive, requiring considerable hardware and laboratory skill.

Primary Cell Cultures

Primary cell cultures are derived from progenitor muscle cells that are usually taken from the hindlimbs of foetal or neonatal rodents. These cells are then cultured in a growth medium for several days until the so-called *myoblasts* (primitive muscle cells with one nucleus per cell and very sparse contractile apparatus) cover the bottom of the culture dish – the condition known as 'confluence'. Media usually include salts, nutrients, buffers, antibiotics, antifungal agents and serum. This medium provides an environment that will enable myoblast division (or 'proliferation'). Once cells have grown to confluence, serum is reduced and altered in source (for example from 20% foetal calf serum to 10% adult horse serum) which will stimulate the differentiation of myoblasts into so-called *myotubes*. During this process mononucleated myoblasts fuse and form multinucleated myotubes which are similar to muscle fibres.

Secondary Cell Cultures

Secondary cell cultures are grown from established cell lines which were usually first derived decades ago and since kept in liquid nitrogen for re-use again and again. Thus, secondary cell culture is easier than primary cell culture, and no further animals need to be sacrificed. These cell lines are well characterized because they are used by many researchers and they are cheap to obtain but still expensive to maintain. The most widely used skeletal muscle cell lines are the rat L6 and mouse C2C12 cell lines. The culturing is similar to that of primary cultures: first, myoblasts are stimulated to proliferate in high serum (for example 20% calf serum) and serum is then reduced (for example to 2% horse serum) to stimulate myotube formation.

Primary and secondary myotubes are especially useful to acutely study the effect of factors such as insulin, myostatin, IGF-1 or of stretch on signal transduction pathway activation and acute outcomes such as protein synthesis and gene expression (Baar et al 2000). Long-term studies are currently limited to primary muscle cell culture studies because established cell lines can usually not be maintained for long in a differentiated state. In addition no good established cell line exercise model exists; electrical stimulation often causes these cells to detach from their surface, resulting in cell death.

A common research strategy in muscle culture experiments is to use pharmacological inhibitors to test whether the response to a stimulus is mediated by a certain signal transduction pathway. For example, we could use cyclosporine A to inhibit calcineurin and investigate the effects on transcription, translation, phenotype, growth and function.

Cell culture models are ideal to test such hypotheses because pharmacological inhibitors would affect many other organs in whole animals unless the drug's target was solely expressed in skeletal muscle. However, pharmacological inhibitors have to be used with great care because many of them inhibit various signal transduction proteins rather than just one. The Cohen group at Dundee have carried out extensive experiments characterizing the specificity of various pharmacological inhibitors and their papers should be read by all who consider using such agents (Bain et al 2003, Davies et al 2000).

Satellite Cell Culture

Satellite cells are mononucleated, muscle-specific stem cells. They are the source of nuclei for growing muscle fibres and play an important function in skeletal muscle repair after injury. Nuclei inside muscle fibres can not proliferate anymore and thus the nuclear DNA would be 'diluted' during fibre hypertrophy if no mechanisms existed that could link muscle fibre volume to the number of nuclei inside a fibre. Satellite cells have this function: muscle growth stimuli make satellite cells proliferate. Some of the daughter satellite cells differentiate and fuse with the existing muscle fibres resulting in an increase in the number of muscle fibre nuclei. The proliferation and differentiation is almost certainly important for skeletal muscle hypertrophy because hypertrophy cannot occur when satellite cell function has been inhibited by irradiation (Rosenblatt et al 1994). Primary cultures of satellite cells are derived by enzymatically and mechanically removing them from their location between muscle fibre plasmalemma and the external lamina ('sarcolemma'). Cells can then be cultured and studied as mononucleated satellite cells or differentiated like the other cell models, by reducing the serum content in the medium. Mononucleated satellite cells are suitable for studying the mechanisms that trigger satellite cell proliferation and for identifying the mechanisms of satellite cell proliferation. Figure 4.6 (A) shows mononucleated, rabbit satellite cells and (B) shows the same cells after differentiation as long myotubes.

(A)   (B)

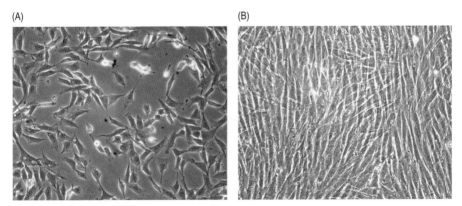

Figure 4.6   Cultured rabbit satellite cells. (A) Mononucleated satellite cells prior to differentiation. (B) Differentiated satellite cells. The cells contain numerous nuclei and are termed myotubes. Pictures were kindly provided by Dr M. Scholz, University of Aberdeen.

Isolated Skeletal Muscle Studies

Isolated skeletal muscle experiments are relatively straightforward if organ baths, stimulators and advice from physiologists are available. One does not usually need an animal license for these experiments if the muscles are removed after humane killing of the animal by a person trained in the techniques. Because there is always a left and a right limb muscle, one can be used as a control and the other one can be treated. Inbred animals (for example Fischer F344 rats) can be used to reduce the genetic variability between animals further and in order to reduce the number of animals needed.

Isolated mammalian skeletal muscles can be maintained in an organ bath for >5 hours (Bonen et al 1994). Excessive stretch during removal from the animal, extensive electrical stimulation and other factors can shorten survival time in the organ bath and activate various signal transduction pathways. Muscles that are suitable for incubation in an organ bath are small, or at least thin in one transverse axis, to allow sufficient O_2 diffusion. (The alternative of perfusing blood or blood substitute through the intramuscular vessels is prohibitively difficult). Suitable muscles are the epitrochlearis, extensor digitorum longus and even soleus muscles if taken from relatively small animals (e.g. rats <250 g body weight). Anatomical knowledge, quick dissection and careful handling of the muscle are essential. The muscle needs to be kept moist with ice-cold Krebs Henseleit buffer and must not be stretched (because this will strongly activate signalling responses and can damage the muscle). Extracted muscles are usually incubated in Krebs Henseleit solution supplemented with mannitol at ~25°C and oxygenated with 95% O_2 and 5% CO_2. A lower tempera-ture will aid oxygenation (Bonen et al 1994) but slows many processes. It may also significantly alter the balance between one and another. An example from normal organ-bath physiology is the inhibition of contraction by protons, which was long considered to be an important mechanism of fatigue, but which turns out to apply in cold-blooded animals and to mammalian muscles at those animals' temperatures but to be of trivial magnitude at mammalian body temperatures (Westerblad et al 1997).

The isolated muscle can then be incubated with pharmacological inhibitors and the diffusion of the inhibitor should not be a problem if the muscle is thin enough for good oxygenation. In addition, the muscles can be hooked to an isometric or isotonic force transducer or length-controlling device. Platinum electrodes and electrical stimulator can be used to elicit contraction.

Using the latter set-up, we have applied two stimulation protocols that mimic endurance and resistance exercise respectively, to try to induce specific signalling responses. The protocols used were derived from work in another laboratory in which these protocols had been used *in vivo* and shown to induce endurance and resistance training-like adaptations (Nader & Esser 2001). The first protocol consisted of 3 hours of stimulation at 10 Hz mimicking endurance training. In the second protocol, muscles were stimulated with 10 sets of six repeated 3-second bursts at 100 Hz mimicking a bout of resistance training. In our studies, the electrical stimulation induced signalling responses that could potentially explain the known specific adaptations to endurance and resistance training (Atherton et al 2005)

In Vivo Animal Experiments

Animal experiments *in vivo* require a Home Office license in the UK. Such experiments must only be carried out if the experimenter is trained in the technique, if there is no alternative way to obtain this information and it must be ensured that the experimental design is sound. Before proposing the experiment, the researcher has to scrutinize whether replacement, reduction or refinement is possible.

Voluntary Running in a Running Wheel

A mild challenge to a rodent is voluntary treadmill running. Running wheels that are free to rotate are placed in the cages of the experimental animals and running wheels that are locked are placed in the cages of the control animals. The distance run over time is recorded. Voluntary running stimulates skeletal muscle adaptations and cardiac hypertrophy similar to those elicited by human endurance training (Houle-Leroy et al 2000). The disadvantages of the technique are that the running distances and speeds will vary and that it is not possible to study the activation of signal transduction pathways or genes after a given period of running at a given pace.

Forced Treadmill Running

Animals can be placed on a motorized treadmill and forced to run at a given pace for given periods of time (Sakamoto et al 2003). In addition, the angle can be varied between uphill, level and downhill running – the latter tending to induce muscle damage because it involves eccentric exercise. Forced treadmill running can be used to study responses to endurance training at different intensities but it is important to familiarize the animals to the treadmill beforehand. Also a licence for it very properly requires a stronger case for the experiments than does voluntary running.

Chronic Electrical Low-frequency Stimulation *in Vivo*

For chronic low-frequency electrical stimulation, miniature stimulators are implanted into the peritoneal cavity and fast muscles (extensor digitorum longus, tibialis anterior) are chronically stimulated at 10 Hz for several weeks. The stimulated muscles can then be compared to the contralateral control muscles. Skeletal muscle responds to chronic low-frequency electrical stimulation with a reversible, fast-to-slow phenotype transformation and weight loss (Brown et al 1989, Pette et al 1992, Salmons et al 1981). Part of the transformation is a very gradual exchange of fast motor proteins with slow motor proteins, best documented by measurements of myosin heavy chain isoforms (Brown et al 1983, Jaschinski et al 1998). Increased mitochondrial biogenesis and other changes in nutrient transporters and enzyme expression shift energy metabolism from glycolysis and glycogen-utilization towards oxidative, fat utilization and glycogen storage (Chi et al 1986, Henriksson et al 1986). Fully conditioned skeletal muscle (for example after about 10 weeks of 24-hour-a-day stimulation in the case of rabbit fast muscle) is energetically similar to heart muscle. In both conditioned skeletal and normal cardiac muscle, increases in contraction frequency or intensity do not lead to phosphocreatine depletion (Balaban et al 1986, Clark et al 1988) which provides a metabolic explanation for the exceptional resistance of both muscle types to fatigue.

Models Inducing Muscle Hypertrophy

Animal models can be used to induce muscle hypertrophy by various forms of muscle overload. The major models have been reviewed recently by Lowe & Alway (2002) and the results of that review are shown in Table 4.3. The table shows that each model

Table 4.3   Outcomes achieved with animal models that induce skeletal muscle hypertrophy.

Variable	Resistance training	High-frequency electrical stimulation	Compensatory overload	Chronic stretch
Duration (weeks)	8–36	6–16	2–12	1–6
Muscle hypertrophy (mass, % increase)	10–30	10–20	50–100	100–300
Fibre hypertrophy (CSA, % increase)	10–30	–	50–100	50–100
Force production (% increase)	10–60	60	40–50	100
Comments	Labour intensive but closest to human resistance training	Equal stimulation of all muscle fibres, small effects	Chronic stimulus, inflammation, oedema	Chronic stimulus, dissimilar to resistance training

CSA cross sectional area. The table is directly taken from Lowe and Always and the comments compiled are based on their review (Lowe & Alway 2002). Resistance training involves stimulating rats to perform resistance exercise by offering rewards. High-frequency electrical stimulation involves the implantation of electrodes and repeated brief, high-frequency stimulations. Compensatory overload can be achieved by removing a synergistic muscle. Chronic stretch is induced by fixing a joint in a position in which the muscle of interest is lengthened.

has advantages and disadvantages and the choice depends on the hypotheses that are to be tested. In the UK, all models require a Home Office license. They can all be used to induce a growth response but compensatory overload and chronic stretch present a constant growth stimulus and the regulatory mechanisms are likely to be somewhat different compared to resistance training and high-frequency electrical stimulation where high-intensity contractile activity and rest periods alternate. Thus, only those two models are adequate models for human resistance training. All increase fibre hypertrophy and are likely to induce satellite cell proliferation and differentiation, which is considered necessary for hypertrophy (Rosenblatt et al 1994).

Transgenic Animals

Important information has been gained from transgenic animals (animals in which the DNA has been manipulated), usually mice. The generation of transgenic mice requires extensive knowledge of and skill in molecular biology. Generally, either *knockouts* (prohibiting the expression of a gene or expression of a mutated product that does not work) or *knock-ins* (promoting the expression of a gene or of an activated product) can be studied. The gene expression can be switched on or off in the whole organism or solely in a particular tissue such as skeletal muscle. Often several isoforms of genes exist and then double or treble knockouts need to be produced in order to study the effect of blocking one signal transduction pathway. A partial reduction of a protein can be achieved by producing heterozygous knockouts where the gene is only knocked out in one allele. Transgenic experiments can also be carried out by injecting DNA constructs into skeletal muscle recovering from chemically-induced injury; more DNA construct will be taken up by muscles recovering from injury (Pallafacchina et al 2002).

There are numerous studies with great relevance for exercise physiology. It has been shown that mice lacking myoglobin expression are viable and have a normal exercise capacity (Garry et al 1998). This one experiment led to a paradigm shift in myoglobin research. Mice overexpressing the transcriptional co-factor PGC-1α have a high mitochondrial content and a muscle phenotype that is 'slower' than usual (Lin et al 2002), confirming that PGC-1α is a muscle fitness gene. In another study, a growth factor that was later named myostatin was knocked out. The mice displayed muscle hypertrophy and hyperplasia, suggesting that myostatin was an inhibitor of muscle growth and a potential mediator of the adaptation to resistance training (McPherron et al 1997).

HUMAN EXERCISE STUDIES

Human studies are necessary to verify findings on other models because we as Sports Scientists or Exercise Physiologists are primarily interested in human beings, not rats or mice. A drawback of human studies is that they usually have to be descriptive (we cannot take out a gene and are usually not able to inhibit a signal transduction pathway in human beings as we can in cell culture) and invasive. Another problem is that experiments on human beings are harder to control than animal studies. Nevertheless, investigators need to try to ensure that they control the experiment especially before and during the intervention. For skeletal muscle studies, subjects should abstain from training at least the day before the experiment and fast overnight (unless their nutrition is tightly controlled). Subjects should be picked up from their homes in order to avoid exercise-activation of signal transduction pathways in their muscles on their way to the experiment. A breakfast will have various effects on skeletal muscle: glucose will stimulate insulin release, which will have an effect on muscle protein metabolism (Rennie et al 2004). Proteins or amino acids will stimulate protein synthesis and the kinase mTOR and via this activate protein synthesis (Proud 2002). Subjects should rest between muscle biopsies, not walk about. In addition, the timing of biopsies is crucial. Some pathways will be activated for hours after an intervention whereas others are only 'acutely' (briefly) activated.

HUMAN MUSCLE BIOPSY

The greatest barrier to molecular exercise physiology research with human beings is that skeletal muscle samples need to be obtained. Skeletal muscle biopsy is a technique that has been 're-discovered' by Bergstrom (1962). About 20–40 mg can be obtained with a standard biopsy needle and more with suction or other biopsy instruments. In our hands, 40 mg of human muscle is sufficient to carry out ~10 Western blotting experiments. Once the muscle is taken out, excessive blood should be removed by washing it in ice cold saline. Blood probably interferes with protein measurements and introduces antibodies which may disturb the subsequent analysis (normally a 'Western blot': see below).

ANALYTICAL METHODS USED IN MOLECULAR EXERCISE PHYSIOLOGY

Molecular exercise physiologists are mainly interested in variations of DNA and concentrations of RNA and proteins. The measurements of these substances are difficult tasks because there is so much different DNA, RNA and protein; to be precise, there are 3.2 Gb of human DNA encoding 25 000 genes (the genome), 50 000–75 000 different mRNAs (the transcriptome) due to alternative splicing and hundred thousand to several million different proteins (the proteome) if one counts all variations such as phosphorylation or the addition of carbohydrate groups. The analytical methods need to be specific and precise enough to detect one of these substances among all the others: it is equivalent to try to count the number of needles in a haystack. In this chapter we will cover DNA, RNA and protein methods commonly used by molecular exercise physiologists.

DNA Methods

Sports scientists and molecular exercise physiologists use DNA methods to search for variations in the human DNA sequence that explain inherited, performance-related traits (Ch. 2).

DNA Extraction

DNA is a robust molecule which can be extracted ideally from blood samples or, non-invasively, from buccal cells obtained by mouth wash (blood sampling is preferred). The cells and nuclei need to be broken up and then DNA is commonly extracted using phenol to separate proteins and lipids from the DNA phase followed by DNA concentration by ethanol precipitation. Because of the toxicity of phenol, alternative methods have been developed. The best option, however, is to use a commercial kit for DNA extraction because it is safer and quicker than manual methods. Some kits allow DNA extraction from blood in 15 minutes.

Polymerase Chain Reaction: Amplification of Specific Stretches of DNA

The great breakthrough in DNA analysis was the polymerase chain reaction (PCR), developed by Mullis in the late 1980s. It does two jobs. First, it amplifies (i.e. increases the concentration of) DNA so that it can be easily analysed. Second, it amplifies only a specific fragment of DNA. DNA variations are much easier to detect in 1 kb than in 3.2 Gb. How does PCR work? During PCR the DNA segment is first demarked by DNA primers. The primers are the DNA selectors: they mark the start and the end point of the piece of double-stranded DNA that will be amplified. The great bioengineering feat of Mullis was to control these reactions simply by temperature rather than adding chemicals. If the reagents are not degraded then the cycle of DNA replication can be repeated many times just by changing temperatures. The final DNA concentration depends on the availability of substrates and on the number of PCR cycles. The three reactions of DNA replication during PCR are:

1. *Denaturation*. The sample is heated to 90–96°C for 30–60 seconds, which separates the two DNA strands.
2. *Annealing*. The sample is cooled down to 40–65°C for 30–45 seconds. At this temperature the forward primer binds to the start point of the chosen fragment on

the first strand and the reverse primer to the end point on the complimentary DNA strand.

3. *Extension.* The temperature is raised again to ~72°C for ~1 minute per 1 kilo base of DNA. At this temperature the *Taq* polymerase replicates DNA from the region marked by the primers in 5'-to-3' direction.

These three steps are now discussed in more detail. DNA is a two-stranded molecule and the strands need to be untangled and separated or denatured before primers can anneal and before replication can occur. Heating the samples to 90–96°C is sufficient to separate DNA; no specific reagents are needed for this step.

PCR primers are ~18–25 nucleotide-long oligonucleotides flanking the DNA fragment of interest. Lowering the temperature to 40–65°C will allow the PCR primers to anneal to the DNA. PCR primers are complimentary to the start or the end of the fragment of interest. The 5' or forward primer will bind to the specific DNA sequence of the first DNA strand: if we add DNA polymerase then DNA will be replicated from the end of the primer in 5'-to-3' direction. The 3' or reverse primer anneals to the other strand and enables DNA polymerase to copy this strand in reverse direction. To illustrate, assume the following, complimentary DNA strands:

5' GGCCACTGTA CCCAGAGATT CAAAACCCCA AACCCGGGAC TTGGGGGCGC 3'

3' CCGGTGACAT GGGTCTCTAA GTTTTGGGGT TTGGGCCCTG AACCCCCGCG 5'

In order to amplify the middle section of the DNA sequence, we need to design one forward or 5' primer that is complimentary to the upper and a reverse or 3' primer that is complimentary to the lower DNA strand. An example for a set of PCR primers is shown below (note that these primers are too short to work well in reality). The primers will anneal to the DNA as follows (the arrows indicate the direction in which DNA replication can occur after primer binding; it always goes in 5'-to-3' direction):

5' GGCCACTGTA CCCAGAGATT CAAAACCCCA AACCCGGGAC TTGGGGGCGC 3'

    GGGTCTCTAA→

                   ← AACCCGGGAC

3' CCGGTGACAT GGGTCTCTAA GTTTTGGGGT TTGGGCCCTG AACCCCCGCG 5'

Another word regarding the design of primers: Primers need to be carefully selected because otherwise they may bind other parts of the genome or bind each other. Online PCR primer design programmes are offered by manufacturers or are available on the internet (www.frodo.wi.mit.edu/cgi-bin/primer3/ primer3 www.cgi). Practical tips for PCR primer design are given in the Appendix.

The third step is the actual DNA amplification for which a DNA polymerase is needed. But what DNA polymerase survives the near boiling of the sample in the denaturation step? Initially, DNA polymerase had to be added after each cycle because it would be destroyed in the denaturation step. However, the breakthrough was the use of DNA polymerase from bacteria which survive in hot wells. A commonly used polymerase is *Taq* polymerase (*Taq* stands for *Thermus aquaticus*, a hot well organism). It is used in the PCR reaction for DNA replication at ~70°C. For this step, Mg^{2+} (necessary for the function of the polymerase) and dNTPs (deoxyribonucleoside triphosphates, the substrates for DNA synthesis: A, G, C and T at concentrations ~200 μM each) must be present.

Taq polymerase then replicates the DNA strand and may overshoot during the first amplification cycles. At the end of the first cycle the fragment might be amplified as follows (the 'overhanging' ends are shown in italics):

5' GGCCACTGTA CCCAGAGATT CAAAACCCCA AACCCGGGAC TTGGGGGCGC 3'

GGGTCTCTAA GTTTTGGGGT TTGGGCCCTG *AA*

TGACAT CCCAGAGATT CAAAACCCCA **AACCCGGGAC**

3' CCGGTGACAT GGGTCTCTAA GTTTTGGGGT TTGGGCCCTG AACCCCCGCG 5'

The overhanging ends occur because DNA polymerase will carry on to replicate DNA until the reaction is terminated. However, after the first cycle, the other primer will bind to the correct end of the amplified sequence and *Taq* polymerase will replicate DNA up to the other end of the template.

GGGTCTCTAA GTTTTGGGGT TTGGGCCCTG *AA*

←**AACCCGGGAC**

GGGTCTCTAA→

TGACAT CCCAGAGATT CAAAACCCCA AACCCGGGAC

Thus, only the correct segment demarked by the two primers will be amplified:

GGGTCTCTAA GTTTTGGGGT TTGGGCCCTG

CCCAGAGATT CAAAACCCCA **AACCCGGGAC**

Extension time needs to be adjusted depending on the size of the DNA fragment. As a rule of thumb, the extension time in minutes should be equal to the number of kilo bases of the product; for example, 2 kb require an extension time of ~2 min during each cycle. If the conditions are right, then DNA will be doubled during each cycle; PCR is thus an exponential reaction. If we start with two DNA copies we will end up with 2^n copies after n cycles. For example, after 10 PCR cycles, we will have amplified two DNA copies into $2^{10} = 1024$ copies. However, at one point the dNTPs will be used up and DNA replication can no longer happen.

DNA Detection

Unless we use quantitative PCR (described under 'RNA methods' below) the outcome of the PCR experiment is unknown because DNA is invisible. The separation of the DNA products and visualization using ethidium bromide staining in UV light is the standard method. The equipment needed is a horizontal electrophoresis system (a vertical electrophoresis system is used for Western blotting) and a power pack.

DNA is separated using agarose gels. The concentration of the agarose will determine the density of the gel: most gels contain between 0.7 and 2% agarose which will make the gels less or more dense, 0.7 % being best for DNA fragments between 5 and10 kb and 2% for fragments below 1 kb.

In order to prepare a 1% minigel, 0.5 g of agarose needs to be dissolved in 50 mL of 0.5 × Tris Borate EDTA buffer (TBE; dissolve 108 g Tris base, 55 g boric acid and 9.3 g EDTA with double-distilled H_2O to make up 1 L of 10 × TBE; '0.5 ×' and '10 ×' mean half and ten times concentrated). Produce the 0.5 × TBE buffer by combining 0.5 part 10 × TBE with 9.5 parts double-distilled water. Microwave the gel solution for 1 minute to dissolve agarose (possibly swirl after 45 seconds) but be careful that it does not boil over. Leave to cool to ~60°C, add 1 μL of a 10 mg mL^{-1} ethidium bromide in water solution and cast the gel. Treat the gel with great care from now on because ethidium bromide is a carcinogen. Add a 'comb' (a plastic template that leaves wells when removed) and remove it once the gel has hardened. Leave it for at least 1 hour and add 0.5 × TBE buffer to the tank to just above the gel.

On parafilm or plastic foil, mix 10 μL of each PCR reaction sample (add more if the bands are faint) with 2 μL of sample buffer (26 mg bromophenol blue, 4 g of sucrose, top up to 10 L with water). Exact, reproducible pipetting is crucial. Load a commercially available DNA 'ladder' size marker (DNA fragments of different size, giving a 'ladder' pattern when separated) into well 1 and the samples in the following wells. Run the gel at 5 V per cm of gel length (i.e. 50 V for a 10 cm gel) and until the marker dye has run 3/4 of the length of the gel. Visualize the gel in UV light. If the DNA bands have the same size as the DNA standards with a similar number of base pairs then it is likely that the PCR amplification was successful.

PCR Applications

PCR can be used for various purposes. Usually, we are not interested in the concentration of DNA but in the variations of DNA between individuals (i.e. their genotype).

PCR can also be used to estimate the concentration of mRNA by converting the mRNA to DNA in a reaction termed reverse transcription. This method will be covered under 'RNA methods' below. Real-time quantitative PCR is a further development of the original technique. Here the concentration of the DNA product is measured during each cycle. The concentration can be determined in various ways; one is to add a fluorescent 'reporter' dye such as Sybr green which binds only to double-stranded DNA (Sybr green becomes fluorescent when that happens). The real-time PCR machine has an inbuilt fluorometer that detects the fluorescence and thus the concentration of double-stranded DNA during each cycle. The cycle in which the fluorescent intensity increases above a threshold level, set just above basal variation, is termed the threshold cycle (C_t); this correlates with the concentration of the original product. The method is often used in combination with a reverse transcription to measure the concentration of mRNA (indicating the expression of a gene). It will be covered in more detail under RNA methods. Measurement of RNA using reverse transcription and real-time quantitative PCR has largely superseded an older method called 'Northern blotting' as the method to quantify mRNAs.

Gene Hunting: Methods for Identifying Polymorphisms Which Determine Inherited Traits

We have explained in Chapter 2 that some physical performance-related traits such as muscle fibre percentage are partially inherited. The aim of this section is to explain strategies that can be used to search for genes that may determine inherited, exercise-related traits. We will first cover some essential vocabulary and concepts.

DNA Polymorphisms

All the DNA of a cell is replicated before cell division with high fidelity but from time to time the mother cell template is incorrectly replicated, resulting in a mutation that will change the DNA sequence of that individual. Also, radiation or some chemicals can mutate DNA. So, by how much does the DNA of two human beings differ? The DNA of any two human beings is >99.9% identical (human DNA differs in, on average, ~1 in every 1200 base pairs) and even between human beings and chimpanzees it is nearly 99% identical. Geneticists use the term 'polymorphism' *(Greek:* many forms) to describe alternative sequences at a given DNA 'locus'. Polymorphisms are thus the results of past mutations. Polymorphisms range from single nucleotide polymorphisms to deletions or additions of large chromosomal areas.

Will all polymorphisms affect our phenotype? No. Many polymorphisms have no effect for two reasons. First, many polymorphisms occur in non-coding regions of the DNA and they will not affect phenotype unless they alter processes like transcription factor binding. Second, we have two copies of the vast majority of genes because 44 out of the 46 human chromosomes occur as pairs (these chromosomes are termed 'autosomes'). Females then have two copies of their 'X' chromosome but males have one 'X' and one 'Y' chromosome as sex chromosomes. If, for example, one copy of the insulin gene (which is located on chromosome 11, an autosome) was normal on one chromosome but not on the other chromosome then the person would still produce some normal insulin. As we saw in Chapter 2, a geneticist would speak of two insulin 'alleles', one mutated which may be denoted 'i' and one normal allele 'I'. If we have two identical copies of the insulin gene then this would be termed 'homozygous' and if they differ it would be termed 'heterozygous'. Four variations are possible: I|I, i|I, I|i and i|i and only an i|i carrier would not produce any normal insulin.

Traits (especially genetic diseases) can depend on just one polymorphism, in which case they are termed 'monogenic' but most traits depend on many polymorphisms, as noted in Chapter 2. Traits which depend on one or very few genes are often discontinuous with clear differences in between; eye colour (blue, green or brown) is one example. Most traits, however, are 'continuous' or 'quantitative' traits such as height or weight. Height can range from that of a small pygmy to that of a giant basketball player, with no distinctive steps in between. A genetic location that affects continuous or quantitative traits is termed a 'quantitative trait locus' (QTL). Continuous or quantitative traits which form a Gaussian distribution through the population, as height and weight do, can hardly ever be explained by a simple, two-variant polymorphism; instead, they are affected more or less strongly by several loci on the genome.

Experimental Strategies for Identifying Polymorphisms Controlling Performance-related Traits

There are two general strategies for making a connection between a performance-related trait and a particular polymorphism:

1. Formulation, then attempted verification, of the hypothesis of a specific gene–phenotype relationship
2. In the absence of such a 'candidate gene hypothesis', linkage analysis studies.

Both types of analysis are follow-up studies, which should only be conducted if a high probability has been established that the trait under scrutiny is inherited (Ch. 2). The chance for discovering causative polymorphisms is much higher in discontinuous traits that have a high heritability.

Verification of Gene-phenotype Hypotheses: Three Studies to Highlight Methodologies

In Chapters 5 and 6 we review genes that have effects on the size or other properties – the phenotype – of a muscle. This knowledge allows researchers to test gene or phenotype-based hypotheses. Here, we describe the experimental approaches used in studying polymorphisms of the angiotensin-converting enzyme (ACE) (Jones et al 2002) to give an idea of a suitable general strategy. A 'gene map' reporting performance and health-related fitness phenotypes is published annually in the journal *Medicine and Science in Sports and Exercise* and describes progress in the field (Wolfarth et al 2005).

ACE Polymorphism and Physical Performance

In the first relevant study the presence of a polymorphism in the antiogensin-converting enzyme (ACE) gene was detected (Rigat et al 1990). The authors used restriction enzymes to cut DNA at specific sites. Rigat et al (1990) used this method to identify a 287 base-pair insertion in intron 13 of the ACE gene that is present in one allele and absent in another (allele I for 'insertion' and D for 'deletion'). Since we have two alleles of each gene the possible allele combinations for this ACE polymorphism are I|I, I|D (or D|I) and D|D. The authors showed that subjects with the I|I genotype had the lowest mean ACE concentration in their serum, subjects with the D|D genotype the highest mean and the heterozygous I|D subjects were in between. Thus, the deletion of this particular 260 base-pair sequence in one of the ACE gene introns leads to increased ACE concentrations in the serum.

ACE is an enzyme that converts angiotensin I into angiotensin II. Angiotensin II causes constriction of blood vessels but also stimulates heart growth and has effects on muscle. With this information, one can hypothesize that the aforementioned ACE polymorphism will affect heart or muscle in a way that influences performance. Montgomery and colleagues tested this hypothesis in several studies by determining relevant performance measures and the ACE genotype. In an early study, Montgomery et al (1997) demonstrated a correlation between the ACE I/D polymorphism and the change in ventricular mass resulting from physical training. The study demonstrated that subjects with D|D and D|I alleles on average increased heart mass by an estimated ~40 g in response to 10 weeks of military training whereas subjects with an I|I genotype increased their cardiac mass by less than 10 g. The ACE I/D genotype was detected by extracting DNA from blood and then by amplifying the DNA using PCR with three primers which amplify an 84-base-pair product for the ACE D allele and a 65-base-pair product for the ACE I allele. The amplified products were then separated on a polyacrylamide gel and visualized. The 65-base-pair DNA fragment was lower on the gel and corresponded to the D allele whereas the 84-base-pair produced was higher and corresponded to the I allele. Thus D|D subjects have one low band, I|I subjects one high band and D|I subjects both a high and a low band. While our purpose here is chiefly to describe methods, it should be noted that some subsequent studies on larger numbers of people have not supported a relationship between ACE genotype and endurance performance parameters whether in sedentary or athletic subjects (Rankinen et al 2000).

Linkage Studies

It is possible to identify candidate regions of a chromosome for genotypes controlling inherited traits even without any *a priori* knowledge of the individual candidate genes.

The method is termed 'linkage analysis'. It works by scanning DNA markers over the whole genome. A DNA marker can be any locus where human beings are polymorphic. There are several classes of genetic markers, including single nucleotide polymorphisms (SNPs), complex loci, major histocompatibility complex loci, allozyme loci and variable number of tandem repeat (VNTR) markers. So what is a marker? All markers have in common that a 'significant' part of the population differs from the rest. SNPs just affect one base pair and they are thus the simplest form of a genetic marker. There are ~10 million SNPs in the human genome. For example, we might find a CAC allele in 40% of the chromosomes and a CCC allele in 60% of the chromosomes. Frequencies for SNPs in different populations can be found on the 'HapMap' website (www.hapmap.org). Other important markers are VNTRs which can be subdivided into microsatellites (~2–6 base pair-long repeats or 'DNA stutters') and minisatellites (~15–70 base pair-long repeats). For these markers, individuals have different numbers of copies. For example, an individual might have a 'TAGTAG' (two repeats of a TAG motif) alelle on one chromosome 2 and a 'TAGTAGTAGTAG' allele (four repeats) on the other chromosome 2. The DNA of such a locus can be amplified with PCR using primers starting in the flanking region (which is identical between individuals) of the VNTR. The PCR will amplify DNA fragments of different lengths. The DNA fragment can then be separated using gel or capillary electrophoresis. The 'TAGTAG' fragment will appear as a lower band on the gel than the 'TAGTAGTAGTAG' fragment. There are other methods to detect such markers but the amplification of DNA by PCR is usually the starting point.

If a marker correlates significantly with a phenotype then it is likely that the polymorphism locus responsible for the trait lies in the vicinity of the marker. Imagine a family in which some members have 100% type II muscle fibres in all muscles (a thought experiment; no such individuals are known). For a linkage analysis study we would determine the fibre types in all members of that family and take a DNA sample from all subjects willing to participate. We would then genotype random markers (i.e. polymorphic DNA loci) spread across the genome. Marker and PCR primer lists can be found on websites listed on www.gdb.org/hugo. Assuming we discovered that nearly all subjects with 100% type II fibres had an AGA allele (but not an AAA allele) on both chromosomes 20, then this would suggest that there is a polymorphism on that chromosome responsible for the inheritance of type II fibres. It is unlikely that the AGA allele itself causes the phenotype (this would be an extremely lucky find). The more conservative conclusion is that the causative polymorphism is likely to lie close to the AGA allele on chromosome 20.

Why do genetic markers inform us about the chromosome regions in which we might find polymorphisms controlling an inherited trait? The secret is that polymorphisms on one chromosome often go against Mendel's second law (that genetic characters segregate independently) by being 'co-inherited'. In order to understand the concept of co-inheritance we will need to cover some basic genetics: Our father and mother have two copies of each autosome (all chromosomes other than X and Y) in their cells. During normal meiosis, each chromosome pair is split and only one chromosome out of the pair enters the oocyte or spermatozoon. Oocyte and spermatozoon merge and the fertilized oocyte has again two copies of each chromosome, one from the mother and one from the father. During meiosis an event termed 'homologous recombination' can occur, producing 'recombined' chromosomes. This happens when homologous chromosomes touch each other, forming a 'chiasma', and exchange homologous parts of their DNA strands. Imagine that the lower third of the first chromosome 20 was replaced with the lower third of the second chromosome 20 by homologous recombination. The resultant chromosome 20 would then be a hybrid containing the upper two-thirds of the first chromosome 20 and the lower third of the second chromosome 20. Now let us go back to the '100% type II fibre polymorphism' and assume that this polymorphism was located on the upper two-thirds of the first chromosome 20. The 100% type II fibre polymorphism would then be linked to all the markers on that section of chromosome 20, but there would be only a random correlation (i.e. no linkage) with markers on the lower third.

Recombination over several generations will turn our chromosomes into patchworks made from all of our ancestors' chromosomes. Recombination is more likely to occur between distant ends of a chromosome than between proximal loci. Because of that, two loci close together are more likely to originate from the same chromosome (and so to be co-inherited) than two loci far apart. As a result, DNA distance, recombination and the resultant inheritance are linked together. If we should discover a marker, say on chromosome 20, whose inheritance pattern nearly always matched the inheritance pattern of the '100% type II fibre' trait, this would suggests that the phenotype and its marker stem from an ancient patch of DNA which has not yet been separated by recombination. We can conclude that the polymorphism that causes the '100% type II fibre phenotype' is close to the marker. The relationship between DNA distance and recombination frequency has been used to produce genetic maps. The unit, a 'Morgan' (M) is defined as the length of DNA that on average has experienced one crossover event per meiosis; more often used in practice is the centi-Morgan (cM), the length of DNA that has experience 0.01 crossover events per meiosis. Genotyping of markers on each chromosome has allowed researchers to produce 'genetic maps' which show distances on chromosomes in cM rather than base pairs which are the unit of so-called 'physical maps'. A list of different genetic maps for all human chromosomes can be found on www.gdb.org/hugo.

How do we practically hunt for a genetic polymorphism responsible for an inherited phenotype? We would carry out a 'family-linkage' study. For this we need to obtain, from a multi-generation family, (a) DNA samples and (b) reliable information about the trait's occurrence in a range of individuals. The first step would then be to use information about the trait to construct a pedigree informing us about the inheritance pattern. Such a pedigree has been constructed for the family of the 'myostatin toddler', a boy in which a polymorphism in the myostatin gene results in an unusually large muscle mass (Schuelke et al 2004). The DNA samples are then used to genotype numerous markers on all chromosomes. Once a genome-wide marker set has been used to screen a family with an inherited phenotype then linkage is estimated by calculating the *lod* (likelihood odds) score. The recombination fraction can vary between 0 (no recombination between phenotype and marker; all subjects with the 100% type II fibre phenotype have the CAC marker) and 0.5 (50% of subjects with the 100% type II fibre phenotype have a CAC marker and the other 50% a CCC marker, indicating that phenotype and marker are not linked at all). Lod scores are then calculated on the assumptions of different linkage values and the maximum result suggests the most likely value for linkage. There is evidence for linkage (indicating that the marker lies close to the polymorphism responsible for the trait) if the lod score is greater than 3. An easy-to-understand description of such a 'gene hunt' has been published for non-geneticists (Aydin 1999).

RNA Methods

Sports scientists and molecular exercise physiologists measure the concentration of mRNA in order to see whether a gene is 'switched on' or 'switched off'. For example, we may wish to investigate the hypothesis that a special form of strength training increases the expression of the muscle growth promoter insulin-like growth factor 1 (IGF-1). This would allow us to judge whether that form of training activates a major muscle growth pathway. So, how do we go about measuring the concentration of mRNA? RNA is much more fragile and harder to extract than DNA because of ribonucleases (RNase). RNase occurs nearly everywhere, are exceptionally stable and degrade RNA quickly. RNA degradation by RNasees can be prevented by keeping samples at −80°C, wearing gloves at all times and using RNase inhibitors, diethylpyrocarbonate (DEPC-) treated water and RNase-free pipette tips. A protocol for the extraction of RNA and subsequent RT-PCR can be found in the Appendix.

RNA Extraction From Skeletal Muscle

The classical method for RNA extraction is the acid guanidinium thiocyanate-phenol-chloroform method (Chomczynski & Sacchi 1987). Mixtures of guanidinium thiocynate and phenol (two of the three substances needed) are commercially available under the trade-names 'Trizol' or 'Tri-reagent'. Chloroform, the third substance, needs to be purchased additionally. All plasticware and equipment needs to be treated with RNAse inhibitors to prevent degradation of the RNA. Usually 20–100 mg of muscle frozen at −80 °C are homogenized in Trizol. Chloroform is then added, the sample is centrifuged and the supernatant is added to an RNAse-free tube. The RNA is recovered after addition of isopropanol and dissolved in diethylpyrocarbonate (DEPC) treated water. The RNA now needs to be quantified and quality-tested. RNA is measured by spectrophotometry and its quality is tested by running a denaturing agarose gel or using an RNA analyser.

Quantitative RT-PCR

Until recently, the standard method of measuring the relative concentrations of mRNA species was the Northern blot. However, a refinement of the PCR methods allows us today to semi-quantify tiny amounts of RNA. The method works by reverse transcribing RNA into cDNA which is then amplified using quantitative real time PCR (see 'DNA methods' for a description of basic PCR). The RNA extract is first treated with DNAse to break down genomic DNA which can interefere with the quantification of RNA by RT-PCR. In the second step, reverse transcriptase, an enzyme that converts RNA into a complimentary copy of DNA, is added and the reaction is allowed to proceed until all RNA is converted into cDNA. The cDNA is then amplified and quantified using real time, quantitative PCR. A typical result is shown in Figure 4.7.

DNA Microarrays

RT-PCR is used to quantify the mRNA for one gene. In other words, it is used to see whether a gene is switched on (i.e. expressed) or off. By contrast, DNA microarrays are used to see whether any of tens of thousands of genes are switched on or off. Current DNA microarrays are capable of detecting expression changes for almost every gene in an organism's genome. They are used in molecular exercise physiology for example to identify the genes that change their expression in response to exercise.

The technique has been described above but we give a more methodological description here. All mRNAs of a sample are reverse transcribed into cDNAs and the cDNAs are all marked with a fluorescent dye. The cDNAs are then incubated with a slide carrying thousands of DNA probes. The cDNAs then bind to their complimentary

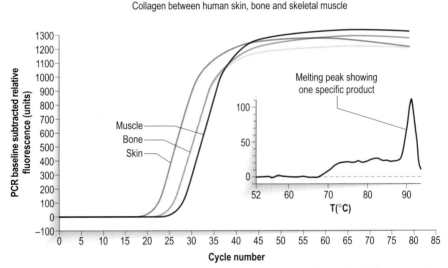

Figure 4.7   The amplification of cDNA reverse transcribed from collagen I mRNA extracted from skin, bone and muscle tissue. The concentration of the cDNA of the skin samples increases earlier than the cDNA in bone than muscle. This suggests that more collagen I mRNA was in the skin sample than in bone and muscle. The insert shows a melting curve analysis where the temperature is increased from 50 to 100°C. The peak occurs at the same temperature which indicates that the PCR products are probably identical.

DNA probes on the slide and fluoresce. The brighter the light emitted from one probe, the more mRNA of that species was in the sample. The method is described in more detail below:

1. Obtain one control (for example resting muscle) and one experimental sample (for example muscle 1 hour after exercise). Extract mRNA from both samples.
2. Reverse transcribe all control and experimental mRNA into cDNA. Also attach a green fluorescent dye to all newly formed control cDNA and a red fluorescent dye to all experimental cDNAs.
3. Mix green control cDNA and red experimental cDNA and incubate with DNA microarray. Each single cDNA will hybridize with complimentary DNA on the microarray (i.e. complimentary bases will pair and form a double strand).
4. Green dots (i.e. only control mRNA present in original samples) indicate that a gene was switched off by the intervention. Red dots (i.e. only experimental mRNA present in original samples) indicates that the gene was switched on by intervention. Yellow dots (green and red at similar intensities) indicate that the expression of the gene has not been affected, while no fluorescence on a dot indicates that the gene is not expressed in the tissue investigated (for example brain genes in skeletal muscle).

A black and white figure of a detail of a processed microarray is shown below (Fig. 4.8).

DNA microarrays are produced via two methods. The first one is to print cDNA probes for each gene on a glass slide using a very precise printer similar to those used for printing computer chips. These arrays are termed 'spotted' or cDNA arrays. The second technique involves the production of synthetically produced oligonucleotide

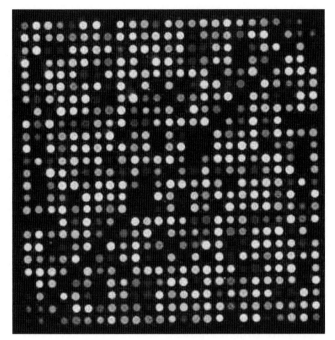

Figure 4.8 Detail of a DNA microarray result. Dots containing probes against specific genes are printed on the slide and hybridized with cDNA obtained from two muscle samples. The intensity of the dot indicates the expression level. Dots were red and green, indicating whether there was a difference in the expression of the gene between muscles.

arrays (short single-strand DNA chains). The oligonucleotides can be synthesized first, then printed on the chip, or synthesized directly on the chip. A common technique involves activation of reactions by photolithographic masks, UV-light and flushes with single nucleotides.

Protein Methods

Sports scientists and molecular exercise physiologists measure proteins to investigate the outcome of an intervention (for example, whether a particular type of endurance training has changed the myosin heavy chain isoform composition of a muscle) or to test a signal transduction hypothesis (for example, whether a certain kinase was activated in a stretched muscle). The first step is the extraction of proteins which depends on the intended use of the protein extract. A protocol describing the extraction of proteins from muscle and the determination of their relative concentration can be found in the Appendix.

Protein Extraction for Western blotting

About 20 mg of rat or human skeletal muscle are the minimal amounts for comfortably extracting proteins for at least 5 Western blots. The concentration of most signalling proteins appears to be lower in human skeletal muscle than in rodent muscle. A solution is to load more protein per lane and/or to extract human proteins at a higher concentration. The extraction medium is a buffer with detergents which contains protease inhibitors. If phosphorylated proteins are being investigated then phosphatase inhibitors against Ser/Thr phosphatase (for example β-glycerophosphate or okadaic acid) and/or Tyr phosphatase (such as sodium orthovanadate) are added. It is not necessary to add a Tyr phosphatase inhibitor if the phosphorylation of a Ser site is investigated – and conversely. The muscle is then minced on ice with scissors (which are very effective) or with a Polytron homogenizer (use flat bottomed vials; the process does not work in Eppendorf vials). The extract can be put on a shaker in a cold room/fridge for up to one hour which will improve extraction of proteins but it might allow some limited protein breakdown and dephosphorylation.

Overall protein content is then measured using a Bradford assay on a small aliquot. Presence of protein will change the colour of the Bradford assay from brown to blue and the intensity of the blueness is measured at 595 nm in a spectrophotometer.

The proteins in the main sample now need to be broken up and to be given negative charges so that they will migrate towards the positive electrode (anode) during electrophoresis. The key substance is sodium dodecyl sulphate, SDS, an anionic detergent (Laemmli 1970). Boiling the protein extract in SDS will break up their secondary and tertiary structures (the equivalent of turning a kitchen into a flatpack). Because SDS is negatively charged and binds to most soluble proteins, the treated proteins will also migrate towards the anode during electrophoresis.

Protein Extraction for Other Purposes

Proteins can also be extracted for other purposes which include:

1. Enzyme (e.g. kinase, phosphatase and ATPase) assays
2. Protein–protein interaction assays
3. Measurement of the binding of transcription factors to DNA by electromobilitiy shift assay (EMSA)
4. Western blotting of unusual proteins (proteins requiring different extraction methods or treatments) such as myosin heavy chains (Talmadge et al 1993).

Usually the basic extraction buffer is similar for all proteins but the subsequent treatment is different. Enzymes need to be extracted intact and ideally the test tube environment should be as similar as possible to the cellular environment. Some enzymes need to be concentrated or isolated from the first extract. This can be achieved by immunoprecipitation (IP). A specific antibody bound to beads is used to capture the enzyme and the enzyme is then washed off into a fresh medium containing no other proteins.

Western Blotting

A detailed protocol for this technique can be found in the Appendix. The term 'Western blotting' is a word play. In 1975, an eminent researcher called Southern had reported a technique for detecting DNA fragments by first separating the fragments by gel electrophoresis, then transfering them on a membrane and subsequently detecting them by using specific probes. Doing the same trick for proteins was termed Western blotting whereas doing it for RNA was termed Northern blotting. Western blotting is the major technique for investigating signal transduction in skeletal muscle. It is a complicated technique and sports scientists untrained in Western blotting will easily spend half a year if they have to get the technique going without help. However,

Western blotting has become much easier over the years due to ready-made gels and improved detection techniques.

The actual Western blot is usually a 2-day procedure. The first step involves loading the protein–SDS–glycerol extract onto an acrylamide gel on which the protein samples are run in several parallel lanes. The first lane is reserved for weight marker proteins. The weight of proteins is measured in kilo Daltons (kDa) and most proteins weigh between 15 and 200 kDa. Ideally the weight markers are pre-stained so that a yellow band will appear at 20 kDa at the bottom of the gel and a blue 180 kDa band will appear at the top of the gel. The following lanes are then loaded with the samples. Usually 20 μg of protein (20 μL of a 1 μg/μL protein extract) are loaded per lane, using pipettes with special loading tips. However, after some training, normal tips can suffice.

The gel consists of two parts: a stacking layer which will concentrate the protein in a sharp band on the border between stacking and separation layers and a fibrous separation layer where the proteins are separated according to their size. The higher the percentage of acrylamide in a gel, the denser the fibrous acrylamide mesh and the better for separation of small proteins. For example, proteins between 30 and 200 kDa can be resolved well on a 7.5–10% gel. The acrylamide percentage is increased up to 12.5% or even 15% for proteins that are lighter than 30 kDa. The proteins that have been made negative by SDS will migrate towards the anode. The acrylamide mesh in the separation layer provides a barrier which slows down the migration of heavier proteins more than of light ones. The gels are immersed in an 'SDS-PAGE running buffer', which can be made in bulk ten-fold concentrated and an aliquot diluted every day. The buffer contains Tris to keep the pH stable, glycine for focussing proteins in the stacking gel and SDS to ensure that high-molecular-weight proteins remain soluble.

Once the bromophenol blue (a dye used to trace the movement of the quickest proteins) front is running off the bottom of the gel, the gel is taken out of the tank. The separated proteins immersed inside the gel now need to be transferred onto a surface such as a polyvinylidene fluoride (PVDF) or nitrocellulose membrane. This process is termed the transfer. The gel is placed on top of the PVDF membrane. Now the cathode is on the gel side and the anode is on the PVDF side. The negatively charged proteins will migrate out of the gel and will be deposited onto the surface of the PVDF membrane. The transfer buffer contains Tris buffer to keep the pH at ~8.3, glycine to carry the current from the gel to the membrane and methanol to avoid swelling of the gel and to strip SDS from the protein – an action which improves the binding of the protein to the PVDF membrane.

If the transfer of proteins onto the membrane was successful then all proteins can be stained with Ponceau red. The weight marker protein will appear in lane one. Sometimes, some of the heaviest proteins (>150 kDa) are still partially in the gel whereas the lighter ones have transferred completely. This is only a problem if you wish to do a Western blot for large proteins; a longer transfer time is the solution.

The membrane now needs to be 'blocked'. Normally antibody would bind unspecifically to many parts of the PVDF membrane because the PVDF membrane is designed to bind proteins and antibodies are proteins. This can be avoided by incubating the PVDF membrane with a lot of non-specific protein so that this, instead of the antibody, occupies the protein-binding sites on the membrane surface. Non-fat dry milk powder or bovine serum albumin (more expensive) is usually used, in Tris-buffered saline solution supplemented with 0.1% Tween-20, a detergent. Thereafter, the membrane is first incubated with a primary antibody (which ideally only binds to the protein of interest) usually at concentrations between 1:500 (20 μL of antibody in

10 mL of buffer) to 1:2000 (5 μL of antibody in 10 mL of buffer). Most workers start with a 1:1000 concentration.

There are two types of antibodies. Polyclonal antibodies are derived from injecting an antigen (the protein of interest or a part of that protein) into another animal and then obtaining the serum of that animal once it has produced the antibody. The immune system of the animal, however, will produce not only one but numerous antibodies against various regions of the same protein. Such antibodies are termed *polyclonal*. However, a single or *monoclonal* antibody can be isolated from the supernatant of a co-culture of spleen cells from an immunized mouse and myeloma cells. An agent is used to fuse the spleen cells with the myeloma cells; some of the resultant cells will then produce the monoclonal antibody. Monoclonal antibodies are often more specific than polyclonal antibodies. However, if the amino acid sequence of the protein which has been the antigen is similar to that of other proteins then even a monoclonal antibody may detect the other proteins as well. Also, monoclonal antibodies could have a poor affinity for their protein. Thus monoclonal antibodies are often but not always better than polyclonal antibodies.

Finding the best antibody is the crucial step. The golden rule is: a Western blot is only as good as the primary antibody. The antibodies from some producers such as Cell Signaling (New England Biolabs) are usually very good whereas the antibodies from other producers are sometimes less reliable. Check the catalogue for an example blot. If it exists then there is a good chance that the antibody will work. Many primary antibodies can be frozen and re-used several times. If the antibody works after the 10th round then there is nothing wrong with using it an 11th time.

Polyclonal antibodies are best diluted in 5% bovine serum albumin Tris-buffered saline buffer with Tween-20, whereas monoclonal antibodies seem to work best diluted in the normal blocking buffer containing milk. One normally incubates the PVDF membrane overnight at 4°C on a rocker. However, shorter incubation times (a Western blot in a day) may be possible if the antibody has a strong affinity for the substrate.

PVDF membranes are then cleaned in a wash buffer before being incubated for 1 hour with blocking buffer containing the secondary antibody conjugated with a detection enzyme. The secondary antibody has been raised against antibodies of the species which was the source of the first antibody. For example, if the first antibody was raised in sheep then an anti-sheep antibody raised in rabbit is used as a secondary antibody.

A commonly used detection protein is the enzyme horseradish peroxidase (HRP). HRP breaks down a peracid into water and O_2^{2-}. O_2^{2-} then activates luminol, a substance which starts to emit light at the position where the primary and secondary antibody are bound. An X-ray film is then positioned on top of the membrane in a cassette in a dark room and the emitted light will expose the X-ray film. The film is then developed and can be scanned using a commercial scanner. An example for a typical Western blot result is shown in Figure 4.9.

BIOINFORMATICS: MOLECULAR EXERCISE PHYSIOLOGY USING COMPUTERS

The 'Dolly the sheep' experiment shows that one copy of its entire DNA (its genome) contains sufficient information to reproduce an organism. Any single copy of Dolly's genome contains all information for development, muscle mass and the responses to environmental stimuli such as exercise. An important task will be to develop

TSC2 Thr1462 phosphorylation

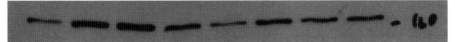

Figure 4.9 Scan of an exposed X-ray film at the end of a Western blot experiment in which extracts obtained from human muscle biopsies were used. The antibody was a tuberin (TSC2) Thr1462 antibody. The molecular weight of TSC2 is 200 kDa and the '160' indicates the position of a marker protein with this molecular weight. The thickness of the bands indicates different amounts of phosphorylated TSC2 Thr1462. The blots need to be normalized against a standard, either by doing a total TSC2 blot or by doing a blot against a general marker such as actin.

computational and other tools that allow us to 'translate' DNA sequences into a model of a living organism. The field which has this among its aims is called 'bioinformatics'. Bioinformatics has been defined as: *Research, development, or application of computational tools and approaches for expanding the use of biological, medical, behavioural or health data, including those to acquire, store, organize, archive, analyse, or visualize such data* (adapted from the National Institutes of Health website).

Sports scientists can use bioinformatic tools in order to address questions such as:

1. What variations in DNA sequence determine physical performance or trainability?
2. What regulatory mechanisms mediate an adaptation to exercise?
3. What are the properties of genes that are up- or down-regulated in response to exercise?

Genome Browsing

Genome browsers are Internet tools, and are usually easy to use after an introduction. The two major browsers are the European Ensembl (www.ensembl.org) and the American National Centre for Biotechnology Information (NCBI) database (www.ncbi.nlm.nih.gov). Both databases link 'raw' DNA sequences to the genes and proteins they encode. Other links contain information about the function of the gene/protein, relation to disease, genetic variations in the human population, similarity (homology) of the DNA sequence between species and papers published on the gene or its product.

Example: Zambon et al found in a microarray experiment that the expression of 'zinc finger protein 151 (pHZ-67)' changed significantly in skeletal muscle after resistance exercise (Zambon et al 2003). The obvious task is to obtain information on the gene and its protein in order to attempt to understand its role in the muscle's response to exercise. The task can be tackled as follows:

1. Enter the Ensemble website (www.ensembl.org) and click on 'human' (www.ensembl.org/Homo_sapiens).
2. In the box after Search for 'anything' enter 'Zinc finger protein 151' and click 'lookup'. A list of entries occurs; the first one is 'Zinc finger protein 151'. Follow this link.
3. The website show the genomic location at ~16 Mb on human chromosome 1.
4. 'Export Data' allows exporting the DNA sequence of the gene or the amino acid sequence of the protein.

5. Clicking 'transcript information', 'exon information' and 'peptide information' shows that the gene has 16 exons which encode 803 amino acids weighing ~88 kDa.
6. Clicking 'Gene variation info' allows seeing bases in the gene that differ between humans, and so constitute what geneticists term alleles (Ch. 2). Such variations are likely to be responsible for variations in the function or expression of gene products.

All this information can be used to generate hypotheses regarding the regulation and function of zinc finger protein 151 after resistance training. Other information is useful to develop techniques to measure zinc finger protein 151 mRNA or protein. The information is also handy for writing essays or papers on that protein! Because gene entries in Ensembl and NCBI are linked to a vast amount of information, one needs several hours' practice before being able to quickly navigate these websites.

KEY POINTS

1. DNA is made out of the following bases: adenine (A), guanine (G), cytosine (C) and thymine (T). The human genome (i.e. all human DNA) contains 3.2 Giga base pairs and 5% of it encodes the total of roughly 25 000 genes.
2. DNA is transcribed by RNA polymerase II into pre-mRNA. pre-mRNA is spliced into mRNA, modified and then translated by the ribosome (rRNA, acting synergistically with tRNA) into protein. The transcription and translation of many genes is changed in response to exercise.
3. The adaptation to exercise is mediated by signal transduction pathways which consist of sensor, signal transduction and effector proteins. The key mechanism of signal transduction is the phosphorylation of proteins by protein kinases at Thr, Ser or Tyr residues and the dephosphorylation by protein phosphatases. All the signal transduction proteins form a signal transduction network that computes signals and regulates specific adaptive responses by affecting transcription, translation and other cell functions.
4. Facts regarding the signal transduction network in human cells: we have ~500 protein kinases, probably a similar number of protein phosphatases, and ~30% of all proteins are phosphorylated; we have ~2000 transcription factors, several translational regulators and numerous other regulatory proteins.
5. Muscle cell culture, isolated muscle, *in vivo* animal experiments and human muscle biopsy studies are muscle models that are used in molecular exercise physiology research.
6. PCR is a method for amplifying specific fragments of DNA. RT-PCR is used to measure mRNA concentrations and Western blotting is used to measure protein concentrations. DNA microarrays are used to compare mRNA concentrations genome-wide.

References

Alonso A, Sasin J, Bottini N et al 2004 Protein tyrosine phosphatases in the human genome. Cell 117(6): 699–711

Atherton P J, Babraj J A, Smith K et al 2005 Selective activation of AMPK-PGC-1alpha or PKB-TSC2-mTOR signaling can explain specific adaptive responses to endurance or resistance training-like electrical muscle stimulation. FASEB Journal 19(7):786–788

Aydin A 1999 How to map a gene. Journal of Molecular Medicine 77(10): 691–694

Baar K, Torgan C E, Kraus W E et al 2000 Autocrine phosphorylation of p70(S6k) in response to acute stretch in myotubes. Molecular Cell Biology Research Communications 4(2): 76–80

Bain J, McLauchlan H, Elliott M et al 2003 The specificities of protein kinase inhibitors: an update. Biochemical Journal 371(Pt 1): 199–204

Balaban R S, Kantor H L, Katz L A et al 1986 Relation between work and phosphate metabolite in the in vivo paced mammalian heart. Science 232(4754): 1121–1123

Bergstrom J 1962 Muscle electrolytes in man determined by neutron activation analysis on needle biopsy specimen: a study in normal subjects, kidney patients, and patients with chronic diarrhoea. Scandinavian Journal of Clinical and Laboratory Investigation 14(suppl 68): 1–110

Bonen A, Clark M G, Henriksen E J 1994 Experimental approaches in muscle metabolism: hindlimb perfusion and isolated muscle incubations. American Journal of Physiology 266(1 Pt 1): E1–E16

Booth F W 1988 Perspectives on molecular and cellular exercise physiology. Journal of Applied Physiology 65(4): 1461–1471

Brown J M, Henriksson J, Salmons S 1989 Restoration of fast muscle characteristics following cessation of chronic stimulation: physiological, histochemical and metabolic changes during slow-to-fast transformation. Proceedings of the Royal Society London B Biological Sciences 235(1281): 321–346

Brown W E, Salmons S, Whalen R G 1983 The sequential replacement of myosin subunit isoforms during muscle type transformation induced by long term electrical stimulation. Journal of Biological Chemistry 258(23): 14686–14692

Buckingham M, Bajard L, Chang T et al 2003 The formation of skeletal muscle: from somite to limb. Journal of Anatomy 202(1): 59–68

Carson J A, Wei L 2000 Integrin signaling's potential for mediating gene expression in hypertrophying skeletal muscle. Journal of Applied Physiology 88(1): 337–343

Chi M M, Hintz C S, Henriksson J et al 1986 Chronic stimulation of mammalian muscle: enzyme changes in individual fibers. American Journal of Physiology 251(4 Pt 1): C633–C642

Chin E R, Olson E N, Richardson J A et al 1998 A calcineurin-dependent transcriptional pathway controls skeletal muscle fiber type. Genes & Development 12(16): 2499–2509

Chomczynski P, Sacchi N 1987 Single-step method of RNA isolation by acid guanidinium thiocyanate-phenol-chloroform extraction. Analytical Biochem 162(1): 156–159

Clark B J, III, Acker M A, McCully K et al 1988 In vivo 31P-NMR spectroscopy of chronically stimulated canine skeletal muscle. American Journal of Physiology 254(2 Pt 1): C258–C266

Cohen P 2002 The origins of protein phosphorylation. Nature Cell Biology 4(5): E127–E130

Davies S P, Reddy H, Caivano M et al 2000 Specificity and mechanism of action of some commonly used protein kinase inhibitors. Biochemical Journal 351(Pt 1): 95–105

Garry D J, Ordway G A, Lorenz J N et al 1998 Mice without myoglobin. Nature 395(6705): 905–908

Gollnick P D, Saltin B 1983 Skeletal muscle adaptability: significance for metabolism and performance. In: Peachey L D, Adrian R H, Geiger S R (eds) Handbook of physiology. Skeletal muscle. Baltimore, Williams & Wilkins, p 555–579

Hameed M, Orrell R W, Cobbold M et al 2003 Expression of IGF-I splice variants in young and old human skeletal muscle after high resistance exercise. Journal of Physiology 547(Pt 1): 247–254

Henriksson J, Chi M M, Hintz C S et al 1986 Chronic stimulation of mammalian muscle: changes in enzymes of six metabolic pathways. American Journal of Physiology 251(4 Pt 1): C614–C632

Holloszy J O, Booth F W 1976 Biochemical adaptations to endurance exercise in muscle. Annual Review of Physiology 38: 273–291

Houle-Leroy P, Garland T Jr, Swallow J G et al 2000 Effects of voluntary activity and genetic selection on muscle metabolic capacities in house mice *Mus domesticus*. Journal of Applied Physiology 89(4): 1608–1616

Jarvis J C, Mokrusch T, Kwende M M et al 1996 Fast-to-slow transformation in stimulated rat muscle. Muscle Nerve 19(11): 1469–1475

Jaschinski F, Schuler M, Peuker H et al 1998 Changes in myosin heavy chain mRNA and protein isoforms of rat muscle during forced contractile activity. American Journal of Physiology 274(2 Pt 1): C365–C370

Jones A, Montgomery H E, Woods D R 2002 Human performance: a role for the ACE genotype? Exercise and Sport Science Reviews 30(4): 184–190

Knighton D R, Zheng J H, Ten Eyck L F et al 1991 Crystal structure of the catalytic subunit of cyclic adenosine monophosphate-dependent protein kinase. Science 253(5018): 407–414

Kouzarides T 2000 Acetylation: a regulatory modification to rival phosphorylation? EMBO Journal 19(6): 1176–1179

Kubis H P, Scheibe R J, Meissner J D et al 2002 Fast-to-slow transformation and nuclear import/export kinetics of the transcription factor NFATc1 during electrostimulation of rabbit muscle cells in culture. Journal of Physiology 541(Pt 3): 835–847

Laemmli U K 1970 Cleavage of structural proteins during the assembly of the head of bacteriophage T4. Nature 227(5259): 680–685

Lim L P, Lau N C, Garrett-Engele P et al 2005 Microarray analysis shows that some microRNAs downregulate large numbers of target mRNAs. Nature 433(7027): 769–773

Lin J, Wu H, Tarr P T et al 2002 Transcriptional co-activator PGC-1 alpha drives the formation of slow-twitch muscle fibres. Nature 418(6899): 797–801

Louis M, Becskei A 2002 Binary and graded responses in gene networks. Science Signal Transduction Knowledge Environment 2002(143): E33

Lowe D A, Alway S E 2002 Animal models for inducing muscle hypertrophy: are they relevant for clinical applications in humans? Journal of Orthopaedic & Sports Physical Therapy 32(2): 36–43

Manning G, Whyte D B, Martinez R et al 2002 The protein kinase complement of the human genome. Science 298(5600): 1912–1934

Maxwell P H, Wiesener M S, Chang G W et al 1999 The tumour suppressor protein VHL targets hypoxia-inducible factors for oxygen-dependent proteolysis. Nature 399(6733): 271–275

McKinsey T A, Zhang C L, Olson E N 2001 Control of muscle development by dueling HATs and HDACs. Current Opinion in Genetics & Development 11(5): 497–504

McPherron A C, Lawler A M, Lee S J 1997 Regulation of skeletal muscle mass in mice by a new TGF-beta superfamily member. Nature 387(6628): 83–90

Messina D N, Glasscock J, Gish W et al 2004 An ORFeome-based analysis of human transcription factor genes and the construction of a microarray to interrogate their expression. Genome Research 14(10B): 2041–2047

Montgomery H E, Clarkson P, Dollery C M et al 1997 Association of angiotensin-converting enzyme gene I/D polymorphism with change in left ventricular mass in response to physical training. Circulation 96(3): 741–747

Nader G A, Esser K A 2001 Intracellular signaling specificity in skeletal muscle in response to different modes of exercise. Journal of Applied Physiology 90(5): 1936–1942

Pallafacchina G, Calabria E, Serrano A L et al 2002 A protein kinase B-dependent and rapamycin-sensitive pathway controls skeletal muscle growth but not fiber type specification, Proceedings of the National Academy of Sciences of the USA 99(14): 9213–9218

Pette D, Vrbova G 1992 Adaptation of mammalian skeletal muscle fibers to chronic electrical stimulation. Reviews of Physiology Biochemistry and Pharmacology 120 115–202

Proud C G 2002 Regulation of mammalian translation factors by nutrients. European Journal of Biochemistry 269(22): 5338–5349

Rankinen T, Wolfarth B, Simoneau J A et al 2000 No association between the angiotensin-converting enzyme ID polymorphism and elite endurance athlete status. Journal of Applied Physiology 88(5): 1571–1575

Rennie M J, Wackerhage H, Spangenburg E E et al 2004 Control of the size of the human muscle mass. Annual Review of Physiology 66: 799–828

Rigat B, Hubert C, Henc-Gelas F et al 1990 An insertion/deletion polymorphism in the angiotensin I-converting enzyme gene accounting for half the variance of serum enzyme levels. Journal of Clinical Investigation 86(4): 1343–1346

Rosenblatt J D, Yong D, Parry D J 1994 Satellite cell activity is required for hypertrophy of overloaded adult rat muscle. Muscle Nerve 17(6): 608–613

Sakamoto K, Aschenbach W G, Hirshman M F et al 2003 Akt signaling in skeletal muscle: regulation by exercise and passive stretch. American Journal of Physiology 285(5): E1081–E1088

Salmons S, Henriksson J 1981 The adaptive response of skeletal muscle to increased use. Muscle Nerve 4(2): 94–105

Saltin B, Nazar K, Costill D L et al 1976 The nature of the training response; peripheral and central adaptations of one-legged exercise. Acta Physiologica Scandinavica 96(3): 289–305

Schuelke M, Wagner K R, Stolz L E et al 2004 Myostatin mutation associated with gross muscle hypertrophy in a child. New England Journal of Medicine 350(26): 2682–2688

Talmadge R J, Roy R R 1993 Electrophoretic separation of rat skeletal muscle myosin heavy-chain isoforms. Journal of Applied Physiology 75(5): 2337–2340

Vattem K M, Wek R C 2004 Reinitiation involving upstream ORFs regulates ATF4 mRNA translation in mammalian cells. Proceedings of the National Academy of Sciences of the USA 101(31): 11269–11274

Wackerhage H, Woods N M 2002 Exercise-induced signal transduction and gene regulation in skleletal muscle. International Journal of Sports Science and Medicine 4: 103–114

Wasserman W W, Sandelin A 2004 Applied bioinformatics for the identification of regulatory elements. Nature Reviews Genetics 5(4): 276–287

Watson J D, Crick F H 1953 Molecular structure of nucleic acids; a structure for deoxyribose nucleic acid, Nature 171(4356): 737–738

Westerblad H, Bruton J D, Lannergren J 1997 The effect of intracellular pH on contractile function of intact, single fibres of mouse muscle declines with increasing temperature. Journal of Physiology 500 (Pt 1): 193–204

Wolfarth B, Bray M S, Hagberg J M et al 2005 The human gene map for performance and health-related fitness phenotypes: the 2004 update. Medicine and Science in Sports and Exercise 37(6): 881–903

Woods Y L, Rena G 2002 Effect of multiple phosphorylation events on the transcription factors FKHR, FKHRL1 and AFX. Biochemical Society Transactions 30(4): 391–397

Wray G A, Hahn M W, Abouheif E et al 2003 The evolution of transcriptional regulation in eukaryotes. Molecular Biolology and Evolution 20(9): 1377–1419

Xie X, Lu J, Kulbokas E J et al 2005 Systematic discovery of regulatory motifs in human promoters and 3′ UTRs by comparison of several mammals. Nature 434(7031):338–45

Zambon A C, McDearmon E L, Salomonis N et al 2003 Time- and exercise-dependent gene regulation in human skeletal muscle. Genome Biology 4(10): R61

Chapter 5

Adaptation to endurance training

Henning Wackerhage

LEARNING OBJECTIVES:

After studying this chapter, you should be able to . . .

1. Describe endurance training methods, explain the rationale for each training method and explain how these training methods may induce specific adaptations.
2. Describe the regulation of a partial or complete fast-to-slow muscle fibre phenotype transformation in response to endurance exercise.
3. Explain how endurance exercise regulates mitochondrial biogenesis.
4. Give a brief overview of the mechanisms that control the growth of the muscular capillary network and the heart in response to endurance exercise.

INTRODUCTION

A key question in molecular exercise physiology is 'Why do endurance and resistance training induce different muscle adaptations?'. Endurance training or chronic, electrical stimulation of a muscle stimulate an exchange of faster with slower motor proteins resulting in a decreased contraction speed and maximal rate of ATP hydrolysis (slow fibres can hydrolyse about 1/3 as much ATP per unit of time as fast fibres); at the same time mitochondrial biogenesis increases and the greater number of mitochondria augments the capacity for regenerative ATP synthesis. Metabolism shifts from predominantly glycolytic towards a more oxidative, fat-combusting ATP generation, which preserves the limited glycogen stores and relies more on the plentiful fat reserves. All of these changes require a transcriptional or translational regulation of the proteins that constitute the motor of the muscle or transfer the chemical energy in nutrients to ATP.

Therefore, endurance trained or electrically stimulated muscles have a lower maximal contraction speed but fatigue later during long-duration exercise. Non-muscle cells inside muscle adapt as well: capillaries sprout and form a more extensive circulatory network which aids the delivery of oxygen to muscle fibres. However, endurance training does not normally promote net muscle growth as is evident, for example, from long-distance runners. They have small muscles with no sign of hypertrophy. In contrast, resistance training has only small effects on motor proteins and metabolism but instead increases protein synthesis for up to 48 hours. The increased protein synthesis as a consequence of resistance training will, over time, cause a growth of the muscle fibres and result in muscle hypertrophy.

It is a unique property of muscle to respond differentially to what essentially seem to be the same set of signals. Both endurance and resistance exercise cause increases in muscle calcium and tension, deplete nutrients, lead to 'energy stress', and so on. However, although the signals seem largely identical the duration and intensity of these signals vary: endurance exercise and the cellular signals that are induced by it are mostly mild but long whereas resistance exercise is intense but short. Can such differences in signal intensity or duration potentially induce different signalling responses and muscle adaptations? Dolmetsch et al (1997) were the first to demonstrate this concept, in showing that two concentration–time patterns of cellular calcium could activate different signalling and cellular responses. Their study was conducted on immune cells but it nevertheless established the principle that variations of one signal (as they occur when training for endurance or strength) can potentially activate different signal transduction pathways and cellular responses. Another possibility is that there is a threshold for the activation of signal transduction pathways. For example, only the high signal intensity associated with resistance training may activate signalling necessary for increased muscle protein synthesis whereas low-intensity endurance training may not activate a pathway at all.

Several of the signals and signal transduction pathways that control muscle adaptation have been discovered in the last 10 years. We now know several uninterrupted chains of events that link an exercise-induced signal to the activation of a signal transduction pathway and an adaptive response. In other cases far less is known. For example, we still know very little about the primary signal that leads to the signalling necessary for increased protein synthesis after resistance training.

In Chapters 5 and 6 we focus mainly on the signals and the signal transduction pathways that regulate the specific adaptations to endurance and resistance exercise, respectively. Chapter 5 is subdivided into four sections which are: (1) Practical endurance training; (2) Fibre phenotypes and regulation of fast-to-slow fibre phenotype conversions by endurance training; (3) Regulation of metabolic enzymes and mitochondrial biogenesis by endurance training; and (4) Other topics: stimulation of angiogenesis and cardiac hypertrophy by endurance training.

PRACTICAL ENDURANCE TRAINING

Advice on endurance training can be found in various manuals (Ackland 1999). Nearly all endurance athletes train using mixtures of intensities and volumes. Traditionally, training volume is increased in the preparatory period. Nearer the competitive period, volume is somewhat decreased and intensity is increased. Athletes then have a tapering period before competitions where the total amount of training is systematically decreased, which allows recovery. In all training periods several training methods are employed. The most common training methods for endurance athletes are: (1) long slow distance (LSD) training; (2) medium and high-intensity continuous training and (3) interval and fartlek training.

A key element of endurance training is the amount of chemical energy that is converted into mechanical energy (i.e. work) and heat by muscle. During running, energy expenditure per unit of time depends roughly linearly on the running speed and it is related to oxygen uptake (Leger & Mercier 1984). We have calculated energy expenditure and oxygen uptake values using Leger & Mercier's 'best fit' equation in order to give an idea about the energy expenditures during typical endurance training at different intensities (Table 5.1).

Long Slow Distance (LSD)

Athletes train continuously at a constant, low intensity which is typically 50–60% of their maximal oxygen uptake. This training is often the bulk training during the preparatory training period, especially for events in the hour to several hours range. The main effect of this type of training is a high total energy consumption and a high amount of fat and glycogen is utilized. One main objective is to achieve a high rate of fat combustion in order to stimulate adaptations of fat metabolism hoping that Roux's functional adaptation theory applies (i.e. that the activation of a system causes its adaptation). Indeed, it has been shown that a period of endurance training increases

Table 5.1 Relationship between body weight, running speed, energy expenditure and oxygen uptake calculated using the prediction equation by Leger & Mercier (1984).

Running speed[1]	Energy expenditure in kJ h^{-1} (kcal h^{-1})			Oxygen uptake (l min^{-1})		
	70 kg	80 kg	90 kg	70 kg	80 kg	90 kg
9.0 km h^{-1}	2577 (617)	2945 (705)	2698 (793)	2.2	2.5	2.8
10.8 km h^{-1}	3055 (731)	3492 (835)	3313 (940)	2.6	2.9	3.3
12.6 km h^{-1}	3534 (845)	4038 (966)	3928 (1087)	2.9	3.4	3.8
14.4 km h^{-1}	4012 (960)	4585 (1097)	4543 (1234)	3.3	3.8	4.3
16.2 km h^{-1}	4490 (1074)	5132 (1228)	5158 (1381)	3.7	4.3	4.8
18.0 km h^{-1}	4968 (1189)	5678 (1358)	6388 (1528)	4.1	4.7	5.3

[1]Running speed can be converted into miles h^{-1} by dividing the km h^{-1} values in column one by 1.61.

fat utilization which reduces glycogen usage during a given bout of exercise (Hurley et al 1986). The rate of fat oxidation depends on the percentage fat combustion (as estimated by measuring the RQ or RER) times total energy expenditure (as can be estimated from the $\dot{V}O_2$). The rate of fat oxidation is highest in starved, resting subjects and decreases with exercise intensity to close to zero at maximal intensity. However, because energy expenditure increases with exercise intensity, the maximal *rate* of fat combustion is usually reached at medium exercise intensities where the *percentage* of fat combustion is already lower than at rest (Romijn et al 1993, van Loon et al 2001). Fat utilization also increases with the duration of an exercise bout because muscle glycogen decreases over time, tilting the balance towards fat metabolism.

Medium and High-Intensity Continuous Training

Athletes often add training above 60% of their maximal oxygen uptake. At higher intensities athletes will probably activate and thus train additional, and possibly, faster motor units compared to slow distance training. Athletes will also use a muscle recruitment pattern that is closer to the one used at the intensity of the competition. Finally, glycogen will be used at the expense of fat and this should promote specific adaptations which may increase the capacity for ATP production by that pathway.

Interval and Fartlek Training

An infinite number of combinations of high- to maximal-intensity, low-intensity and rest periods are possible. An exercise bout where intensity is varied is called fartlek training. Fartlek is a Swedish word which is translated into 'speed play' and is less structured than interval training and there are usually no real breaks. During fartlek training, athletes may, for example, use uphill parts of a course to run at high intensity and downhill parts to run at a low intensity. A bout of interval training is more structured than fartlek training and there are passive breaks. Usually, athletes warm-up and then complete repetitions of a set distance with passive breaks in between. The intensity of exercise, number of sets and repetitions per set, duration or distance of the interval, duration and activity level during the break can all be varied. When doing fartlek or interval training the fibre recruitment, ventilation, oxygen uptake and glycolytic rate are often close to the intensity of the competition. The relative and absolute amount of carbohydrate (glycogen) metabolism via glycolysis and oxidative phosphorylation increases above medium intensity and reaches near 100% at intensities where the maximal oxygen uptake is reached. During very high intensities growth signalling may be activated, resulting in increased protein synthesis; this is discussed in Chapter 6.

What Determines the Overall Training Load?

The training volume differs perhaps surprisingly between individual endurance events. Endurance sports can be split into two groups with respect to the training volume that is tolerated by world-class athletes: swimmers, cyclists, rowers, canoeists and triathletes train at high volumes. For example, some Ironman triathletes train for up to 40 hours per week – an average of almost 6 hours per day. Assuming a maximal oxygen uptake of 6 L and an average training intensity of 60% of the maximal oxygen uptake, that amount of training is equivalent to an energy turnover of (~42 000 kcal (~172 800 kJ)) per week, which does not include the energy necessary to cover expenditure during the non-training time. This amount of energy is equivalent to the oxidation of ~10 kg of glycogen (oxidation of 1 g of carbohydrate or protein yields 17 kJ of energy) or ~4.5 kg of fat (oxidation of 1 g of fat yields 38 kJ of energy) per week. No wonder that triathletes and Tour de France cyclists can eat enormous amounts of food and do not put on weight.

In contrast, a world class marathon runner is unlikely to run much more than 2 hours daily (or 14 hours per week). The explanation of the large difference in training volumes is probably that running involves a significant eccentric component and high volumes of running have been shown to cause histologically identifiable muscle damage (Hikida et al 1983) and considerable wear and tear on joints. It is likely that the training volume of an endurance athlete is limited by muscle and joint damage and – if damage is low – by factors other than muscle overexertion, then skeletal muscle can tolerate and still adapt even to permanent contractile activity. This is evident from experiments where skeletal muscles are stimulated chronically at low frequency (usually 10 Hz) for weeks *in vivo* (Henriksson et al 1986, Salmons & Henriksson 1981).

FIBRE PHENOTYPES AND REGULATION OF FAST-TO-SLOW FIBRE PHENOTYPE CONVERSIONS BY ENDURANCE TRAINING

The concepts of 'slow' (type I) and 'fast' (type II) muscle fibre (pheno-)types and changes of muscle fibres and their proteins in response to endurance exercise, chronic electrical stimulation and denervation (i.e. muscle fibre plasticity) have been discussed in Chapter 3. The most important observations are summarized here but the focus of this section is to attempt to explain the mechanisms that are responsible for a fibre phenotype and for changes in fibre proteins in response to endurance training. For simplicity, we use the terms 'slow' or 'fast' genes (or proteins) to denote genes that are more expressed in muscle fibres with a type I or II phenotype, respectively. Increased muscle activity promotes the exchange of faster with slower motor proteins. Several months of endurance exercise decrease the percentage of muscle fibres that express predominantly fast IIx myosin heavy chain (MHC) (and IIb MHC in species other than human) and increase the percentage of the intermediate IIa MHC isoform. Such training does not induce measurable II-to-I MHC isoform exchanges. However, increasing the stimulus by using chronic electrical muscle stimulation stimulates a complete or near complete exchange of type II with type I MHC isoforms in several species. In contrast, the inactivity of a muscle induced by denervation results in most cases in a I-to-II MHC isoform expression change. To summarize, a positive dose–response relationship exists between the amount of muscle contractile activity and the expression of slower MHC isoforms which is reversible. The relationship between the amount of contractile activity and the expression of faster proteins is negative. MHC proteins are a common marker but many other proteins with slow and fast isoforms respond in the same manner.

Regulation of Fast-to-Slow Fibre Phenotype Conversions

The key question for the molecular exercise physiologist is 'how is the (pheno-) type of a muscle fibre regulated by endurance training or chronic electrical stimulation?'. Molecular exercise physiologists attempt to identify mechanisms which must be continuous chains of events linking endurance training signals (such as a rise of cytosolic calcium over a longer period of time or muscle glycogen depletion) to the activation of signal transduction pathways which regulate known adaptations to endurance training.

The landmark study in this field was published by Eva Chin and co-workers (Chin et al 1998). In their study they discovered a continuous chain of events linking calcium to the up-regulation of several 'slow' genes. They identified calcium as the exercise-related signal, calcineurin and the nuclear factor of activated T-cells (NFAT, a transcription factor) as the signalling pathway that was activated by calcium and the increased expression of slow marker genes by NFAT as the adaptation that is known to occur in response to endurance training. An overview about the mechanism by which calcineurin may control adaptations to endurance training is given in Figure 5.1.

Chin et al carried out several experiments to identify calcineurin-NFAT signalling as one mechanism that mediates a change of gene regulation in response to endurance training. In the first experiment rats were treated for 6 weeks with 5 mg kg^{-1} of cyclosporin A, a pharmacological inhibitor of the calcineurin pathway. As a result, the number of type II fibres determined by ATPase histochemistry increased significantly in the soleus muscle (Fig. 5.2).

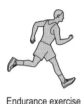

Endurance exercise

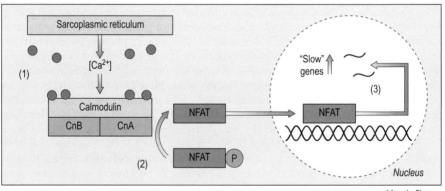

Figure 5.1 Schematic drawing of the calcineurin-mediated adaptation to a rise in cytosolic calcium during endurance exercise. (1) Muscle contraction during endurance exercise occurs when calcium is released from the sarcoplasmic reticulum into the cytosol. A second effect of the cytosolic rise of calcium is the binding of calcium to calmodulin, causing its activation. (2) Calmodulin in turn activates calcineurin which consists of a regulatory (CnB) and catalytic (CnA) subunit. Calcineurin is a protein phosphatase, i.e. an enzyme that dephosphorylates other proteins. Activated calcineurin dephosphorylates the transcription factor NFAT which exposes its so-called nuclear localization signal (NLS) to the machinery that imports proteins into the nucleus. NFAT then enters the nucleus. (3) Inside the nucleus NFAT binds to transcription factor binding sites of slow genes such as slow troponin or myoglobin. The increased expression of such proteins is a known adaptation to endurance training and the final link in the continuous chain of events between endurance training and the expression of slow genes.

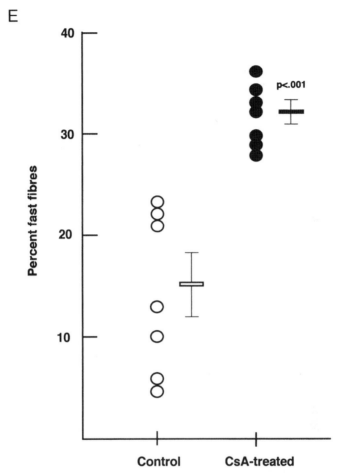

Figure 5.2   Fibre composition of soleus muscles from intact rats treated with cyclosporin (*E*). Circles represent individual animals. (○) Vehicle-treated; (●) cyclosporin A-treated and mean values in each group (± S.E.) are shown as horizontal lines. The difference in group means was highly significant (*P* <0.001 by unpaired Student's *t*-test). Figure and legend reproduced from Chin et al (1998), with permission from Cold Spring Harbor Laboratory Press.

These data suggested that the active calcineurin pathway promotes the formation of slow fibres and inhibits that of fast fibres. This experiment indicated that a blockade of calcineurin affected ATPase activity (which is measured in the fibre typing experiment) but it does not indicate whether all genes with a fibre-type specific expression pattern were affected.

The authors carried out various other experiments in order to gain more insight. They showed that constitutively active calcineurin increased the expression of the slow-fibre specific troponin I and of the myoglobin gene in cultured muscle cells (higher levels of myoglobin and slow-fibre specific troponin I can be found in slow, oxidative fibres). They also identified NFAT binding sites in the promoter region of some slow genes. Chin et al (1998) then concluded: 'These results identify a molecular mechanism by which different patterns of motor nerve activity promote selective changes in gene expression to establish the specialized characteristics of slow and fast myofibres'.

The paper of Chin et al (1998) was the start of the new era in muscle adaptation research that followed the era in which researchers such as Saltin, Gollnick and Holloszy had discovered the muscle adaptations to endurance exercise (Gollnick & Saltin 1983, Holloszy & Booth 1976). The classical exercise physiology researchers had described the adaptations to exercise in muscle and Chin et al as some of the first representatives of the molecular exercise physiology era identified a mechanism by which known adaptations can be explained. We should like to point out that Saltin, Holloszy and Booth (Gollnick died in 1991) all have now authored molecular exercise physiology papers.

Was Chin's paper the complete explanation for skeletal muscle fibre type adaptation? No. Two papers in particular showed that calcineurin is not the sole explanation for muscle fibre phenotype changes in response to endurance exercise: First, Swoap et al (2000) showed that calcineurin did not only activate 'slow' muscle gene promoters but also the promoters of some 'fast' muscle genes in cultured muscle cells. In other words Swoap et al showed that calcineurin could increase the transcription of genes that are more expressed in fast muscle fibres which directly contradicts the hypothesis of Chin et al. However, Swoap et al obtained their data in cultured muscle. Cultured muscle cells are not fully mature and the results may have to be viewed with caution. Nonetheless the DNA of cultured muscle cells is identical to the DNA of living animals and the muscle-making programme (which is termed myogenesis) is switched on in the cultured cells. The second paper was a paper that reported that the extracellular signal regulated-kinase 1/2 (ERK1/2) pathway was also activated by muscle contraction and could upregulate slow genes (Murgia et al 2000); we will discuss the function of this pathway later.

Another twist was added to the calcineurin story when two groups reported that IGF-1 could induce hypertrophy by activating the calcineurin pathway in skeletal muscle (Musaro et al 1999, Semsarian et al 1999). These papers in *Nature* were probably a follow-up to an important paper in *Cell* that showed that an activation of calcineurin promoted cardiac hypertrophy in the heart. Thus, does calcineurin control the phenotype of muscles or their size, or both? A common strategy in molecular biology is to create transgenic animals in order to assess the *in vivo* function of an activated or inhibited pathway. For example, calcineurin could be modified so that it is constantly activated (knock-in mutant) in skeletal muscle or calcineurin could be knocked out by deactivating the gene. Calcineurin knockout mice have been created for the calcineurin A and B forms. The effect of the knockout on these mice suggests that calcineurin is probably not a major growth regulator in skeletal muscle, but confirms that calcineurin controls the fibre (pheno-)type of a muscle fibre (Bodine et al 2001, Parsons et al 2004).

To conclude, calcineurin is likely to be activated by muscle contractions because of the rise of calcium during contraction. There are few experimental data because there are no phospho-specific NFAT antibodies against the muscle form of NFAT and because current calcineurin assays do not work well. Researchers have used the bandshift of NFAT (different bands may indicate NFATs with different phosphorylation states), NFAT localization (active NFAT is nuclear) and genes up-regulated by NFAT as indicators of calcineurin activity mainly in cultured cell models. It is currently unclear whether calcineurin is more activated by endurance than resistance exercise. Results from studies where calcineurin activity was changed by pharmacological inhibitors or transgenic intervention show that activated calcineurin will regulate some 'slow' genes and will change the percentages of fibre types as measured by ATPase or MHC assays. However, these assays only measure one protein and a muscle fibre is made up of thousands of proteins. DNA microarray experiments are needed to identify the genes that are regulated by calcineurin. In addition, experimenters should also verify that NFAT (the calcineurin-regulated transcription factor) binds to the promoter of those genes. More recent papers have shown that calcineurin is not the sole signal transduction pathway that regulates muscle fibre phenotype in response to endurance exercise or chronic electrical stimulation.

If calcineurin is not the only regulator of fibre phenotype in response to endurance training then other signal transduction pathways must contribute to this process. Generally, two research tasks need to be carried out in order to test the hypothesis that a signal transduction pathway mediates the adaptation to exercise. The two research tasks are:

1. Researchers need to demonstrate that the pathway is activated by endurance exercise before the adaptation occurs.
2. Researchers then need to show that changes in the activation of the pathway by means other than exercise (for example, by pharmacological inhibitors or genetic modification) affects proteins or cellular functions that are known to adapt to exercise.

If that had been established, then researchers need to demonstrate an uninterrupted chain of events starting with an exercise-related signal and ending with the regulation of a known adaptation to exercise. Finally, the activation of the pathway by exercise also needs to be demonstrated for human beings and there should ideally be some evidence that the activation of the pathway will have the same effect in human beings. There are some large differences between rodents and human beings. For example, protein turnover is very roughly 5- to 10-fold higher in a rat muscle than in a human muscle. However, it is likely that the differences between humans and rodents are mainly quantitative and do not result from different signalling processes. Many signal transduction pathways are highly conserved between rat and human skeletal muscle.

Points (1) and (2) have also been demonstrated for the extracellular signal-regulated kinase (ERK1/2) pathway. This pathway belongs to the group of signal transduction pathways that are termed mitogen-activated protein kinases (MAPKs). MAPK pathways are kinase cascades in which one kinase phosphorylates and activates its downstream kinase. The whole kinase cascade functions like a chain of falling dominos. MAPK pathways have three central kinases plus some upstream and downstream elements. The general structure of a MAPK pathway is: activating signal → MAPKKK → MAPKK → MAPK → cellular effect. In the ERK1/2 pathway, kinases such as Raf-1 are the MAPKKK, MEK1/2 is the MAPKK and ERK1/2 is the MAPK.

Numerous studies have demonstrated an increase in ERK1/2 phosphorylation and activity in response to electrical muscle stimulation and exercise in rodents and human beings (Widegren et al 2001). The activation of ERK1/2 by exercise is much easier to demonstrate than the activation of calcineurin because phospho-ERK1/2 and total ERK1/2 antibodies work well. The phosphorylation of ERK1/2 at the two specific phosphorylation sites often increases manifold in response to exercise. The exercise-related signal that leads to ERK1/2 activation, however, is currently unknown.

A transgenic experiment was carried out in order to investigate the function of ERK1/2 pathway activation on muscle phenotype and size. In that experiment, DNA encoding constitutively activated forms of the signalling protein RasV12 (which activates ERK1/2) was injected into muscles. Researchers often use existing DNA constructs that they get from past experiments or collaborators rather than trying to develop entirely new DNA constructs for each experiment. This may explain why a

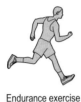

Endurance exercise

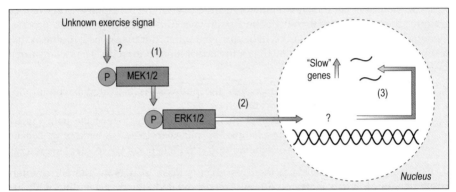

Muscle fibre

Figure 5.3 Schematic drawing of ERK1/2-mediated adaptation to endurance exercise.
(1) Increases in ERK1/2 phosphorylation are well documented but the mechanism by which
exercise activates the ERK1/2 signalling cascade is unknown. The ERK1/2 pathway is a kinase
cascade where upstream kinases phosphorylate and activate their downstream kinase targets. In
the ERK1/2 pathway MEK1/2 is the upstream kinase for ERK1/2. (2) Phosphorylated ERK1/2 is
imported into the nucleus. (3) Because ERK1/2 is not a transcription factor (i.e. it does not bind
DNA) the ERK1/2-dependent up-regulation of slow genes must occur via an unknown mechanism.

RasV12 construct has been used instead of an activated ERK1/2 DNA construct. The
DNA constructs were injected into a muscle that was recovering from chemical injury
and acted to significantly increased the expression of the slow myosin heavy chain
isoforms and the percentage of slow muscle fibres (Murgia et al 2000). The ERK1/2
pathway is shown in Figure 5.3.

So, if calcineurin and ERK1/2 are both involved in regulating slow genes in
response to endurance exercise, then do they regulate the same genes? We have carried out a study together with the University of Copenhagen in which we have
investigated this question. Cultured, primary muscle cells were incubated with an
inhibitor of calcineurin (cyclosporin A) or an inhibitor of the ERK1/2 pathway
(U0126). We then measured the mRNA for multiple MHCs (Fig. 5.4). The data for
MHC IIb show that only U0126 affected MHC IIb expression whereas the expression
of MHC IIx responded to both U0126 and cyclosporin A. The conclusion of this study
is that calcineurin and ERK1/2 affect fast and slow genes differentially: activated
ERK1/2 down-regulates MHC IIx and IIb mRNA (because ERK1/2 inhibition activates
the MHC isoforms) and calcineurin down-regulates only MHC IIx but not MHC IIb.

The regulation of fast and slow genes in response to exercise and chronic electrical
stimulation is therefore probably regulated gene for gene via different mechanisms.
Thus, the model 'endurance exercise signal → activation of signal transduction
pathway → activation of a transcription factor → up-regulation of all slow genes and
down-regulation of all fast genes' is too simplistic.

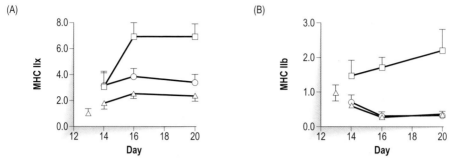

Figure 5.4 Relative amounts of myosin heavy chain (MHC) isoform mRNA (mean ± SEM, n = 4) over time in cultured muscle cells. (A) MHC IIx. (B) MHC IIb. ▲ = control; ● = cyclosporin A-treated (calcineurin inhibition); ■ = U0126-treated (ERK1/2 pathway inhibition). Reproduced from Figure 2c, d of Higginson J et al Blockades of mitogen-activated protein kinase and calcineurin both change fibre-type markers in skeletal muscle culture. Pflugers Archiv 2002, with kind permission of Springer Science and Business Media.

LOCATION AND REGULATION OF MHC ISOFORM GENES

The expression of MHC isoforms is probably also related to their genomic location and we leave the calcineurin-ERK1/2 story briefly to focus on the genomic location of MHC isoform genes. The major MHC isoforms expressed in skeletal and cardiac muscle are (we have added the abbreviation under which these genes can be found in the Ensembl genome browser: www.ensembl.org and a brief description of the iso-form): MHC Iβ (MYH6; main slow muscle isoform); MHC Iα (MYH6; major cardiac isoform); MHC IIa (MHC2; intermediate isoform); MHC IIx/d (MYH1; the main human fast isoform); MHC IIb (MYH4; fastest isoform but not expressed in human locomotory muscles). Furthermore, there are developmental isoforms which are denoted MHC embryonic (MYH3) and MHC perinatal (MYH8). A very fast isoform is expressed in some extraocular muscles and is termed MHC extraocular (MYH13). Finally, there is an MHC pseudogene which is expressed in non-human but not in human masticatory muscle and it has been hypothesized that the loss of expression of this isoform was important for human evolution (Stedman et al 2004).

The locations of functionally related genes such as the genes encoding glycolytic enzymes are often spread all over our genome. Sometimes, however, one ancestor gene duplicates and the new genes may obtain slightly different functions. This has probably occurred in the case of MHC genes resulting in a large MHC gene family. Interestingly, the major skeletal muscle human and mouse MHC genes are clustered as a fast/developmental (MHC IIa, IIx/d, IIb, embryonal, perinatal, extraocular on human chromosome 17) and a slow/cardiac gene cluster (MHC Iα; Iβ on human chromosome 14) (Weiss et al 1999). The genomic location of major skeletal muscle MHC genes in the human and mouse genome is shown in Table 5.2.

It is striking that function and genomic location are so closely related. Not only do the fast/developmental and slow/cardiac genes occur in two different locations but the IIa, IIx/d and IIb genes are arranged from intermediate to fastest in both the human and mouse genome.

Has the genomic location of MHC isoform genes something to do with their regulation? Little is known but there are parallels between the MHC genomic loca-tions and their regulation by increased amounts of contractile activity and the globin (a major part of haemoglobin) gene isoform locations and their sequential expression

Table 5.2. Genomic locations (chromosome; followed by location in mega bases (Mb) on that chromosome) of skeletal and cardiac muscle human myosin heavy chain (MHC) genes and their orthologues in mouse (*Mus musculus*).

Species Cluster	MHC Iα (*MYH6*) Slow/cardiac	MHC Iβ (*MYH7*)	MHC IIa (*MYH2*)	MHC IIx/d (*MYH1*) Fast/developmental	MHC IIb (*MYH4*)
Human	14; 22.92Mb	14; 22.95Mb	17; 10.37Mb	17; 10.34Mb	17; 10.29Mb
Mouse	14; 46.91Mb	14; 46.91Mb	11; 66.78Mb	11; 66.83Mb	11; 66.87Mb

pattern during development (Weiss et al 1999). There are two globin gene clusters, an α-globin family with three genes and four pseudogenes (DNA sequences that look like genes but that are not expressed) located on chromosome 16 and a β-globin family with five genes and one pseudogene on chromosome 11. The location of these genes from 5′ (upstream, left) to 3′ (downstream, right) corresponds with their sequence of expression during development. During development the most 5′ isoform is expressed first, followed by intermediate form and development ends when the most 3′, adult α-globin and β-globin genes are expressed. The β-globin genes are partially regulated via a so-called locus control region and it is an intriguing possibility that the myosin heavy chain isoform genes are regulated by similar mechanisms. To conclude, the genomic location of major skeletal and cardiac MHCs needs to be taken into account when investigating the regulation of these genes in response to physical training by pathways such as the calcineurin or ERK1/2 pathways.

MORE SIGNAL TRANSDUCTION PATHWAYS ARE ACTIVATED DURING EXERCISE

Since the landmark study of Chin et al, many signal transduction pathways have been shown to be activated either by muscle contraction or to induce endurance training-like adaptations or both. Pathways that have been shown to be activated by muscle contraction and potentially mediate change to a slower phenotype include AMP-activated kinase (AMPK), peroxisome proliferator-activated receptor γ coactivator 1α (PGC-1α), the protein kinase B (PKB or Akt) pathway, protein kinase C (PKC), MAPKs such as p38 (p38 indicates the weight of this MAPK which is 38 kDa), c-Jun-N-terminal kinase (JNK) and nuclear factor-κB (NF-κB). Every reader must surely be confused by names such as 'nuclear factor-κB' but this list simply shows that many signal transduction pathways are activated by muscle contraction.

How can we interpret the aforementioned evidence for a signal transduction 'jungle' that appears to be activated by endurance exercise and regulates specific adaptations to it? First, these findings force us to conclude that the research-fostering hypothesis of Chin et al does not stand up: it is probably not just one or two pathways but rather a *signal transduction network* which regulates the adaptation of skeletal muscle to endurance exercise (Wackerhage & Woods 2002). The bottom line is that the Chin et al hypothesis is too simplistic. This is no critique because the formulation of that hypothesis was justified on the bases of their data. Hypotheses must be challenged and a good hypothesis will stimulate good research, even if the final hypothesis is different. We need such hypotheses in order to scrutinize them and to develop the field of research. The Tim Noakes 'Challenging beliefs: ex Africa semper aliquid novi' hypothesis on the control of maximum oxygen uptake is another example for a hypothesis that stimulated much debate, research and that provided the material for many undergraduate exercise physiology essays.

How can we develop the hypothesis of Chin et al? As was mentioned above, we need to see the adaptation-mediating system as a signal transduction network which is capable of sensing numerous exercise-related signals, to compute this information and to regulate fast and slow genes via several mechanisms. An analogy to the nervous system can be made: few outputs are based solely on one sensory input like a sound, a flash of light or a change of temperature. Our brain computes all the sensory input. Similarly, cells never just respond only to low glucose, a stretch, change of temperature or a rise in calcium. They constantly sense all these signals and many outputs (i.e. the expression of a gene, protein synthesis or other cellular functions) depend on a combination of signals. Exercise changes many variables and therefore the adaptations to exercise depend partially on calcium and the calcineurin pathway but other signals such as hypoxia, stretch and immune cell interactions which will activate other pathways and contribute to the adaptive response.

Food for thought: Wilma Rudoph (100 m, 200 m and 4 × 100 m gold medalist Rome 1960) and Peter Radford (British 100 m, 4 × 100 m bronze medalist Rome 1960) both had debilitating diseases so that they had to use a wheelchair in their childhood. Did the inactivity of their leg muscles and a sprinter genotype promote the expression of fast genes enhancing their sprinter muscle phenotype? Professor Sharp has suggested this idea during the revision of this chapter.

ACTN3 POLYMORPHISM

In this chapter we focus mainly on signal transduction and gene regulation related to exercise rather than on polymorphisms that regulate fibre phenotype and physical performance. An overview over gene variations linked to performance and health-related fitness phenotypes is published annually in the journal *Medicine and Science in Sports and Exercise* (Wolfarth et al 2005) and the ACE genotype was covered in Chapter 4.

Here, we review information on the α-actinin (ACTN) genotype. ACTNs anchor actin to the Z-line in between sarcomeres. There are two types in skeletal muscle, ACTN2 which occurs in all muscle fibres and ACTN3 which is expressed only in fast type II fibres. In their study, a 'nonsense' mutation was detected in the ACTN3 gene (North et al 1999) which explained why some patients with muscle disease and normal subjects do not express function ACTN3 at all (not even in type II fibres). North et al (1999) used RT-PCR to amplify mRNA obtained from muscle samples of patients with myopathies and controls. They amplified ACTN3 mRNA fragments that span bases 24-2852 of the ACTN3 mRNA. The mRNA was reverse transcribed into cDNA and then amplified and sequenced. It showed an C→T mutation at position 1747 in exon 16 that converted a codon into a stop codon. Thus, transcription stopped earlier, resulting in a shorter mRNA and non-functional protein. The authors then showed that this would result in an ACTN3 R577X mutation (X stands for a stop codon) in the protein. That means that the mutated protein stops at position 577 but not in the normal protein where it is an arginine (abbreviated R). 96% of the subjects that do not express ACTN3 at all are homozygous for the 577X X genotype. Based on the identification of this loss of function polymorphism and on the selective expression of the ACTN3 gene in type II muscle fibres, Yang et al (2003) hypothesized 'that deficiency of ACTN3 would reduce performance in sprint/power events and

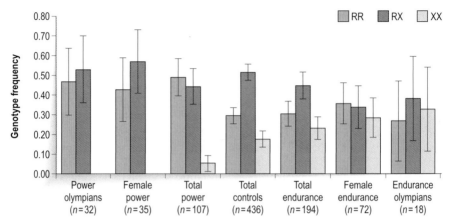

Figure 5.5   ACTN3 genotype frequencies in different power athletes, endurance athletes and controls. RR = 'normal genotype'; RX = 'one normal allele, one premature stop codon' XX = 'both alleles have the premature stop codon'.

would therefore be less frequent in elite sprint athletes'. The strength of the study is the quality of the subjects tested and the size of the sample. The researchers tested 107 specialist sprint/power athletes versus 194 specialist endurance athletes versus 436 controls. Athletes were recruited at the Australian Institute of Sport and the population included several subjects that competed in Olympic games. Thus, because the athletes were among the best in their sport one could assume that the groups included few 'little talent-lots of training' subjects but subjects that have larger than normal talent (which can be interpreted as more than average genetic predisposition). Surprisingly, neither the genotyping method nor the source of DNA are given in the paper. The authors were, however, likely to obtain genomic DNA from buccal cells obtained by mouthwash or from blood and used PCR to amplify the ACTN3 DNA. Using suitable primers allows the investigators to distinguish between a 577XX genotype (one band), 577RR genotype (band in a different position than 577XX band) and two bands for the heterozygous 577RX genotype. The results show that none of the Power Olympians have the 577XX phenotype and only few of all the power athletes (Fig. 5.5).

The ACTN3 study is a study which is do-able for 'normal' sports scientists because the PCR genotyping method can be copied from the original paper and because PCR can be learned within a week. The study also highlights the requirement for hundreds of 'high quality' volunteers in such studies in order to filter out genetic effects. There is no doubt that the genetic contribution to performance in sprint/power, endurance and other sports is polygenic. Thus, the continuous/quantiative nature of such traits and the effect of several polymorphisms implies that large numbers of subjects are needed to filter out the effect of one polymorphism.

REGULATION OF METABOLIC ENZYMES AND MITOCHONDRIAL BIOGENESIS BY ENDURANCE TRAINING

An increase in the capacities for oxidative phosphorylation and fat metabolism is a major adaptation to endurance exercise. The higher enzyme activities largely result from an increased synthesis of mitochondria – termed *mitochondrial biogenesis*. We discuss mitochondrial biogenesis in a separate part of this chapter because its regulation is rather distinct from other adaptive responses to endurance training.

The mitochondrial content of muscle is unlikely to limit the maximal oxygen uptake of a trained athlete; the maximal cardiac output is probably the main limiting factor (Bergh et al 2000). Nonetheless, an increased mitochondrial content has several consequences that will increase endurance exercise performance. The most important consequences are:

1. More mitochondria mean that more pyruvate (i.e. the end product of glycolysis) can be oxidized. This will result in lower pyruvate concentrations at a given exercise intensity. Pyruvate is linked to lactate via the lactate dehydrogenase reaction. Thus, lower pyruvate means lower lactate concentrations at given exercise intensities.
2. More mitochondria will increase the capacity for efficient oxidative ATP synthesis: >30 mol of ATP are produced by oxidative phosphorylation per mol of glycogen (or, more correctly, per mol of glycosyl units). In contrast, only 3 mol of ATP per mol of glycogen are generated by glycolysis per mol of glucose. Thus, the increased capacity for oxidative phosphorylation will contribute to saving glycogen.
3. More mitochondria also mean a higher capacity for fat oxidation which can explain the increased fat oxidation at a given exercise intensity after a period of endurance training (Hurley et al 1986). Higher fat combustion will contribute to glycogen saving and will enable the endurance-trained athlete to exercise for longer at a given (low to medium) intensity.

Adaptation of Oxidative Enzymes to Endurance Exercise

In the exercise field, Gollnick and Saltin found higher succinate dehydrogenase activities (succinate dehydrogenase is a mitochondrial enzyme and can be used as a marker for mitochondrial content or oxidative capacity) in the vastus lateralis muscles of endurance-trained subjects (Gollnick et al 1972), suggesting that training is linked to a higher activity of oxidative enzymes. In a second, longitudinal study, the authors investigated the effect of training directly. They showed that 5 months of endurance training (1-hour training on 4 days per week) increased the succinate dehydrogenase activity in vastus lateralis from 4.65 ± 1.15 to 9.06 ± 1.60 μmol g^{-1} min^{-1} and maximal oxygen uptake by 15% (Gollnick et al 1973). Gollnick and Saltin have summarized their data concerning the effect of training status on succinate dehydrogenase activity and maximal oxygen uptake in a review chapter in the *Handbook of Physiology* (Gollnick & Saltin 1983). The table is reproduced here (Table 5.3).

Table 5.3 shows that succinate dehydrogenase activity and maximal oxygen uptake are correlated which does, however, not suggest that a higher succinate dehydrogenase activity determines maximal oxygen uptake. It also shows that whole muscle succinate dehydrogenase activity differs ~five-fold between detrained and trained endurance athletes and ~three-fold between untrained subjects and endurance athletes. Much of this difference is likely to be due to the endurance training because a doubling of succinate dehydrogenase activity can be achieved with just 5 months of 4 hours per week endurance training (Gollnick et al 1973). Much larger increases in the activities of mitochondrial enzymes result from chronic electrical low-frequency stimulation of fast rodent muscle. We should like to stress again that the protein turnover of rodents is 5–10 times higher and thus the magnitude of response may be different if electrodes attached to the sciatic nerve stimulated human leg muscles.

Table 5.3   Overview of the relationship between maximal oxygen uptake and the activity of a mitochondrial marker enzyme, succinate dehydrogenase (in $\mu mol\ g^{-1}\ min^{-1}$) in different muscle fibre phenotypes and whole muscle (Gollnick & Saltin 1983).

Conditioning state	Maximal oxygen intake (ml kg^{-1} min^{-1})	Muscle fibre type			Whole muscle
		I	IIa	IIx[1]	
			($\mu mol\ g^{-1}\ min^{-1}$)		
Detrained	30–40	5.0	4.0	3.5	4.0
Untrained	40–50	9.2	5.8	4.9	7.0
Endurance training	45–55	12.1	10.2	5.5	11.0
Endurance athlete	> 70	23.2	22.1	22.0	22.5

[1]These fibres were originally named IIb fibres but it has more recently been shown that MHC IIb is not normally expressed in human locomotor muscles.

Adaptation of Fat Metabolism

Another adaptation to endurance training is an increase in the activity of enzymes that facilitate fatty acid transport and catalyse β-oxidation (fats consist of a glycerol and three fatty acids; β-oxidation is the breakdown of fatty acids for oxidative phosphorylation) and other steps in fat metabolism. A landmark study was carried out by Mole et al (1971) who discovered that the activity of several enzymes involved in palmitate (a fatty acid) oxidation in rats was doubled after a period of endurance training. The finding was supported by one in human beings where endurance training caused an increase in the activity of another fat-metabolizing enzyme, 3-hydroxyacyl-CoA-dehydrogenase, in the trained muscles and increased whole-body fat oxidation at a given exercise intensity (Hurley et al 1986). The increased fatty acid metabolism is important for long-distance endurance events because it reduces the use of the limited muscle and liver glycogen reserves. It has a disadvantage, however, which was pointed out by Professor Sharp during the revision of this chapter. The energy yield per litre oxygen is about 19 kJ per litre O_2 for fat and 21 kJ per litre O_2 for carbohydrates. In other words we use (8–9% more oxygen for fat than for carbohydrate oxidative phosphorylation. Thus, the heart and lungs need to work harder for a given rate of aerobic energy production when we oxidize fat compared to carbohydrates.

Regulation of Mitochondrial Biogenesis

Mitochondrial biogenesis is a unique situation because mitochondria have their own DNA which we inherit from the mitochondria inside our mothers' oocytes. The sequencing of the 16 569 base pairs of human mtDNA by a Cambridge team was not only the first breakthrough in the mitochondrial biogenesis field but also in the field of genome sequencing. mtDNA encodes a few subunits of electron transport complexes, as shown in Table 5.4, but the majority of mitochondrial proteins are encoded in nuclear DNA (nDNA). Table 5.4 indicates the numbers of subunits of electron transfer chain complexes encoded in mtDNA and nDNA respectively (Poyton & McEwen 1996).

The origin of mtDNA can be explained by the endosymbiosis hypothesis that was first proposed by Lynn Margulis. According to her hypothesis, mitochondria and

Table 5.4   Numbers of subunits of electron transfer chain complexes encoded in either mtDNA or nDNA (Poyton & McEwen 1996).

Electron transfer chain complex	mtDNA	nDNA
I NADH dehydrogenase complex	7	>25
II Succinate dehydrogenase	–	4
III Cytochrome bc1 complex	1	10
IV Cytochrone c oxidase	3	10
(V) F_0F_1 ATP synthase	2	11

their DNA evolved from bacteria with a precursor form of oxidative metabolism. These bacteria entered eukaryotic host cells which at that period had no mitochondria, and over time evolved into eukaryotic cells with both glycolytic and oxidative metabolism (Gray et al 1999, Margulis & Bermudes 1985). The typhus agent *Rickettsia prowazekii* is possibly the closest relative of the mitochondria that once (thankfully) invaded our cells.

Regulation of Mitochondrial Biogenesis by Endurance Exercise

So how does endurance exercise increase mitochondrial biogenesis in muscle? Research in recent years has led to the identification of many signalling events that are involved in mitochondrial biogenesis. On the basis of these findings, we propose a three-step model to explain how endurance training may activate mitochondrial biogenesis (Fig. 5.6):

1. Increased peroxisome proliferator-activated receptor γ coactivator 1α (PGC-1α) expression and activation by endurance exercise-activated signal transduction pathways;
2. PGC-1α-dependent transcription factor activation leads to the increased expression of nuclear respiratory factors (NRF-1,2) and mitochondrial genes encoded in nDNA;
3. PGC-1α and NRF-1 increase the expression of mitochondrial transcription factor A (Tfam) which binds to mtDNA and activates the transcription and replication of mitochondrial genes encoded in mtDNA followed by mitochondrial assembly.

The three steps of the mitochondrial biogenesis model proposed are now discussed in greater detail.

Increased PGC-1α Expression and Activation by Endurance Exercise-Activated Signal Transduction Pathways

PGC-1α is the master regulator of mitochondrial biogenesis. In this section we will discuss the mechanisms that lead to the increased expression and activation of PGC-1α. Three exercise-activated kinases are thought to be responsible for this:

1. AMP-dependent protein kinase (AMPK)
2. Calmodulin-dependent kinase (CamK)
3. p38 (a MAPK with the molecular weight of 38 kDa).

AMPK is particularly important. It is the primary sensor of the energy status of the cell and activates numerous short- and long-term responses if the energy status of a

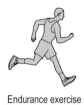

Endurance exercise

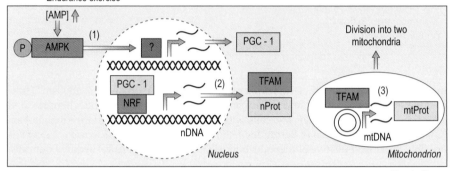

Muscle fibre

Figure 5.6   Schematic drawing of AMPK-PGC-1α (the CamK and p38 pathways are also involved but not shown in this figure) induced mitochondrial biogenesis in response to endurance exercise. (1) The increased energy turnover leads to an increased concentration of AMP during endurance exercise. Elevated AMP concentrations lead to an increased phosphorylation of AMPK by its upstream kinase. Phosphorylated and activated AMPK does increase the expression of the transcriptional co-factor PGC-1α via a yet unknown mechanism. PGC-1α does not bind DNA but transcription factors such as NRF and greatly enhances their effect. (2) PGC-1α bound to NRF and other transcription factors increases the expression of TFAM and mitochondrial proteins encoded in nuclear DNA (nProt). (3) TFAM migrates to the mitochondrion, binds to mtDNA and increases the expression of proteins encoded in mtDNA (mtProt) and the replication of mtDNA (doubling of mtDNA, not shown. Once the mitochondrion components of the mitochondrion (mtDNA, nuclear and mitochondrion-encoded proteins, membranes and so forth) have been synthesized, mitochondria divide.

muscle is low. Activated AMPK reduces non-vital energy consumption, activates ATP synthesis and increases mitochondrial biogenesis. AMPK is activated primarily by [AMP] (the square brackets indicate a concentration) which depends on the concentrations of ATP and ADP. The ATP concentration is approximately 5–8 mM in muscle cytosol and the estimated ADP concentration is probably 100–1000 times lower, probably in the region of 10 μM. The ATP concentration probably decreases only minimally even during fatiguing exercise. Some biopsy studies contradict this statement but in many fatiguing ^{31}P-NMR (a method to measure [ATP] in human muscle *in vivo*) we have never observed a decrease of more than ~20%. The freezing of muscle biopsies is possibly too slow to maintain a constant ATP. Once ATP is split to ADP and P_i it is immediately regenerated by the transfer of a phosphate group from phosphocreatine to ADP, backed up by glycolysis and oxidative phosphorylation. In this system, a hardly detectable decrease of ATP from 8 mM to 7.9 mM is equivalent to a 10-fold increase of ADP from 10 μM to ~100 mM simply because the resting concentration of ADP is that much lower. ADP is a regulator of glycolysis and of oxidative phosphorylation. Oxidative phosphorylation is very sensitive to [ADP] but glycolysis is only activated at the high ADP concentrations that occur during intense exercise (Mader 2003).

The increase of [ADP] during exercise is directly linked to an increase in [AMP] via the adenylate kinase (this enzyme is also known as 'myokinase') reaction: ADP → AMP + ATP. Increased [AMP] then stimulates the phosphorylation of AMPK at site Thr172 (Thr172 denotes the amino acid that is phosphorylated, threonine, and the location of the amino acid in the protein, number 172) by its upstream kinase. Various studies show that exercise does indeed increase AMPK Thr172 phosphorylation and AMPK activity (the rate at which AMPK phosphorylates its target proteins) in skeletal muscles of rodents and human beings (Hardie 2004).

A glycogen-binding domain has been recently discovered in the β-subunit of AMPK (Hudson et al 2003). This finding can explain the inhibitory effect of muscle glycogen on AMPK activity in muscle that was previously reported. Therefore, is mitochondrial biogenesis more activated if athletes train in a glycogen-depleted state? This question shows that the signal transduction is not just academic but leads to some intriguing suggestions with practical relevance. If this hypothesis was true then, in future, endurance athletes may train on a low carbohydrate diet to achieve further AMPK activation and mitochondrial biogenesis for a while before embarking on a carboloading strategy to recover for a competition. Training in a low-glycogen state, however, has numerous drawbacks such as lower glycolytic rates and fatigue which may weigh in more than the potential benefit of an increased AMPK activation.

The link between AMPK activation and increased PGC-1α expression has been demonstrated but it is unclear how the activity of AMPK is exactly linked to PGC-1α expression (i.e. we do not know the transcription factors involved). Several studies shows that treatment with the AMPK-activator AICAR increases PGC-1α expression and mitochondrial biogenesis in rodent muscle. These data are evidence that energy stress sensed by AMPK can lead to an increased expression of PGC-1α and mitochondrial biogenesis.

AMPK appears to be the major regulator of mitochondrial biogenesis but there are other signals. Calcium can increase the activities of both calcineurin and calmodulin-dependent kinase (CamK; several isoforms exist). The activation of CamK by exercise has not been experimentally demonstrated yet, probably because a CamK assay rather than a Western blot using a phospho-specific antibody is necessary. Nonetheless, because CamKs are calcium/calmodulin-activated it seems likely that CamKs are more active during exercise. Increased activity of CamK has been shown to increase PGC-1α expression and mitochondrial biogenesis (Wu et al 2002). Finally, p38 has been identified as a kinase that is activated by some forms of contractile activity. Active p38 has been shown to be capable of phosphorylating and activating PGC-1α.

PGC-1α-Dependent Transcription Factor Activation Leads to the Increased Expression of Nuclear Respiratory Factors (NRF-1,2) and Mitochondrial Genes Encoded in nDNA

AMPK, CamK IV and p38 are all activated in response to exercise and increase the expression or activation of peroxisome proliferator-activated receptor γ coactivator 1α PGC-1α) as was discussed above. PGC-1α is the master regulator of mitochondrial biogenesis: it triggers the specific signalling cascade that controls the various jobs that need to be done for producing additional mitochondria. In step 2 we will discuss the regulation and function of PGC-1α and its relation to nuclear respiratory factors 1 and 2 (NRF-1, 2) which are all involved in the up-regulation of mitochondrial genes expressed in nDNA.

PGC-1α   PGC-1α was originally discovered as a regulator of adaptive thermogenesis, i.e. increased heat production in response to a cold stimulus. Specifically, it was shown to activate mitochondrial biogenesis in brown fat and skeletal muscle and its expression increased in response to cold. PGC-1α was then found to strongly stimulate the expression of the NRF-1 and NRF-2, which are known regulators of mitochondrial biogenesis. The overexpression of PGC-1α in muscle leads to 'redder' (i.e. more myoglobin containing), slower muscle fibres with more mitochondria. This suggests that PGC-1α is not only a specific regulator of mitochondrial biogenesis but also controls other genes that are part of a slower muscle phenotype (Lin et al 2002). Muscle PGC-1α is up-regulated in response to swimming exercise in rats and in response to cycling exercise in human beings. The likely cause are an increase in AMPK, CamK and p38 activities in response to endurance exercise.

PGC-1α is not a transcription factor but a transcriptional co-factor. That means that PGC-1α itself does not bind to DNA; instead it binds and further activates transcription factors resulting in an increased expression of their target genes. PGC-1α also acts as a 'magnet' for proteins that are involved in opening up DNA for transcription.

Interestingly, PGC-1α can be linked to type 2 diabetes: two papers suggest a decreased expression of PGC-1α and PGC-1α-dependent genes in type 2 diabetic muscle. A lower expression of PGC-1α was also noted in skeletal muscle of obese subjects and in some studies PGC-1α polymorphisms were found to be associated with diabetes. The PGC-1α link may at least partially explain the effectiveness of endurance exercise for treating type 2 diabetes mellitus.

NRF-1, NRF-2   The Scarpulla group was responsible for the characterization of transcription factors involved in mitochondrial biogenesis before the discovery of PGC-1α. A major breakthrough was the identification of a binding site via which the mitochondrial cytochrome c promoter and other mitochondrial genes were activated. They named the transcription factor bind to this site 'nuclear respiratory factor-1' which is abbreviated as NRF-1. NRF-1 can activate many genes in nDNA that encode building blocks for a mitochondrion (Scarpulla 2002). The importance of NRF-1 for mitochondrial biogenesis is demonstrated by the fact that NRF-1 knockout mice die while still embryos because of a severe defect in mitochondrial biogenesis. Shortly after the discovery of NRF-1, the Scarpulla group identified NRF-2 as another transcription factor that up-regulated other mitochondrial genes in nDNA (Scarpulla 2002).

Putting the data discussed under points (1) and (2) together, this suggests that AMPK, CamK and p38 first increase the expression and activation of PGC-1α. PGC-1α then binds to yet unknown 'first stage' transcription factors which stimulate the expression of the 'second stage' transcription factors NRF-1 and NRF-2. PGC-1α also binds to and activates NRF-1 and NRF-2. This then stimulates the expression of mitochondrial genes encoded in nDNA.

PGC-1α and NRF-1 Induce Mitochondrial Transcription Factor A (TFAM) Which in Turn Activates the Transcription and Replication of Mitochondrial Genes Encoded in mtDNA Followed by Mitochondrial Protein Import and Assembly

The increased expression of mitochondrial genes encoded in nuclear DNA by PGC-1α and NRF-1,2 is not sufficient. The information also needs to be communicated from the nucleus to the mitochondrion in order to express the genes encoded in mtDNA. Moreover the mtDNA – which itself is an essential part of a mitochondrion – needs to be replicated.

The crucial nucleus-to-mitochondrion messenger is mitochondrial transcription factor A (Tfam; also known as mtTFA). Tfam was identified as a transcription factor encoded in nDNA that could bind the promoter of mtDNA. In another experiment Tfam was shown to be essential for mitochondrial biogenesis because its knockout is lethal during embryogenesis. Mice without Tfam die because of severe mtDNA depletion and a lack of oxidative phosphorylation, suggesting that it is necessary for replication of mtDNA and for the synthesis of functional mitochondria. So, how does Tfam fit into the overall picture of mitochondrial biogenesis?

Virbasius and Scarpulla discovered binding sites for NRF-1 and NRF-2 in the upstream region of the Tfam gene, suggesting that Tfam is up-regulated in response to NRF-1 and NRF-2. Another group discovered that PGC-1α co-activates and amplifies the effect of NRF-1, resulting in a higher expression of Tfam. The model is thus that exercise induces PGC-1α, NRF-1 and NRF-2 first and that these transcriptional regulators then increase the expression of Tfam. The increase in Tfam expression in response to exercise has been demonstrated in electrically stimulated muscle and an 85% increase in Tfam mRNA has been observed after a 16-week aerobic exercise programme in human skeletal muscle (Short et al 2003). Tfam must then somehow migrate to the mitochondrion and bind to the promoter of mtDNA causing the expression of its genes and the replication of mtDNA. The mRNAs are then translated and the mtDNA-encoded proteins can be used for mitochondria building

At this stage, mitochondrial genes encoded in nDNA and mtDNA are produced and mtDNA is doubled. The mitochondrial proteins encoded in nDNA need to be shipped to the mitochondrion, pass the membrane and form complexes. Many more events need to be controlled: the non-protein building materials such as phospholipids for the mitochondrial membrane need to be synthesized by proteins and the splitting process from one mitochondria into two needs to be co-ordinated. One can imagine that a huge amount of regulatory co-ordination is necessary to drive all these events.

To conclude, we now know many major parts in the long chain of events that links endurance exercise to increased mitochondrial biogenesis. AMPK but also CamK and p38 sense endurance training signals and increase the expression of, or activate PGC-1α which is the master regulator of mitochondrial biogenesis. PGC-1α bound to 'first stage' transcription factors induces the 'second stage' transcription factors NRF-1 and 2. PGC-1α also binds and activates NRFs resulting in the up-regulation of mitochondrial genes encoded in nuclear DNA and Tfam. Tfam then migrates to the mitochondrion and activates the expression of genes encoded in mitochondrial DNA (mtDNA) as well as the replication of mtDNA. Finally, non-protein building blocks of the mitochondrion need to be synthesized and new mitochondria need to be assembled.

ENDURANCE EXERCISE-INDUCED ANGIOGENESIS

Another function stimulated by exercise is the formation of new capillaries in parallel with the existing capillaries; this process is termed 'angiogenesis' (Prior et al 2003). Exercise-induced angiogenesis can be measured in cross-sections as (a) an increased capillary-per-fibre ratio, (b) a higher number of capillaries around muscle fibres (capillaries can touch more than one fibre) or (c) a higher number of capillaries per unit area (misleading if fibre size changes). For example, the average number of capillaries around a muscle fibre was 4.76, 4.84 and 2.94 in untrained and 7.79, 6.63 and 4.5 in endurance training subjects for type I, IIa, and 'IIb' fibres (the latter were probably what we would now call IIx fibres) respectively, in human muscle (Ingjer 1979). These data demonstrate two things: first, slow and intermediate fibres have more capillary contacts than fast fibres, and second, endurance-trained subjects have more capillary contacts per fibre than untrained subjects. Twenty-four weeks of endurance training increased the number of capillaries per muscle fibre by nearly 30%, demonstrating that angiogenesis is highly stimulated by endurance training in human beings. Chronic low-frequency electrical stimulation causes an even more pronounced increase in angiogenesis.

How do the signals associated with exercise regulate the growth of the capillary network in skeletal muscle? The growth of capillaries is an important research area in cancer research and developmental biology. Cancers do not grow without the presence of blood vessels and therefore stopping the growth of new vessels seems a feasible therapeutic intervention. Angiogenesis is also important in the development of multicellular organisms. Every tissue needs to receive oxygen and nutrients via its blood vessels and thus the organism can only grow because of an ever expanding network of vessels. In recent years, exercise scientists have applied this knowledge to exercising muscle. Exercise-induced angiogenesis can be described as a two-step process:

1. Up-regulation of angiogenic growth factors by exercise signals
2. Angiogenic growth factors then stimulate capillary formation and maturation.

Up–regulation of Angiogenic Growth Factors by Exercise Signals

The key specific angiogenic factors are vascular endothelial growth factor (VEGF; the 'master' regulator), angiopoietins and ephrins; different isoforms of these factors and their receptors exist (Yancopoulos et al 2000). It was recently shown that many of these angiogenic growth factors respond to exercise training in rat skeletal muscles, showing that not only VEGF is affected. In this part of the chapter we will first introduce the angiogenic regulators, then review the signals that may control these regulators before finally discussing how vascular growth is regulated by angiogenic regulators.

Regulation of Angiogenic Growth Factors and Angiogenesis by Hypoxia

One candidate signal for exercise-induced angiogenesis as well as other muscular adaptations is hypoxia. Severe hypoxia occurs at high altitude, for example when trying to climb the high peaks of the Alps, Andes or the Himalaya. In muscle, hypoxia can also occur if we exercise hard or if we exercise in altitude training camps at moderate altitudes such as 2000–2500 metres. Hypoxia will increase energy stress and thus raise [AMP]. Higher [AMP] will activate the AMPK pathway as was explained in the section of mitochondrial biogenesis. However, there is also a direct sensing system for hypoxia. This system involves the oxygen-sensing van Hippel-Lindau (VHL) protein and a transcription factor that is termed 'hypoxia-induced factor-1' (HIF-1). At normal oxygen VHL is bound to HIF-1; VHL is a cellular 'death row warden': it holds HIF-1 for destruction by a protein breakdown machine which is termed the proteasome. The concentration of HIF-1 is low at normal oxygen because HIF-1 is constantly broken down under these conditions. Once oxygen decreases, VHL detaches from HIF-1 and the degradation of HIF-1 is slowed down. The HIF-1 concentration increases as a result.

More HIF-1 then directly binds to the promoter of the master angiogenic regulator VEGF and increases the expression of VEGF. VEGF then stimulates angiogenesis. This mechanism is probably responsible for the development of collateral vessels if a blood vessel is blocked. The blockade will reduce blood flow and induce hypoxia, resulting in increased HIF-1 and VEGF concentrations and the latter will stimulate the development of new blood vessels.

The up-regulation of VEGF by hypoxia in the exercising muscles sounds like a good explanation for exercise-induced angiogenesis. However, it is currently unclear whether this is the major mechanism by which angiogenesis increases in response to endurance exercise. An increase in VEGF expression was found after normoxic and hypoxic exercise in human beings but there was no significant relationship between the level of oxygen and VEGF expression. These data suggest that an exercise signal other than oxygen is the main factor driving VEGF expression (Richardson et al 1999). So, what could the other exercise signal be?

Up-regulation of Angiogenic Growth Factors and Angiogenesis by Mechanical Signals

Shear stress and wall tension within capillaries are two mechanical signals that may regulate angiogenesis. Exercise increases cardiac output from a resting value of ~5 l min^{-1} up to maxima of ~40 l min^{-1} in highly trained endurance athletes (Ekblom 1968). Nearly all of this extra cardiac output flow is directed towards the working skeletal muscles (Armstrong 1988). As a result, much more blood will flow through the arteries, arterioles, capillaries, venules and veins of a working muscle. Blood flow has been estimated to increase ~100-fold from rest to peak effort in exercising knee-extensor muscles (Saltin et al 1998). This means a change from a trickle to a torrent for the capillaries within exercising muscle. However, an increase in blood flow will also open more capillaries so that the increase is considerably less than 100-fold for each capillary.

An elevation of blood flow due to pharmacological treatment with either dipyridamole or the α-sympathetic blocker prazosin is sufficient for increased capillary growth in rat skeletal muscle. Increased blood flow increases shear stress as is shown in the following formula:

$$\tau = \eta \cdot \frac{4V_{RBC}}{r}$$

in which τ = shear stress; η = viscosity; V_{RBC} = velocity of red blood cells; r = vessel radius.

Arterioles can compensate the exercise-induced increase in shear stress by changing their diameter through vasodilation. Capillaries, however, cannot change their diameter and thus will be exposed to the increased shear stress during exercise. Little is presently known about the mechanisms by which shear stress activates the transcription of angiogenic factors. One factor involved might be nitric oxide (NO). Muscle NO bioavailability increases in response to shear stress and physical training. Blockage of NO synthase by feeding N(G)-nitro-l-arginine (l-NNA) to rats was used to inhibit NO release and reduce NO levels. Hindlimbs were then electrically stimulated and the l-NNA treatment abolished the increase in capillary-to-fibre ratio by stimulation (Hudlicka et al 2000). These data suggest that shear stress-dependent release of NO may be a crucial mechanism by which exercise-induced angiogenesis can be initiated.

The shear stress hypothesis sounds as plausible as the hypoxia hypothesis but there is a caveat as well. Flow or shear stress-mediated angiogenesis is probably due to a process called intussusception in this context (the splitting of the capillary by formation of a wall through the lumen of one original capillary, as opposed to capillary sprouting) (Zhou et al 1998). However, exercise-induced angiogenesis occurs largely as sprouting which is a different mechanism. To conclude, it is currently unclear whether hypoxia, shear stress or another signal are responsible for the up-regulation of VEGF by endurance exercise. However, VEGF and many other angiogenic growth factors and their receptors change their expression in response to exercise.

Up-regulation of Angiogenic Growth Factors and Angiogenesis by Energy Stress

Very recently it was demonstrated that AMPK and the p38 MAPK (which are both implicated in the regulation of mitochondrial biogenesis, see above) could also up-regulate VEGF mRNA and protein in cultured C2C12 cells. AICAR treatment (which increased both AMPK and p38 phosphorylation) also increased VEGF mRNA and protein in ischemic hindlimbs of mice (Ouchi et al 2005). These data suggest that AMPK and p38 are not only involved in the regulation of mitochondrial biogenesis but that they are also important for the increased expression of VEGF.

Up-regulation of Capillary Formation and Maturation by Angiogenic Growth Factors

Angiogenic growth factor expression has been discussed under step 1. Under step 2, we first discuss the angiogenic growth factors VEGF and angiopoietins and then try to show how an increased expression of angiogenic growth factors regulates angiogenesis.

VEGF and VEGF Receptors

VEGF appears to be the most critical initiator of angiogenesis. It regulates the proliferation, migration, elongation, network formation, branching and leakiness of endothelial cells. Various VEGF isoforms and VEGF receptors exist (Yancopoulos et al 2000). We know that VEGF is essential for angiogenesis because homozygous and even heterozygous VEGF knockout mice die during gestation with an abnormal formation of blood vessels. Similarly, knockout of VEGF receptor isoforms die in utero with defects in angiogenesis.

Angiopoietins and Tie Receptors

Angiopoietins are a second class of angiogenesis regulators (Yancopoulos et al 2000). The major isoforms are angiopoietin1 (Ang1) and angiopoietin2 (Ang2). Ang1 knockout mice die *in utero*; the phenotype suggests that the Ang1 regulates late events during angiogenesis. Overexpression of Ang1 leads to larger, leakage-resistant vessels. In contrast, Ang2 was discovered as an antagonist of Ang1 that was only expressed at sites of vascular remodelling. Transgenic overexpression of Ang2 disrupts blood vessel formation in the embryo. Thus, Ang2 may be a vessel-destabilizing factor that is necessary for vascular remodelling. Therefore, the ratio between Ang2/Ang1 is probably important for the leakiness of blood vessels. Higher An2/Ang1 ratios will result in more leaky vessels which are needed for a remodelling of the vascular system. In muscle, the Ang2/Ang1 ratio was increased when angiogenesis was induced by exercise training (Lloyd et al 2003), which is in line with this hypothesis.

THE COMPLETE PICTURE

Exercise induces various signals in skeletal muscle. Of these, hypoxia via HIF-1, and shear stress (possibly via NO production) regulate the expression of angiogenic factors such as VEGF, Ang1 and Ang2. A second event is the increased expression of matrix metalloproteinases, which are proteases that pave a path for new capillaries through the thicket of collagens, fibronectins and laminins that constitute the basement membrane and extracellular matrix. It is evident that matrix metalloproteinases are essential because the inhibition of these proteases with the inhibitor GM6001 prevents capillary growth (Haas et al 2000). Increased VEGF then initiates capillary sprouting through the extracellular matrix and increased Ang2/Ang1 ratio is necessary to make existing vessels more leaky, which is necessary for the sprouting process. An overview over this process is given in Figure 5.7.

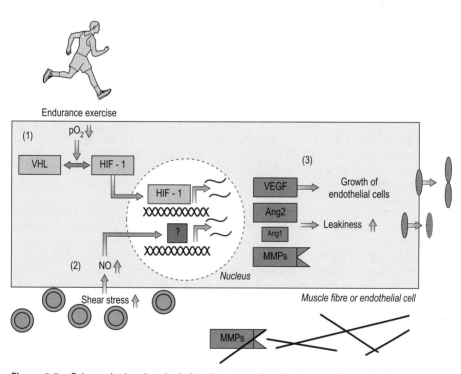

Figure 5.7   Schematic drawing depicting the events that increase angiogenesis in response to endurance training. (1) Intramuscular hypoxia is likely to reduce HIF-1 degradation mediated by VHL (the death row warden for HIF-1). HIF-1 increasingly expresses factors involved in angiogenesis. (2) The increased blood flow during exercise will increase shear stress and probably NO synthesis in endothelial cells. NO via an unknown mechanisms is also likely to affect factors involved in angiogegenesis. (3) Exercise via (1) and (2) and possibly other mechanisms will induce VEGF, the key growth factor for endothelial cells. It will increase the proliferation and growth of these cells which is necessary for the growth of capillaries. The An2/Ang1 ratio increases which will increase the leakiness of vessels. Increased leakiness facilitates angiogenesis. MMPs pave a path through the thicket of the extracellular matrix that surrounds all muscle cells. This is necessary for the growth of capillaries into this space.

Development of the Athlete's Heart

In this section we deviate slightly from the skeletal muscle theme by discussing the athlete's heart, which is a key adaptation to endurance training. The easy-to-measure consequence of an athlete's heart is a lower resting heart rate: endurance athletes have resting heart rates down to 30 beats min^{-1} which is at about half the normal resting heart rate. Assuming a similar resting cardiac output of ~ 5 L min^{-1} this would indicate that the resting stroke volume of the athlete's heart is ~170 mL, which is twice the stroke volume of a normal heart. The endurance athlete's heart is modified from normal by a left ventricular hypertrophy, allowing the heart to generate a higher stroke volume. Because maximal heart rate is only slightly lower in endurance trained athletes, the higher stroke volume allows a higher cardiac output during exercise where a maximal cardiac output is approached.

In classical studies, Ekblom (1968) showed that highly endurance trained subjects can increase their cardiac output from ~5 L min^{-1} at rest to ~40 L min^{-1} during maximal exercise. In contrast, normal subjects can increase their cardiac output from ~5 L min^{-1} at rest only to ~20 L min^{-1} during maximal exercise. Cardiac output and maximal oxygen uptake correlate strongly (Ekblom 1968) and together with other evidence this suggests that the pumping performance of the heart (i.e. the maximal cardiac output) probably determines the maximal oxygen uptake (Bergh et al 2000).

The athlete's heart embodies a *physiological* form of cardiac hypertrophy. In contrast, there are several forms of *pathological* cardiac hypertrophy that can occur in response to the overload induced by myocardial infarction, inflammation hypertension, valve disease or mutations in myofibrillar proteins. There are often two phases of pathological cardiac hypertrophy: the first phase is an asymptomatic cardiac hypertrophy (or asymptomatic left ventricular dysfunction) and the heart then decompensates during the second phase, resulting in heart failure. It was shown in the Framingham study that left ventricular hypertrophy is associated with more clinical events and an increased mortality (Levy et al 1990).

There are two major questions for the molecular exercise physiologist: (1) 'What are the signal transduction events that link the increased cardiac performance during exercise to eccentric left-ventricular cardiac hypertrophy?' and (2) 'Why does exercise cause physiological cardiac hypertrophy whereas disease stimuli cause pathological forms of cardiac hypertrophy that often result in heart failure?'.

In the last 10 years, much research has been carried out in order to identify the signal transduction pathways that regulate cardiac hypertrophy in response to cardiac overload. A landmark paper was published in 1998 (Molkentin et al 1998). In that paper a link is demonstrated for the first time between a signal associated with increased cardiac work and the activation of a signal transduction pathway that is capable of inducing cardiac hypertrophy. The authors first carried out a yeast two-hybrid screen in order to identify proteins that can bind to the transcription factor GATA4 (the factor is named after the DNA sequence, 'GATA' to which it binds). The yeast two-hybrid screen was used to discover binding partners for GATA4 in order to expand the chain of events linking disease stresses to cardiac hypertrophy. One GATA4 binding partner identified was nuclear factor of activated T cells 3 (NFAT3; note that the heart isoform of this protein is different from the muscle isoform). The authors knew from other papers that NFAT transcription factors regulated changes in gene expression in response to calcium in T-cells. NFAT3 may thus be the missing link between $[Ca^{2+}]_i$, GATA4 and cardiac hypertrophy. The authors then went on to test this hypothesis in detail. First, they showed that B-type natriuretic peptide (BNP; a marker gene that is switched on during cardiac hypertrophy) was strongly up-regulated when the calcineurin-NFAT3-GATA4 signalling axis was activated in cultured heart muscle cells. In another experiment they showed that inhibition of calcineurin-NFAT3 signalling prevented the heart muscle hypertrophy that is normally induced by the pharmacological agents angiotensin II or phenylepinephrine. Finally, they produced transgenic mice in which active calcineurin or NFAT3 were overexpressed in heart muscle *in vivo*. Both types of transgenic mice displayed cardiac hypertrophy and several mice died prematurely. Finally, cardiac hypertrophy induced by overexpression of active calcineurin in heart muscle was prevented by treating these mice with the calcineurin inhibitor cyclosporin A.

Was the discovery of the '$[Ca^{2+}]_i\uparrow$ (in a harder working heart) $\rightarrow$ calcineurin $\rightarrow$ NFAT3 $\rightarrow$ cardiac hypertrophy' signalling cascade the complete explanation for the development of cardiac hypertrophy in response to physiological or pathological cardiac overload? No. Many papers subsequently showed the activation of signalling pathways by cardiac hypertrophy stimuli and the development of cardiac hypertrophy when these signalling proteins were activated (Molkentin & Dorn II 2001, Ruwhof & van der Laarse 2000). However, not all pathways cause a decompensation of the heart such as often occurs in pathological but not physiological cardiac hypertrophy. Researchers were also cautioned by the finding that the overexpression of green fluorescent protein alone (a protein without an effect on heart function) led to cardiac hypertrophy. This suggested that the overexpression of a foreign protein independent of its function could stimulate cardiac hypertrophy. Thus the results obtained from previous transgenic mouse models had to be interpreted with caution.

Several papers suggest that calcineurin does not regulate exercise-induced or physiological cardiac hypertrophy. First, calcineurin inhibition with cylclosporin A fails to prevent exercise-induced cardiac hypertrophy (Hainsey et al 2002). Second, it was shown that exercise models inducing cardiac hypertrophy do not activate NFAT-dependent gene expression in mice (although such activation was achieved by pathological stimuli) (Wilkins et al 2004). These results suggest that calcineurin-NFAT signalling does not mediate physiological cardiac hypertrophy (i.e the athlete's heart), at least in rodents. The calcineurin pathway may therefore be specific for pathological cardiac hypertrophy.

Current research suggests that the phosphatid inositol-3-kinase (PI3K)-protein kinase B (PKB)-mammalian target of rapamycin (mTOR) signalling cascade may specifically regulate exercise-induced, physiological hypertrophy of the heart muscle as it does in skeletal muscle (see extensive discussion of this pathway in Chapter 6). Knockout of a PI3K isoform in the heart prevents cardiac hypertrophy in response to exercise but not to a pathological stimulus such as pressure overload (McMullen et al 2003). PI3K is a known activator of PKB whose cardiac overexpression also induces cardiac hypertrophy. More studies are needed to pinpoint the different mechanisms by which exercise or pathological stimuli induce different stimuli. At this stage, it seems likely that the activation of PI3K-PKB (McMullen et al 2003) and possibly of ERK1/2 signalling (Bueno et al 2000) may specifically regulate exercise-induced, physiological hypertrophy i.e. development of the athlete's heart. In contrast, calcineurin-NFAT3 signalling and other pathways seem to regulate the development of pathological cardiac hypertrophies that often lead to heart failure (Wilkins et al 2004).

KEY POINTS

1. Intramuscular calcium is increased during endurance exercise. This will activate calmodulin and calcineurin. Calcineurin dephosphorylates the transcription factor NFAT which exposes the nuclear localization signal of NFAT to the cellular

transport system. NFAT will be imported into the nucleus, bind to the promoters of 'slow' genes and increase their expression. The calcineurin pathway is an uninterrupted chain of events linking signals associated with endurance exercise to specific adaptations (i.e. the up-regulation of slow genes). Subsequent research has shown that many more signal transduction pathways are activated by endurance exercise and that the adaptive response is regulated by a signal transduction network rather than by one or two signal transduction pathways.

2. The increase in mitochondria after endurance training is termed mitochondrial biogenesis. Endurance exercise activates signal transduction pathways such as the energy status-sensing AMPK pathway which induce the transcriptional co-factor PGC-1α. PGC-1α is the master regulator of mitochondrial biogenesis. PGC-1α will induce and further activate NRFs which increase the expression of genes encoded in nDNA. PGC-1α and NRFs will also induce the transcription factor Tfam which migrates to the mitochondrion and binds to the promoter of mtDNA. Tfam activates the expression and replication of mtDNA. Finally mitochondria are assembled from all the building blocks.

3. Endurance exercise increases the sprouting of capillaries, resulting in more capillary contacts per muscle fibre. Hypoxia, shear stress (the latter probably via the expression of NO) and energy stress increase the expression of the master regulator VEGF. VEGF increases the growth of capillary cells. The Ang2/Ang1 ratio increases which aids vascular remodelling. MMPs will be increasingly expressed and pave a path through the thicket of the extracellular matrix for the sprouting capillaries.

4. Cardiac hypertrophy can occur in response to pathological and physiological (i.e. endurance exercise) stimuli. The calcineurin pathway is probably a major regulator of pathological cardiac hypertrophy and the PI3K-PKB-mTOR pathway is involved in mediating the specific form of physiological cardiac hypertrophy that is known as 'the athlete's heart'.

References

Ackland J 1999 The complete guide to endurance training. A&C Black, London

Armstrong R B 1988 Distribution of blood flow in the muscles of conscious animals during exercise. American Journal of Cardiology 62(8): 9E–14E

Bergh U, Ekblom B, Astrand P O 2000 Maximal oxygen uptake 'classical' versus 'contemporary' viewpoints. Medicine and Science in Sports and Exercise 32(1): 85–88

Bodine S C, Stitt T N, Gonzalez M et al 2001 Akt/mTOR pathway is a crucial regulator of skeletal muscle hypertrophy and can prevent muscle atrophy in vivo. Nature Cell Biology 3(11): 1014–1019

Bueno O F, De Windt L J, Tymitz K M et al 2000 The MEK1-ERK1/2 signaling pathway promotes compensated cardiac hypertrophy in transgenic mice. EMBO Journal 19(23): 6341–6350

Chin E R, Olson E N, Richardson J A et al 1998 A calcineurin-dependent transcriptional pathway controls skeletal muscle fiber type. Genes & Development 12(16): 2499–2509

Dolmetsch R E, Lewis R S, Goodnow C C et al 1997 Differential activation of transcription factors induced by Ca^{2+} response amplitude and duration. Nature 386(6627): 855–858

Ekblom B 1968 Effect of physical training on oxygen transport system in man. Acta Physiologica Scandinavica 328(suppl): 1–45

Gollnick P D, Armstrong R B, Saltin B et al 1973 Effect of training on enzyme activity and fiber composition of human skeletal muscle. Journal of Applied Physiology 34(1): 107–111

Gollnick P D, Armstrong R B, Saubert C W et al 1972 Enzyme activity and fiber composition in skeletal muscle of untrained and trained men. Journal of Applied Physiology 33(3): 312–319

Gollnick P D, Saltin B 1983 Skeletal muscle adaptability: significance for metabolism and performance. In Handbook of Physiology. Skeletal Muscle. Editors Peachey L D, Adrian R H, Geiger SR, p. 555–579. Williams & Wilkins, Baltimore

Gray M W, Burger G, Lang B F 1999 Mitochondrial evolution. Science 283(5407): 1476–1481

Haas T L, Milkiewicz M, Davis S J et al 2000 Matrix metalloproteinase activity is required for activity-induced angiogenesis in rat skeletal muscle. American Journal of Physiology 279(4): H1540–H1547

Hainsey T, Csiszar A, Sun S et al 2002 Cyclosporin A does not block exercise-induced cardiac hypertrophy. Medicine and Science in Sports and Exercise 34(8): 1249–1254

Hardie D G 2004 AMP-activated protein kinase: a key system mediating metabolic responses to exercise. Medicine and Science in Sports and Exercise 36(1): 28–34

Henriksson J, Chi M M, Hintz C S et al 1986 Chronic stimulation of mammalian muscle: changes in enzymes of six metabolic pathways. American Journal of Physiology 251(4 Pt 1): C614–C632

Hikida R S, Staron R S, Hagerman F C et al 1983 Muscle fiber necrosis associated with human marathon runners. Journal of Neurological Sciences 59(2): 185–203

Holloszy J O, Booth F W 1976 Biochemical adaptations to endurance exercise in muscle. Annual Review of Physiology 38: 273–291

Hudlicka O, Brown M D, Silgram H 2000 Inhibition of capillary growth in chronically stimulated rat muscles by N(G)-nitro-l-arginine, nitric oxide synthase inhibitor. Microvascular Research 59(1): 45–51

Hudson E R, Pan D A, James J et al 2003 A novel domain in AMP-activated protein kinase causes glycogen storage bodies similar to those seen in hereditary cardiac arrhythmias. Current Biology 13(10): 861–866

Hurley B F, Nemeth P M, Martin W H, III et al 1986 Muscle triglyceride utilization during exercise: effect of training. Journal of Applied Physiology 60(2): 562–567

Ingjer F 1979 Capillary supply and mitochondrial content of different skeletal muscle fiber types in untrained and endurance-trained men. A histochemical and ultrastructural study. European Journal of Applied Physiology and Occupational Physiology 40(3): 197–209

Leger L, Mercier D 1984 Gross energy cost of horizontal treadmill and track running. Sports Medicine 1(4): 270–277

Levy D, Garrison R J, Savage D D et al 1990 Prognostic implications of echocardiographically determined left ventricular mass in the Framingham Heart Study. New England Journal of Medicine 322(22): 1561–1566

Lin J, Wu H, Tarr P T et al 2002 Transcriptional co-activator PGC-1 alpha drives the formation of slow-twitch muscle fibres. Nature 418(6899): 797–801

Lloyd P G, Prior B M, Yang H T et al 2003 Angiogenic growth factor expression in rat skeletal muscle in response to exercise training. American Journal of Physiology 284(5): H1668–1678

Mader A 2003 Glycolysis and oxidative phosphorylation as a function of cytosolic phosphorylation state and power output of the muscle cell. European Journal of Applied Physiology 88(4–5): 317–338

Margulis L, Bermudes D 1985 Symbiosis as a mechanism of evolution: status of cell symbiosis theory. Symbiosis 1: 101–124

McMullen J R, Shioi T, Zhang L et al 2003 Phosphoinositide 3-kinase(p110alpha) plays a critical role for the induction of physiological, but not pathological, cardiac hypertrophy. Proceedings of the National Academy of Sciences of the USA 100(21): 12355–12360

Mole P A, Oscai L B, Holloszy J O 1971 Adaptation of muscle to exercise. Increase in levels of palmityl Coa synthetase, carnitine palmityltransferase, and palmityl Coa dehydrogenase, and in the capacity to oxidize fatty acids. Journal of Clinical Investigation 50(11): 2323–2330

Molkentin J D, Dorn II G W 2001 Cytoplasmic signaling pathways that regulate cardiac hypertrophy. Annual Review of Physiology 63 391–426

Molkentin J D, Lu J R, Antos C L et al 1998 A calcineurin-dependent transcriptional pathway for cardiac hypertrophy. Cell 93(2): 215–228

Murgia M, Serrano A L, Calabria E et al 2000 Ras is involved in nerve-activity-dependent regulation of muscle genes. Nature Cell Biology 2(3): 142–147

Musaro A, McCullagh K J, Naya F J et al 1999 IGF-1 induces skeletal myocyte hypertrophy through calcineurin in association with GATA-2 and NF-ATc1. Nature 400(6744): 581–585

North K N, Yang N, Wattanasirichaigoon D et al 1999 A common nonsense mutation results in alpha-actinin-3 deficiency in the general population. Nature Genetics 21(4): 353–354

Ouchi N, Shibata R, Walsh K 2005 AMP-activated protein kinase signaling stimulates VEGF expression and angiogenesis in skeletal muscle. Circulation Research 96(8):838–46

Parsons S A, Millay D P, Wilkins B J et al 2004 Genetic loss of calcineurin blocks mechanical overload-induced skeletal muscle fiber-type switching but not hypertrophy. Journal of Biological Chemistry 279(25): 26192–26200

Poyton R O, McEwen J E 1996 Crosstalk between nuclear and mitochondrial genomes. Annual Review of Biochemistry 65: 563–607

Prior B M, Lloyd P G, Yang H T et al 2003 Exercise-induced vascular remodeling. Exercise and Sport Science Reviews 31(1): 26–33

Richardson R S, Wagner H, Mudaliar S R et al 1999 Human VEGF gene expression in skeletal muscle: effect of acute normoxic and hypoxic exercise. American Journal of Physiology 277(6 Pt 2): H2247–H2252

Romijn J A, Coyle E F, Sidossis L S et al 1993 Regulation of endogenous fat and carbohydrate metabolism in relation to exercise intensity and duration. American Journal of Physiology 265(3 Pt 1): E380–E391

Ruwhof C, van der L A 2000 Mechanical stress-induced cardiac hypertrophy: mechanisms and signal transduction pathways. Cardiovascular Research 47(1): 23–37

Salmons S, Henriksson J 1981 The adaptive response of skeletal muscle to increased use. Muscle Nerve 4(2): 94–105

Saltin B, Radegran G, Koskolou M D et al 1998 Skeletal muscle blood flow in humans and its regulation during exercise. Acta Physiologica Scandinavica 162(3): 421–436

Scarpulla R C 2002 Nuclear activators and coactivators in mammalian mitochondrial biogenesis. Biochimica et Biophysica Acta 1576(1-2): 1–14

Semsarian C, Wu M J, Ju Y K et al 1999 Skeletal muscle hypertrophy is mediated by a Ca^{2+}-dependent calcineurin signalling pathway. Nature 400(6744): 576–581

Short K R, Vittone J L, Bigelow M L et al 2003 Impact of aerobic exercise training on age-related changes in insulin sensitivity and muscle oxidative capacity. Diabetes 52(8): 1888–1896

Stedman H H, Kozyak B W, Nelson A et al 2004 Myosin gene mutation correlates with anatomical changes in the human lineage. Nature 428(6981): 415–418

Swoap S J, Hunter R B, Stevenson E J et al 2000 The calcineurin-NFAT pathway and muscle fiber-type gene expression. American Journal of Physiology 279(4): C915–C924 van Loon L J, Greenhaff P L, Constantin-Teodosiu D et al 2001 The effects of increasing exercise intensity on muscle fuel utilisation in humans. Journal of Physiology 536(Pt 1): 295–304

Wackerhage H, Woods N M 2002 Exercise-induced signal transduction and gene regulation in skleletal muscle. International Journal of Sports Science and Medicine 4: 103–114

Weiss A, McDonough D, Wertman B et al 1999 Organization of human and mouse skeletal myosin heavy chain gene clusters is highly conserved. Proceedings of the National Academy of Sciences of the USA 96(6): 2958–2963

Widegren U, Ryder J W, Zierath J R 2001 Mitogen-activated protein kinase signal transduction in skeletal muscle: effects of exercise and muscle contraction. Acta Physiologica Scandinavica 172(3): 227–238

Wilkins B J, Dai Y S, Bueno O F et al 2004 Calcineurin/NFAT coupling participates in pathological, but not physiological, cardiac hypertrophy. Circulation Research 94(1): 110–118

Wolfarth B, Bray M S, Hagberg J M et al 2005 The human gene map for performance and health-related fitness phenotypes: the 2004 update. Medicine and Science in Sports and Exercise 37(6): 881–903

Wu H, Kanatous S B, Thurmond F A et al 2002 Regulation of mitochondrial biogenesis in skeletal muscle by CaMK. Science 296(5566): 349–352

Yancopoulos G D, Davis S, Gale N W et al 2000 Vascular-specific growth factors and blood vessel formation. Nature 407(6801): 242–248

Yang N, MacArthur D G, Gulbin J P et al 2003 ACTN3 genotype is associated with human elite athletic performance. American Journal of Human Genetics 73(3): 627–631

Zhou A, Egginton S, Hudlicka O et al 1998 Internal division of capillaries in rat skeletal muscle in response to chronic vasodilator treatment with alpha1-antagonist prazosin. Cell Tissue Research 293(2): 293–303

Chapter **6**

Adaptation to resistance training

Henning Wackerhage and Philip Atherton

Philip J Atherton BSc PhD
Research Associate, School of Biomedical Sciences,
University of Nottingham, Derby

CHAPTER CONTENTS

LEARNING OBJECTIVES:

After studying this chapter, you should be able to . . .

1. Apply resistance training methods and nutritional strategies to stimulate muscle growth and increase strength.
2. Explain how resistance training is linked to a subsequent increase of muscle protein synthesis. Describe the regulation and functions of IGF-1 and myostatin.
3. Explain how resistance training stimulates the proliferation and differentiation of muscle satellite cells.

INDUCING SKELETAL MUSCLE GROWTH BY RESISTANCE TRAINING

Resistance training is used to increase muscle mass and strength in athletes such as 100 m sprinters, throwers, bodybuilders and rugby players. Resistance training also has numerous clinical applications as diverse as rehabilitation after trauma, controlling sarcopenia (i.e. the normal loss of muscle during ageing) and treatment of muscle wasting states which can occur because of cancer, HIV, rheumatoid arthritis, burns and sepsis.

Research results since 1995 have given us an idea about how resistance training activates protein synthesis. Some of the regulatory mechanisms involved are well characterized but others – such as the anabolic signal and its sensor – are gaps in our understanding. Before explaining the anabolic signal transduction induced by resistance training, we will first review human studies where protein synthesis and sometimes breakdown have been measured in response to resistance training and nutritional interventions.

RESISTANCE TRAINING IN HUMAN BEINGS

The muscle mass of untrained human beings varies because of a large variation in the number of fibres in a given muscle. Lexell et al (1988) counted between 393 000 and 903 000 skeletal muscle fibres in whole vastus lateralis sections in a group of nine cadavers with a mean age of 19 years. Thus there is a large variation in the numbers of muscle fibres in muscles between individuals. The number of muscle fibres in an adult human muscle is more or less fixed but we can use resistance training to increase the size of our fibres. Because of that, an individual who has small leg muscles implying few muscle fibres will never be able to develop legs like Arnold Schwarzenegger who has many, hypertrophied fibres. For inducing muscle hypertrophy in untrained subjects, 8–12 concentric/eccentric (i.e. shortening/lengthening) repetitions with moderate movement pace per set and ~3-minute breaks between sets are generally recommended (Kraemer et al 2002). In a normal training programme, subjects perform 1–8 sets per exercise and several exercises. Resistance training causes hypertrophy predominantly in type II fibre subtypes and only little or not at all in type I fibres (Hather et al 1991). This might be partially because fast motor units, to which type II fibres belong, are almost only recruited during intense contractions but not during low-intensity contractions such as standing or walking. The behaviour of motor units is explained by Henneman's 'size principle'. Essentially it states that slow motor units have a lower threshold than fast motor units. Because of that we need to lift heavy weights to make our type IIb/x muscle fibres contract. Type II fibres also develop a higher force than the weaker type I fibres. High force might be the critical growth signal and the force of type I fibres might not be high enough to induce muscle growth.

Can we increase the number of muscle fibres (hyperplasia) in adult skeletal muscle? This question has been discussed controversially (Antonio & Gonyea 1993, Matoba & Gollnick 1984). A meta-analysis of 17 studies in animals concluded that hyperplasia can occur in response to overload and especially in response to chronic stretch in several species (Kelley 1996). In human beings, however, it is difficult to investigate whether hyperplasia occurs because muscle biopsy methods do not allow reliable estimates of whole muscle fibre numbers (Sjostrom et al 1991) and post-mortem whole muscle sections cannot be used for longitudinal studies. Limited evidence for hyperplasia in human skeletal muscle comes from a post-mortem whole muscle section study, where the tibialis anterior of the dominant leg (i.e. the leg we use for high and long jumping) had significantly more fibres than the tibialis anterior of the non-dominant leg (Sjostrom et al 1991). This might suggest that loading differences over a long time can eventually cause some hyperplasia. An alternative explanation could be that these differences are due to an asymmetric development. The consensus is that type II fibre hypertrophy is responsible for muscle growth in response to resistance training but limited hyperplasia cannot be excluded.

Why do muscles hypertrophy? Hypertrophy is derived from Greek *hyper* (above, more than normal) and *trophe* (nutrition) but it means in the muscle context an increase of muscle fibre size. Protein is the main building material of muscle and an increase in muscle protein is thus the key requisite for hypertrophy. A hypertrophying muscle accumulates protein or has, in other words, a positive net positive protein balance:

net protein accretion = protein synthesis – breakdown.

Net protein accretion can result from an increase in protein synthesis, a decrease in protein breakdown or any combination thereof resulting in protein accretion. Protein synthesis and breakdown continuously occur in skeletal muscle and vary ~50–100% over the course of a day depending on age, diet and physical activity (Price et al 1994). The protein turnover of a fasted human muscle is 1.5 % per day, which is roughly ten times lower than the protein turnover in liver or white cells (Table 6.1).

Muscle protein synthesis has been directly measured in animal and human muscle using stable isotope-labelled tracer amino acids (Chesley et al 1992). We recently found that myofibrillar muscle protein synthesis increases ~5-fold 3 hours after resistance but not after endurance exercise-like electrical stimulation of an isolated rat muscle (Fig. 6.1). Because this experiment was conducted outside the organism, it demonstrates that some types of muscle contraction can increase protein synthesis without the need for testosterone or growth hormone release.

In human beings, muscle protein synthesis remains elevated following a bout of resistance training for up to 48 hours in trained subjects and for over 48 hours in untrained subjects (Biolo et al 1995, Chesley et al 1992, Phillips et al 1997, Phillips et al 1999, Rennie & Tipton 2000, Yarasheski et al 1992). Post-exercise protein synthesis increases more in untrained subjects than in resistance-trained subjects (Phillips et al 1999) where the adaptive response to resistance training has levelled off. After a bout of resistance exercise, protein breakdown increases as well (Biolo et al 1995, Phillips

Table 6.1   Basal protein and protein turnover data for human tissues.

Tissue	Protein weight (kg)	% turnover (%/day)	Protein weight turnover (g/day)
Skeletal muscle	6	1.5[1]	90
Liver, gut	1	15	150
White cells	0.25	20	50

Cited from a presentation held by M. J. Rennie at the Physiological Society meeting at Cambridge, UK, in December 2003.
[1]Rat skeletal muscle turnover is >5 times higher, which demonstrates the difference between rat and human muscle protein turnover.

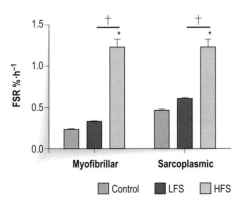

Figure 6.1   The effect of 3 hours of 10 Hz stimulation (LFS; endurance training model) or 60 3-second bursts of 100 Hz stimulation (HFS, resistance training model) on myofibrillar and sarcoplasmic protein synthesis in isolated rat muscle. FSR, fractional (protein-) synthesis rate.

et al 1997) and without food intake, net protein breakdown occurs until we eat again. Thus, resistance training alone increases protein turnover but only an additional meal will cause net protein accretion (Tipton et al 1999). A mixed meal increases the availability of amino acids and glucose and the latter will in turn increase insulin. The increase in amino acids will further increase protein synthesis whereas insulin will mainly reduce protein breakdown (Rennie & Tipton 2000). Recently, two studies suggested that ingestion of a protein meal immediately after severe dynamic or resistance exercise leads to a greater anabolic muscle effect than eating the same meal hours later (Esmarck et al 2001, Levenhagen et al 2001). The amount of essential amino acids needed for maximal stimulation of protein synthesis by nutrition alone is one meal with ~10 g essential amino acids in young subjects (Cuthbertson et al 2004). 10 g of essential amino acids is equivalent to roughly 20 g of total amino acids or protein. Therefore, we would need to drink ~700 ml of milk (which contains ~30 g of protein per litre) to achieve a maximal stimulation of protein synthesis. A pint of skimmed milk or a protein bar will do the trick.

If drinking milk or eating a steak increases protein synthesis, should frequent high-protein snacks not turn us into body builders and solve the sarcopenia problem? No. Feeding protein or amino acids alone stimulates protein synthesis but the effect lasts only for ~2–3 hours (Bohe et al 2001) even if the essential amino acid concentration is kept up by infusion. The muscle might function like a protein-stat to nutrition: protein synthesis shuts down if the bag is full (Millward 1995). In contrast, resistance training stimulates protein synthesis for up to 48 hours as was stated above (Rennie & Tipton 2000). Therefore, eating 10 steaks daily will not turn us into bodybuilders but rather make us obese, whereas resistance training plus a small amount of nutritional protein will stimulate muscle hypertrophy.

How much protein do we need to eat if we plan to use nutrition and resistance training for stimulating muscle growth? Websites targeting bodybuilders advocate ingestion of up to ~5 g of protein kg^{-1} day^{-1}. In contrast, the recommended daily allowance (RDA) is 0.83 g of protein kg^{-1} day^{-1} for the healthy adult population (Rand et al 2003). A re-analysis of nitrogen balance measurement data (the key method to determine protein requirements) suggests that 1.33 g protein kg^{-1} d^{-1} is a 'safe' estimate (meaning on the high side) for the protein requirement of athletes engaging in resistance training (Phillips 2004). Some studies show that training makes protein metabolism more efficient which means that less than the RDA of 0.83 g of protein kg^{-1} day^{-1} would suffice for strength athletes (Rennie & Tipton 2000).

So what should be recommended to strength athletes and bodybuilders? The actual average protein consumption is ~1.5–2 times higher than the RDA in Western Europe and the USA. A normal dietary protein intake should thus cover the protein need of bodybuilders; if proteins are used for weight loss via the 'Atkins' or other high-protein diets in the pre-contest phase, then a high intake with low health risk is probably below 2 g of protein kg^{-1} d^{-1} (Metges & Barth 2000). The take-home message is that the timing of protein feeding is more important than the amount. We should try to better time our meals in dependence of circadian rhythms, fluctuating hormone release patterns and training times rather than overloading our digestive and renal systems with excessive amounts of protein.

OVERVIEW OF SIGNALLING MECHANISMS MEDIATING THE ANABOLIC RESPONSE TO RESISTANCE TRAINING

We have just reviewed the response of muscular protein synthesis to resistance exercise and nutrients. How do these stimuli increase protein synthesis and muscle growth? What are the signals, their sensors and what are the signal transduction pathways that control protein synthesis? Also, protein synthesis is a multi-step process with transcription and translation being the major steps. Do resistance exercise and/or nutrition mainly activate transcription or translation or both? Many questions spring to mind and research in recent years has shown that an intricate cascade of events is involved. We have recently tried to sort relevant research findings and have subdivided the events into five steps (Rennie et al 2004). According to our model, resistance exercise increases muscle growth as follows (Fig. 6.2):

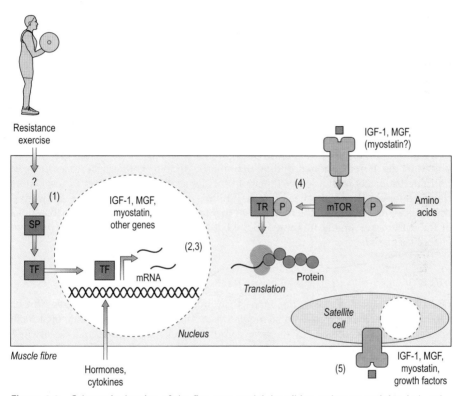

Figure 6.2 Schematic drawing of the five-step model describing resistance training-induced hypertrophy. (1) The resistance training exercise signal(s) is currently unknown. We hypothesize that the signal will be sensed and activate 'upstream' signal transduction proteins (SP) and transcription factors (TF). (2) The upstream signalling will increase the expression of IGF-1, MGF and decrease the expression of myostatin. Hormones such as testosterone and cortisol but also cytokines will further affect the expression of these growth factors. However, it is not entirely clear whether expression changes of muscle growth factors are necessary. (3) 'Upstream' signalling and signalling induced by IGF-1, MGF and myostatin will alter the expression of hundreds to thousands of other genes in skeletal muscle. (4) IGF-1 and MGF will activate the mTOR signal transduction pathway, resulting in the activation of translational regulators (TR) and translation. There is possibly another link between the growth signals and the mTOR signal transduction pathway. Amino acids can further activate mTOR and the timing is important. (5) IGF-1, MGF and myostatin and other growth factors will stimulate satellite cell proliferation and differentiation.

1. Sensing of an anabolic signal associated with resistance exercise
2. Changed expression or release of skeletal muscle growth factors
3. Global transcriptional regulation
4. Activation of the mammalian target of rapamycin (mTOR) signalling cascade resulting in increased protein synthesis
5. Increased satellite cell proliferation and differentiation.
   We will now discuss each of the five steps in more detail.

1. The Search for the Anabolic Signal

Resistance exercise makes type II muscle fibres grow but endurance exercise – at first glance a similar signal – does not. The biggest difference is the intensity of the exercise; thus, one could hypothesize that the 'anabolic signal' is related to the high intensity of resistance exercise. But is 'high intensity' always required for muscle growth? No. For example, habitual or low-intensity physical activity is sufficient to stimulate a muscle re-growth response after cast immobilization (Berg et al 1991). A possible explanation is that there is a 'moving threshold' for the necessary intensity that stimulates muscle growth. This hypothesis predicts that the system is sensitive in atrophied muscle and less sensitive in hypertrophied muscle. Thus, we only need a little activity during spaceflight or after cast immobilization to stimulate growth whereas high-intensity training is needed to stimulate growth in strength athletes. This hypothesis is supported by the aforementioned finding that muscle protein synthesis increases more in untrained subjects with a lower threshold for the anabolic signal than in resistance-trained subjects after resistance exercise (Phillips et al 1999). The identity of the anabolic signal, its sensor and the mechanism that may adjust the sensitivity or threshold of the system are largely unknown. So, what does the literature say about putative anabolic signals?

Stretch?

One possible signal is stretch (i.e. increase in muscle length) which increases protein synthesis and activates translational regulators in cultured muscle cells (Baar et al 2000, Vandenburgh & Kaufman 1979). Passive muscle stretch in normal and denervated rodent muscle also increases muscle protein synthesis *in vivo* (Goldberg et al 1975, Goldspink 1977). However, passive stretch does not increase protein synthesis when compared to control where the same tension is achieved as a result of isometric exercise (Fowles et al 2000). Limited evidence against the stretch hypothesis is the observation that isometric exercise of muscle at resting length (i.e. at short length) does increase myofibrillar protein synthesis ~5-fold 3 hours after stimulation (Atherton et al 2005). Thus stretch does not seem to be the key anabolic signal associated with resistance exercise but it can stimulate a large growth response in rodent muscle.

Swelling?

The cross-sectional area of exercising muscle increases more in response to high-intensity than low-intensity exercise (Nygren & Kaijser 2002). This probably suggests a shift of muscle water into the exercising muscle. According to the cell swelling theory proposed by Häussinger, swelling promotes anabolism whereas cellular shrinkage leads to catabolism (Häussinger et al 1993, Ritz et al 2003). Muscle swelling could thus be a signal that activates protein synthesis in response to resistance training. Swelling is known to increase amino acid transport in cultured muscle fibres (Low et al 1997). Furthermore, an integrin-substrate binding inhibitor (integrins are proteins that bind to the extracellular matrix surrounding muscle fibres and to proteins inside the fibre) was shown to inhibit swelling-induced glutamine uptake (Low & Taylor 1998), suggesting that integrins are involved in sensing the swelling effect. Integrin-related signalling has been hypothesized to be involved in the regulation of muscle hypertrophy in response to exercise (Carson & Wei 2000). Taken together, one might hypothesize that resistance training leads to muscle fibre swelling which, via integrin signalling, increases protein synthesis. This hypothesis has not yet been tested properly.

High Tension?

High muscle tension is an obvious trigger signal candidate that might activate the anabolic signalling cascade. If this were the case, what are possible force or tension sensors and where are they located? All tension sensors must come under load during muscle contraction to be capable of sensing tension. Initially it was thought that the tension generated by the actin and myosin in the sarcomere was transmitted linearly from the tendon of origin to the tendon of insertion. In that case, force sensors must lie in series with the sarcomere because parallel elements will slacken during muscle contraction. Subsequent research shows, however, that much force is transmitted laterally from the force-generating sarcomere (i.e. the M- and Z discs) via so-called costameres to the mesh of stringy proteins (i.e. collagen, laminin) that constitutes the extracellular matrix of a muscle. The tension is then linearly transmitted via these extracellular matrix proteins from tendon to tendon. Tension can be sensed any-where in this system. Titin kinase is a putative tension sensor. When muscle tension increases, titin kinase 'opens' at its catalytic site which will affect the activity of titin kinase (Grater et al 2005). It has recently been shown that titin kinase interacts with various proteins in a load-dependent manner. In denervated muscle titin kinase con-trols the translocation of muscle specific ring finger 2 (MuRF2) into the nucleus result-ing in a repressed transcription of genes that are up-regulated in cardiac hypertrophy (Lange et al 2005). The study also showed that a human mutation in the titin protein kinase domain causes hereditary muscle disease (Lange et al 2005). Tension could also be sensed by proteins that are part of so-called costameres that connect the sarcomere to the extracellular matrix. These proteins include integrins and dystrophin which are known to be linked to signalling proteins such as focal adhesion kinase (FAK) (Carson & Wei 2000). If this system came under load one could envisage how integrins or dystrophin trigger a signalling response that leads to increased protein synthesis.

Muscle Damage?

It is unclear whether exercise and particularly eccentric exercise leads to microscopic muscle damage such as Z-disc streaming (Clarkson & Hubal 2002) or whether appar-ent damage signs are normal physiological adaptations instead (Yu et al 2004). Muscle damage activates protein synthesis linked to repair (Vierck et al 2000) but it is unclear whether damage is the signal that stimulates protein synthesis in response to resist-ance training. An argument against this hypothesis is that Marathon running appears to induce marked muscle damage (Hikida et al 1983) but the muscles of Marathon runners do not adapt with hypertrophy to that stimulus. To conclude, damage may occur after resistance training but it is unlikely to be the signal that stimulates muscle hypertrophy in response to resistance training.

To conclude, there are several candidate signals and sensors which may potentially be responsible for initiating the signalling responses necessary for muscle growth after resistance training. More research is needed to identify the actual signal and sensor.

2. Links to Skeletal Muscle Growth Factors and Other Signalling Events

The still unconfirmed anabolic signal must be linked to the expression or release of known muscle growth factors such as IGF-1 or myostatin, or must activate protein synthesis and satellite cell proliferation via a different mechanism. We know little about the connecting link between the sensor of the anabolic signal and the expression or release of muscle growth factors. In one paper it had been shown that the phosphorylation of c-Jun-N-terminal kinase (JNK, a MAP kinase, see Ch. 5) is quantitatively related to the tension generated (Martineau & Gardiner 2001). However, JNK phosphorylation also increases in response to limb immobilization and it is therefore unlikely that JNK mediates the upstream signalling link between the anabolic signal and muscle growth factors.

By contrast, we know a lot about the response of muscle growth factors to resistance training and other interventions. The two major muscle growth factors constitute a 'yin-yang' system, with IGF-1 being the major muscle growth promoter and myostatin the major muscle growth inhibitor. The regulation of both factors, in particular by resistance exercise, is discussed below.

Growth Hormone and IGF-1

Insulin-like growth factor-1 (IGF-1, previously known as somatomedin C), is part of the growth hormone system that mainly regulates the organisms' growth to adulthood. A growth hormone deficiency causes dwarfism and an excess of growth hormone leads to gigantism, which is also known as acromegaly. An Internet search for human growth hormone and IGF-1 shows that both are advertised as 'anti-ageing' and muscle growth treatments. But research findings contradict these claims. Inhibition rather than activation of the IGF-1 system increases lifespan in several species (Carter et al 2002) suggesting that IGF-1 has a 'quick ageing' rather than the promised 'anti-ageing' effect. Similarly, there is little scientific evidence for the suggested muscle hypertrophy effect if human growth hormone is given to healthy adults (Rennie 2003).

How does growth hormone work? Growth hormone increases IGF-1 expression in the liver but IGF-1 can also be produced by muscle. IGF-1 secreted by liver into the blood stream acts as a growth-stimulating second messenger in several tissues including muscle (Butler & Le Roith 2001). Apart from growth hormone, IGF-1 expression also increases in response to testosterone but decreases in response to factors which are known to cause muscle atrophy. These factors include glucocorticoids such as cortisol or cytokines such as tumour necrosis factor-α (TNF-α). IGF-1 function is modulated by six different IGF-1 binding proteins, IGFBP 1-6, which control the amount of IGF-1 available to bind to its receptors. For example, only the IGFBP 3-IGF-1 complex but not IGF-1 alone increases protein synthesis in muscles of semi-starved rats (Svanberg et al 2000). However, IGF-1 alone is sufficient for an increase of protein synthesis in cultured muscle cells (Rommel et al 2001).

The anabolic effect of IGF-1 on skeletal muscle is well established. Muscles and other organs of mice where the IGF-1 gene is not expressed are smaller than in normal mice and only some of the transgenic mice that lack IGF-1 survive into adulthood. In contrast, IGF-1 infusion into skeletal muscle results in skeletal muscle hypertrophy and skeletal muscle-specific overexpression of IGF-1 causes hypertrophy as well. However, this does not prove that IGF-1 is the growth factor that increases muscle mass after resistance exercise. Some IGF-1 is synthesized in skeletal muscle. Rats in which hypophysectomy (removal of the pituitary gland where growth hormone is made) had been performed still increase muscle IGF-1 expression and display muscle hypertrophy in response to growth stimuli such as muscle stretch. The local muscle response to anabolic signals is at least partially regulated by a changed expression of several IGF-1 splice variants (different sections are spliced out of the full IGF-1 RNA resulting in slightly different isoforms of IGF-1). Yang et al (1996) identified a stretch-responsive isoform in rabbit muscle which was named mechano-growth factor (MGF) and they suspected that this form was important for local muscle growth regulation in response to stretch. MGF mRNA in particular was found to be elevated up to 40 hours after exercise in resistance-trained rat muscles.

The effect of resistance training on IGF-1 splice variant expression in human skeletal muscle is less clear than in rodents. IGF-1 mRNA was significantly elevated 48 hours after eccentric resistance exercise and a trend towards an increase was observed after concentric resistance exercise (Bamman et al 2001). Resistance exercise increased MGF but not IGF-1Ea (i.e. the liver type of IGF-1) significantly 2.5 hours after exercise in young but not old muscle (Hameed et al 2003). Studies by Danish and American groups suggest that IGF-1 splice variants may remain unchanged or even decrease after resistance exercise (Psilander et al 2003). Other studies found no or merely a 20% increase in circulating IGF-1 in response to resistance training. More detailed time course studies – which are difficult to carry out in human beings – are necessary in order to be able to conclusively answer the question whether IGF-1 splice variants or their binding proteins respond to resistance training as they do in rodents.

To summarize, IGF-1 is a muscle growth factor that promotes protein synthesis and hypertrophy in skeletal muscle. IGF-1 is probably involved in the regulation of muscle growth in response to overload and resistance training in rodent models. In human beings, however, the IGF-1 response to resistance exercise and training is not characterized well enough. Moreover, we have little information about the link between the crucial resistance exercise signal and the expression or release of IGF-1. More research, especially in human beings, is needed to advance our knowledge in this area.

Myostatin

Mutations in the myostatin gene give rise to musculous 'mighty mice', double-muscled cattle and 'super toddlers'. Myostatin is part of the growth and development factor (GDF) subfamily which itself is part of the transforming growth factor-β (TGFβ) superfamily. Proteins in this superfamily regulate growth, differentiation and programmed cell death, also known as apoptosis. Myostatin is a GDF whose knockout in mice resulted in skeletal muscle hypertrophy and hyperplasia (McPherron et al 1997). Soon after it was shown that 'double-muscled' cattle breeds such as Piedmontese and Belgian Blue had natural mutations within the myostatin gene. Recently, a myostatin mutation was shown to result in an extraordinarily muscular child (Schuelke et al 2004) shown in Figure 6.3. At 4.5 years of age, the boy was reported to hold two 3-kg dumbbells in horizontal suspension with his arms extended. The quadriceps area of the boy was 6.72 cm^2, which is more than twice the mean of 3.13±0.49 cm^2 of 10 age- and sex-matched controls. The researchers used PCR (the polymerase chain reaction) to amplify the three exons and flanking intron sequences of the myostatin gene. The PCR results suggested a loss-of-function mutation in the myostatin gene in the toddler

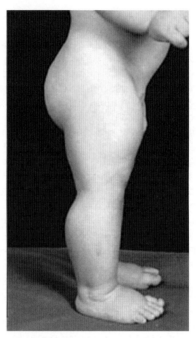

Figure 6.3 Leg phenotype of toddler with a myostatin mutation that results in a shortened, non-functional form of myostatin. Note the size especially of the calf muscles. Reproduced from Schuelke et al (2004), Copyright © 2004 Massachusetts Medical Society. All rights reserved.

and the mother; this mutation was absent in 200 alleles from control subjects with a similar ethnic background. This confirmed that the mutation was rare and affected a muscle growth-controlling gene. The mutation was a G→A mutation in a site in intron 1 that is likely to result in incorrect splicing of the myostatin pre-mRNA.

In contrast, increased systemic myostatin causes muscle wasting as seen in cancer and AIDS. In line with this finding, an increased muscle and serum myostatin concentration was found in HIV-infected men (Gonzalez-Cadavid et al 1998). To conclude, myostatin is a potent, negative regulator of skeletal muscle mass. Natural myostatin polymorphisms occur in cattle and human beings, resulting in individuals with an extremely high muscle mass.

Myostatin is also an important target for drug developers, and trials involving human subjects are currently being carried out; inhibition of myostatin with a specific antibody alleviated many problems seen in mdx mice – which are considered to be a model for human muscular dystrophy (Bogdanovich et al 2002). A myostatin inhibitor is also likely to be an important drug for treating diseases related to a sedentary lifestyle because myostatin knockout mice are also leaner than wildtype controls. Myostatin is a comparatively easy drug target for various reasons. First, it needs to be inhibited, which is usually easier than activating a protein. Second, natural inhibitors (follistatin, gasp-1) exist which can be used as 'templates' for drug design. Third, myostatin is secreted into the extracellular space to act so that a myostatin-targeting drug does not need to cross the cell membrane. Fourth, myostatin action is largely upon muscle and adipose tissue so that few side-effects in other tissues are expected. The downside of such a potentially fitness-inducing, rejuvenating drug is that it would undoubtedly be used as a doping agent by many of those wishing to increase muscle mass and strength for athletic performance.

Several studies suggest that myostatin is regulated by environmental stimuli. In animals myostatin mRNA increases during hindlimb unloading and space flight. In contrast, myostatin decreases during recovery and muscle regrowth after muscle injury. The story is less clear for myostatin expression in response to resistance training in human beings: Some reports suggest that muscle myostatin mRNA or circulating myostatin protein do decrease (Roth et al 2003, Walker et al 2004, Zambon et al 2003) whereas others suggest that it does not (Willoughby 2004). The jury is still out and a high-resolution time course after human resistance exercise and training needs to be obtained in order to see whether there is a regulatory myostatin expression change in response to resistance exercise.

What regulates the expression and release of myostatin? In one study, DNA-binding motifs for glucocorticoid, androgen and thyroid hormone receptors and various transcription factors were predicted (Ma et al 2001), although the prediction of such DNA-binding elements can be unreliable. Of these, the predicted up-regulation of myostatin expression by glucocorticoids was experimentally verified (Ma et al 2003). In another study, growth hormone inhibited the expression of myostatin in growth hormone-deficient patients and in muscle culture (Liu et al 2003). The transcription factor and the binding site by which the growth hormone effect is mediated are currently unknown but IGF-1 could be a mediator. Support for this latter hypothesis comes from the finding that IGF-1/IGFBP-3-complexes reversed an alcohol-induced increase in myostatin expression (Lang et al 2004). The expression of myostatin is apparently fibre-type specific: myostatin expression correlates with the percentage of IIb fibres in mice (Carlson et al 1999).

Myostatin shares the property with IGF-1 of interacting with serum-based factors. Follistatin (Lee & McPherron 2001) and growth and differentiation factor-associated serum protein-1 (gasp-1) (Hill et al 2003) are identified as proteins that can bind and inhibit myostatin. The formation of myostatin-inhibitor protein heterodimers is likely to prevent receptor binding (Groppe et al 2002). Such myostatin-inhibiting proteins could be used to treat muscle-wasting conditions. In addition, resistance training might lead to an increase in the expression of these factors rather than to a reduced expression of myostatin.

A Different Mechanism?

Altered expression of IGF-1, myostatin and their binding proteins is one possible way to explain the increased muscle growth and underlying signalling in response to resistance exercise. The evidence is, however, not entirely convincing. Evidence against an IGF-1-dependent mechanism is that the increase in protein synthesis can also be activated in passively stretched muscles even if the link between IGF-1 and protein synthesis is pharmacologically or genetically inhibited (Hornberger et al 2004). In addition, PKB is activated directly after a brief resistance training-like stimulus (Atherton et al 2005, Bolster et al 2003). If transcriptional up-regulation of IGF-1 and/or down-regulation of myostatin were responsible for these responses then the expression, splicing, secretion and receptor binding of these proteins would have to happen within minutes. It could be that transcriptional regulation of these factors occurs over a longer term but that secretion or localization of IGF-1, myostatin or their binding proteins occurs in the short term. A phenomenon described as 'growth factor shedding' has been observed in mechanically stimulated endothelial cells (Tschumperlin et al 2004). Such a mechanism could explain the rapid increase in growth signalling in skeletal muscle after resistance exercise.

To summarize, IGF-1 is a potent muscle growth activator and myostatin a potent muscle growth inhibitor. Both factors are expressed in skeletal muscle, are secreted, interact with binding proteins and are likely to change their expression in response to at least some general growth factors such as testosterone or inhibitors such as TNF-α. Both IGF-1 and myostatin are likely to regulate transcription via downstream transcription factors, protein synthesis and protein breakdown. There are no entirely convincing data that link an expression change of IGF-1 or myostatin to muscle growth in response to human resistance training.

3. Global Transcriptional Regulation

IGF-1, myostatin and other mechanisms will affect the expression of hundreds if not thousands of genes after resistance training. This conclusion is derived from DNA microarray studies (see Ch. 4 for an explanation of the method) that are increasingly used in exercise research. Here, we focus on how IGF-1 and myostatin might regulate transcription and on the gene clusters whose expression is changed in response to resistance training.

IGF-1 Effect on the Forkhead (FKHR) Transcription Factor

Much of the IGF-1 growth signalling will be discussed in detail under step 4. Briefly, IGF-1 receptor binding will lead to the activation of PKB via an increased phosphorylation of PKB at the two amino acids residues Thr308 and Ser473. This will increase the kinase activity of PKB (i.e. PKB phosphorylates its target proteins more) (Vanhaesebroeck & Alessi 2000). The forkhead transcription factor FKHR has been identified as a transcription factor that can be directly phosphorylated by PKB at Thr24, Ser256, and Ser319 when cells are incubated with IGF-1 (Guo et al 1999, Rena et al 1999). The phosphorylation of FKHR results in exclusion from the nucleus and thus inhibits the transcriptional activity of FKHR. Ser322 and Ser325 were additionally discovered as two phosphorylation sites that were phosphorylated in IGF-1 stimulated cells and were important for the nuclear exclusion of FKHR (Rena et al 2002).

Insulin – which also activates PKB – has been shown to regulate ~800 genes in human skeletal muscle within 3 hours and several of these genes are probably regulated because of a phosphorylation and inactivation of FKHR (Rome et al 2003). One responsive gene cluster consisted of genes regulating protein breakdown via the ubiquitin-dependent proteasome pathway. Recently, it has been shown that this gene cluster is regulated via phosphorylation and deactivation of FKHR (Sandri et al 2004). These findings would suggest that IGF-1 and insulin cannot only stimulate protein synthesis via the PKB pathway (as will be explained under step 4) but also reduce protein breakdown. Attractive as this hypothesis is, it is hard to reconcile with data on human beings where muscle protein synthesis and breakdown seem to be coupled; i.e. they both seem to go up or down in parallel and small differences result in positive or negative protein balances. For example, resistance training increases both protein synthesis and breakdown (Rennie & Tipton 2000) whereas cast immobilization decreases both (Gibson et al 1987).

Myostatin Effect on Smad2/3 and Transcription

Myostatin signalling is described in more detail than IGF-1 signalling here because the endpoint of the pathway, Smad2/3, is a transcription factor and thus myostatin probably achieves its growth effect via transcriptional regulation. The abbreviation 'Smad' stands for '(similar to) mothers against decapentaplegic homolog' and is related to the function of these proteins in fruitflies. The link to protein synthesis, which is mildly inhibited by myostatin at least in cultured muscle cells (Taylor et al 2001), is not yet established. Myostatin dimers bind to the activin receptors IIA and IIB (Lee & McPherron 2001). This event leads to the recruitment of activin type I receptors which are also known as activin receptor-like kinases. In the case of myostatin, these kinases lead to the phosphorylation of the transcription factors Smad2 and Smad3 at Ser465/Ser467 (Bogdanovich et al 2002). The phosphorylation of Ser465/467 is necessary for forming a complex between Smad2 and Smad4 (Souchelnytskyi et al 1997). The gene clusters regulated by myostatin-activated Smads are unknown and a DNA microarray study is highly desirable to shed some light on the mechanism by which myostatin inhibits muscle growth. Some cellular effects of myostatin will be discussed later when we explain the regulation of satellite cell proliferation and differentiation in response to resistance exercise.

DNA microarray studies investigating the effects of resistance exercise on gene regulation have been carried out on rats and human subjects. In rats mRNA and mRNA that was actively translated (i.e. bound to ribosomes) were investigated after a bout of maximal eccentric contractions (Chen et al 2002). The authors identified a cluster of tumour suppressor or antigrowth genes which might keep muscle nuclei post-mitotic (i.e. these myonuclei do not divide anymore) despite the presence of mitogens (factors that stimulate mitosis or cell division). The authors also identified several genes that were translationally regulated (Chen et al 2002). In human beings who had performed a bout of resistance exercise, the expression of circadian clock genes was found to be 'reset' by exercise (Zambon et al 2003). Moreover, a significant decrease of myostatin was observed, supporting the hypothesis that myostatin mediates part of the muscle growth response after resistance exercise. There is much more to explore in the results of both studies and the files have been deposited online so that searches can be carried out.

To conclude, resistance training leads to a changed expression of numerous genes in skeletal muscle. Some of these genes are probably controlled by the inhibition of the transcription factor FKHR by IGF-1 or by the likely decrease of Smad2/3-binding to DNA due to a decrease in myostatin. One effect will be a resetting of the muscle clock, and an anti-growth programme might prevent the division of nuclei within muscle fibres at a time when muscle growth is stimulated.

4. Activation of the mTOR Signalling Cascade and Protein Synthesis

In this part of the chapter we aim to describe how IGF-1 activates protein synthesis. Glancing at Figures 6.2 and 6.5 from time to time will make sense because otherwise it is easy to get lost in this signalling labyrinth.

Initially it was reported that IGF-1 induced skeletal muscle growth via the calcineurin pathway which had been shown to promote cardiac hypertrophy. However, it now seems unlikely that the calcineurin pathway regulates skeletal muscle hypertrophy because pharmacological and transgenic blockade of calcineurin does not prevent hypertrophy in response to synergist ablation (one muscle is removed and the 'overload' of the synergists induces hypertrophy) (Bodine et al 2001, Parsons et al 2004). It seems more likely that activated calcineurin regulates fibre phenotype as discussed in Chapter 5.

In 2001, two papers provided evidence that IGF-1 induced growth via the protein kinase B-tuberin (TSC2)-mammalian target of rapamycin (mTOR) signalling cascade

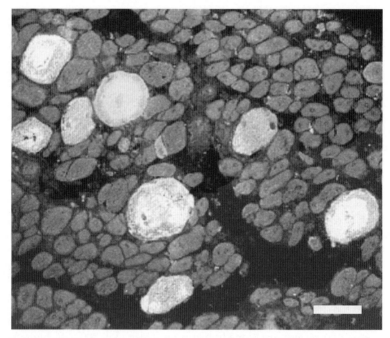

Figure 6.4 Constitutively active PKB induces muscle fibre hypertrophy in regenerating skeletal muscle. Immunofluorescence analysis of a transverse section of regenerating denervated soleus muscle transfected with HA–tagged constitutively active PKB. The HA tag is a part of the influenza hemagglutinin protein; it is used to detect fibres by immunohistochemistry that have taken up and express the constitutively active PKB. Note that transfected fibres are much larger in size than surrounding untransfected fibres. Figure and part of the legend reproduced from Pallafacchina et al (2002), Copyright (2002) National Academy of Sciences, USA.

and translational regulators (Bodine et al 2001, Rommel et al 2001). In 2002, the Schiaffino group showed that expression of constitutively active PKB caused hypertrophy in those muscle fibres that had taken up a PKB DNA construct (Pallafacchina et al 2002) (Fig. 6.4).

Later it was shown that the overexpression of a constitutively active form of PKB induced muscle hypertrophy in mice (Lai et al 2004). These data show that IGF-1 activates protein synthesis via PKB and PKB activation equally stimulates protein synthesis and results in muscle growth.

However, at this stage it is unclear whether resistance training activates this cascade via IGF-1 and PKB or lower down at the level of mTOR (Hornberger et al 2004). The PKB pathway is much studied because it is not only a key growth pathway but also the pathway that mediates muscle glucose uptake and glycogen synthesis in response to insulin. IGF-1 probably specifically activates different isoforms of signalling proteins in this pathway which can explain why IGF-1 has a greater effect on muscle protein synthesis than insulin (which stimulates glucose uptake and glycogen synthesis). An overview over resistance training-induced activation of protein synthesis by the PKB-TSC2-mTPR pathway is given in Figure 6.5.

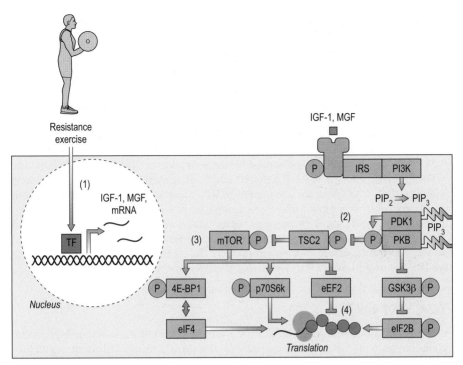

Figure 6.5 Activation of translation (protein synthesis) by resistance training assuming IGF-1 or MGF synthesis as an intermediate step. (1) Resistance exercise will via an unknown signal, signal transduction pathway and transcription factor (TF) increase the expression of IGF-1 and/or MGF. (2) IGF-1 and/or MGF will bind to its receptor, causing its phosphorylation. The scaffolding protein IRS will be recruited, activate PI3K which phosphorylates PIP_2 to PIP_3. PIP_3 binds to the PH domain of PDK1 and PKB, causing PKB phosphorylation by PDK1 and by mTOR associated with Rictor (not shown). PKB activates and inhibits the mTOR-inhibitor TSC2 (thus mTOR is active when PKB is active). (3) mTOR then directly or indirectly affects the phosphorylation of 4E-BP1, p70 S6k and eEF2 causing an increased translation (protein synthesis) via each of these translational regulators. PKB also phosphorylates and inhibits GSK-3β which in turn phosphorylates eIF2B less. Dephosphorylated eIF2B also stimulates translation.

IGF-1 Receptor and IRS1–4

How does IGF-1 activate PKB? IGF-1 can bind to any of three receptors which are members of the so-called tyrosine kinase growth factor receptor family:

1. IGF-1 receptor
2. Insulin receptor
3. IGF-II receptor (also known as mannose 6-phosphate receptor).

The IGF-1 receptor, to which IGF-1 preferentially binds, is shown to be important for organism and muscle growth by the fact that IGF-1 receptor knockout mice die at birth and display a severe growth deficiency and muscle atrophy. Upon IGF-1 binding, the IGF-1 receptor phosphorylates a tyrosine, an amino acid in its structure which is essential for starting the downstream signalling cascade. The autophosphorylated receptor then attracts, by protein–protein interaction, scaffolding proteins which facilitate the activation of specific signal transduction pathways. IGF-1 activates the extracellular signal regulated kinase 1/2 (ERK1/2) and PKB pathways in skeletal muscle via different scaffolding proteins. We will not discuss the ERK1/2 effect in this chapter because the activation of the ERK1/2 pathway is probably more related to muscle fibre phenotype regulation but not as much to growth, as was discussed in Chapter 5.

Insulin receptor substrate (IRS) proteins are the scaffolding proteins that control the activation of the PKB pathway in response to IGF-1, IGF-2 and insulin. There are four IRS isoforms, IRS1–4. IRS isoforms are phosphorylated at tyrosine residues by active IGF-1/insulin receptors. Phosphorylated IRS attract phosphatidylinositol-3-kinase (PI3K) to the receptor which is essential for the activation of PKB further downstream.

The four IRS isoforms all have different functions. Intrauterine growth was reduced by 50% and glucose tolerance is impaired in IRS-1 knockout mice, showing that both growth and glucose metabolism are controlled by IRS-1. In contrast, IRS-2 knockout mice predominantly show changes in reproduction and energy homeostasis, IRS-3 knockout mice show no growth or metabolic defects, and IRS-4 mice have mild growth, reproduction and metabolism defects. Taken together, these studies suggest that IRS-1 is important for IGF-1-stimulated muscle growth.

PI-3K, PDK1 and PKB

All IRS isoforms have binding sites for the aforementioned PI3K. This kinase phosphorylates not proteins but so-called phosphatidylinositols (PtdIns). PtdIns are regulatory lipids that can be phosphorylated and dephosphorylated just like proteins. PI3K uses ATP to phosphorylate $PtdIns(3,4)P_2$ (or shorter PIP2) to $PtdIns(3,4,5)P_3$ (PIP3).

PIP_3 is a 'matchmaker' for PIP_3-dependent protein kinase-1 (PDK1) and PKB. The matchmaking works as follows. Both the PDK1 and PKB proteins have a PIP_3 binding site, named the pleckstrin homology (PH) domain. PIP_3 binds to the PH domain of both kinases and stimulates their translocation from the cytosol to the cell membrane. Once this has happened PDK1 is able to phosphorylate PKB at Thr308 (the Ser473 is phosphorylated by mTOR; see below). Both PDK1 and PKB regulate organ and muscle growth as is evident from muscle growth changes in PDK1 and PKB transgenic mice.

There are three PKB isoforms, PKBα (Akt1), PKBβ (Akt2) and PKBγ (Akt3) and transgenic mice have been generated for each PKB isoform. PKBα knockout mice have defects in foetal and postnatal growth that persist into adulthood. In contrast, PKBβ knockout mice suffer from diabetes, suggesting that PKBα mainly regulates growth whereas PKBβ regulates insulin-activated glucose uptake. PKBγ knockouts display brain defects. The effect of PKB activation on skeletal muscle growth was demonstrated in an experiment where a constitutively active PKB construct was expressed in regenerating skeletal muscle (Pallafacchina et al 2002). Fibres that took up and expressed the construct were roughly twice as large as fibres that did not take up the construct. Mice overexpressing a constitutively active form of PKB develop muscle hypertrophy (Lai et al 2004). Thus, activation of the right PKB isoform in muscle will result in muscle hypertrophy in sedentary (i.e. not resistance training) mice.

The Bit in the Middle: From PKB via TSC2 and Rheb to mTOR

PKB is a major protein kinase which activates protein synthesis by phosphorylating the signalling proteins tuberin (TSC2, which lies on the major signalling route to protein synthesis) and glycogen synthase kinase-3β (GSK-3β; which lies on the major signalling route to glycogen synthesis but also affects protein synthesis). TSC2 was recently discovered as an important, missing link that connects PKB to mTOR and other translational regulators. TSC2 is a negative regulator of protein synthesis: The inhibition of TSC2 by IGF-1 increases protein synthesis and TSC2 activation decreases protein synthesis. PKB phosphorylates TSC2 at Ser939 and Thr1462 resulting in the inhibition of TSC2. The TSC2 protein has a domain that hydrolysis a GTP molecule to GDP on a small protein termed Ras homolog enriched in brain (Rheb). Rheb then transduces the signal downstream.

TSC2 is activated (resulting in less protein synthesis) by the energy stress which occurs during exercise. One signal of energy stress is a rise in [AMP] which is sensed by the [AMP]-activated AMP-dependent protein kinase (AMPK; see Ch. 5). It was recently shown that AMPK could directly phosphorylate TSC2 at Thr1227 and Ser1345 which are different from the Ser939 and Thr1462 sites that have been reported to be phosphorylated by PKB. The AMPK mechanism prevents energy-consuming protein synthesis when a muscle is experiencing energy stress. This mechanism might explain why protein synthesis is inhibited in an exercising muscle (Rennie & Tipton 2000).

How energy-consuming is protein synthesis? Much energy is used to catalyse the elongation of the amino acid chain during protein synthesis. ATP is hydrolysed to AMP and two GTP are hydrolysed to GDP for each amino acid added to growing protein (Browne & Proud 2002). Assuming an average amino acid weight of 135 Da, the production of one millimole of a 50 kDa protein (a protein consisting of ~370 amino acids) requires the use of ~1500 mmol (or 1.5 mol) ATP equivalents. This effect can explain the so-called thermogenesis effect of high-protein diets such as the Aktins diet (Nair et al 1983). The thermogenesis or energy turnover effect of protein feeding is small, however, when compared to exercise. Heart rate and oxygen uptake (indicators of thermogenesis and energy turnover) clearly do hardly increase after a meal that contains a lot of protein and the increase is probably limited to ~2 hours after the meal (Bohe et al 2001).

Back to the signalling: IGF-1 will inhibit TSC2 which will leave Rheb in its active GTP-bound state. Rheb then somehow activates the mammalian target of rapamycin (mTOR) in response to insulin and muscle loading. In these situations, phosphorylation of mTOR at Ser2448 occurs and the activity of this kinase increases. mTOR receives three signalling inputs (also discussed in Ch. 4 as an example for the integration of various signals by signal transduction proteins):

1. IGF-1, IGF-2 or insulin receptor binding (via PKB-TSC2 signalling)
2. Energy stress (via AMPK-TSC2 signalling)
3. Amino acid availability (via an unknown pathway).

Depending on the strength of each of the three inputs, protein synthesis will be either increased or decreased by mTOR-dependent signalling. For example, if, say, IGF-1 is increased after a hard bout of resistance exercise, if the energy status is normal and if drinking a pint of milk has increased the amino acid concentration then protein synthesis will be high. In contrast, if IGF-1 is low in a cast-immobilized leg in a starved subject then protein synthesis will be low.

mTOR is a large serine/threonine kinase that phosphorylates and activates the translational (or protein synthesis) regulators. The kinase activity of mTOR is indicated by the phosphorylation of mTOR on Thr2446 and Ser2448. Phosphorylation of Thr2446 increases when AMPK is activated and is low in response to nutrients and insulin. In contrast, phosphorylation of Ser2448, which is only two amino acids away, is decreased in response to AMPK activation but increased in response to nutrients and insulin. Thus, Thr2446 and Ser2448 seem to be always phosphorylated in opposite directions and the more Ser2448 is phosphorylated the more mTOR stimulates protein synthesis.

The AMPK-effect on TSC2 and protein synthesis has important consequences for athletes: the higher the energy stress (and thus [AMP]) the lower protein synthesis. We do not yet know whether AMPK inhibits protein synthesis for a long time after the energy stress has ended or whether protein synthesis is inhibited only acutely when AMPK is activated. AMPK effects may be partially responsible for lower strength gains after combined resistance and endurance training when compared to endurance training alone (Hickson 1980, Putman et al 2004). In addition, the increase in type I fibres (which are innervated during both endurance and resistance training), was reported to be larger after resistance training alone than after combined endurance and resistance training (Putman et al 2004).

On the basis of our isolated muscle data (Atherton et al 2005), we hypothesize that standard resistance exercise is likely either not to activate AMPK or to only cause a brief AMPK activation whereas endurance exercise is likely to stimulate AMPK for much longer. Especially the long duration of AMPK activation during endurance training is important for AMPK-dependent adaptations. Resistance training is short but sharp with a lot of recovery in between. Especially due to the short duration of a set of resistance exercise the decrease of [phosphocreatine] is probably limited and short. [AMP] is high when [phosphocreatine] is low due to the combined creatine kinase, ATPase and myokinase reactions. We have used ^{31}P-NMR to measure the ATP and phosphocreatine concentrations in the calf muscles of untrained subjects and sprinters carrying out three sets of resistance exercise with 12 repetitions (Fig. 6.6). We found that at the end of each set [phosphocreatine] decreased to ~50% of the resting value in the untrained subjects and ~30% in the trained subjects. These data indirectly suggest that a standard set of resistance training causes only short and limited rises in [AMP] as opposed to exercises with a medium-high intensity that can be maintained for ~1–5 minutes.

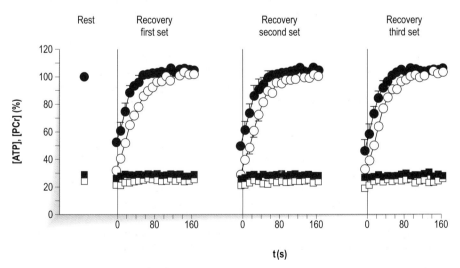

Figure 6.6 Phosphocreatine (PCr) and ATP relative to resting concentrations in sprinters (○, n = 8) and untrained subjects (●, n = 6) during three sets of calf hypertrophy training with 12 repetitions. Data during the sets are not shown because the sets varied in duration (Wackerhage H, Müller K, Zange, K, unpublished).

mTOR is not only activated by IGF-1 and insulin but also by amino acids – as is evident from an amino acid effect on Ser2448 phosphorylation. The amino acid effect has recently been suggested to be mediated at least partially via the mTOR binding proteins regulatory associated protein of TOR (raptor) and G protein β-subunit-like protein (GβL, pronounced 'gable') (Kim et al 2003). Research into the identification of the amino acid-sensing mechanism is currently a major goal.

To summarize, the chain of events up to here is: IGF-1 activates PKB via various steps → PKB phosphorylates and inhibits the GAP activity of TSC2 → Rheb is more in its GTP-bound active state → increased phosphorylation of mTOR at Ser2448 via an unknown mechanism (Fig. 6.5).

The protein kinase mTOR is the main regulator of protein synthesis; it controls the rate of translation initiation (i.e. it controls the rate of mRNA-binding to ribosomes which are the protein synthesis machines of the cell) and elongation (the addition of more amino acids to a synthesized protein; see Ch. 4). Two major targets which are phosphorylated directly or indirectly by active mTOR are p70 ribosomal protein S6 kinase (p70 S6k, also known as S6k1) and 4E-binding protein 1 (4E-BP1).

p70 S6k and 4E-BP1; Regulators of Translation Initiation

One important mTOR target is p70 S6k. p70 S6k can be phosphorylated at several sites by mTOR. Knocking out p70 S6k inhibits animal growth but the explanatory power of this transgenic mouse model is limited because of the up-regulation of a related kinase. Knocking out both kinases results in increased perinatal lethality and the growth defect is similar to that in the p70 S6k knockout mice. The stimulatory effect of p70 S6k (S6k1) on muscle size has recently be demonstrated in a p70S6k knockout model (Ohanna et al 2005).

p70 S6k has previously been shown to regulate the translation of specific mRNAs but this now seems unlikely. The link between p70 S6k and protein synthesis is currently unclear. High-intensity contractions in rats increase p70 S6k activity and translation (Baar & Esser 1999). Resistance exercise also increases phosphorylation of p70 S6k at various sites in human muscle and oral intake of branched-chain amino acids increases the phosphorylation even further (Karlsson et al 2004). It was shown that p70 S6k phosphorylation and protein synthesis increase in parallel for up to 24 hours after resistance exercise in rats (Hernandez et al 2000). The latter finding is an important observation: the regulators of translation initiation and protein synthesis are activated for up to 48 hours but upstream signalling regulators such as PI3K and PKB have long ceased to signal. There must thus be a mechanism that keeps translation and protein synthesis going for up to 48 hours after resistance training.

The second mTOR target is 4E-binding protein 1 (4E-BP1), an inhibitor of translation. 4E-BP1 is normally bound to the eukaryotic translation initiation factor 4E (eIF4E). The phosphorylation of 4E-BP1 at various sites removes 4E-BP1 from eIF4E, allowing eIF4E to participate in initiating translation. 4E-BP1 knockout mice display an interesting but unexpected phenotype: the mice are of normal size but have smaller fat pads than wild-type animals. These mice also have an increased expression of PGC-1 (see Ch. 5) in white adipose tissue which has been discussed as a regulator of mitochondrial biogenesis. The reason for this finding and for the lack of a growth effect is unknown.

Another Path to Translation Initiation: GSK-3β and eIF2B

PKB regulates protein synthesis not only via the TSC2-Rheb-mTOR-p70 S6k (4E-BP1) connection but also by branching out via a glycogen synthase kinase-3β (GSK-3β) and eukaryotic initiation factor 2B (eIF2B) link (Fig. 6.5). GSK-3β is, among other things, a regulator of glycogen and protein synthesis. PKB inhibits GSK-3β by phosphorylating it on Ser9 and the phosphorylation of this amino acid increases when IGF-1 is added to muscle cells. The inhibition of GSK-3β with the not very specific inhibitor lithium chloride has been shown to induce hypertrophy in cultured muscle cells. GSK-3β inhibition due to PKB-phosphorylation decreases the phosphorylation of eIF2B at Ser535, another regulator of translation initiation. Less phosphorylated eIF2B promotes initiation of translation. We observed a decreased phosphorylation of eIF2B at Ser535 after resistance training-like electrical stimulation of an isolated muscle (Atherton et al 2005).

Translation Elongation: Control by eEF2

Translation elongation also depends on mTOR. mTOR activates p70 S6k as described above which, in turn, can phosphorylate and deactivate the eukaryotic elongation factor 2 kinase (eEF2k) which then decreases the phosphorylation of eukaryotic elongation factor 2 (eEF2) at Thr56. Dephosphorylated eEF2 is more active and promotes the elongation of the nascent peptide during translation. Similar to the regulators of translation initiation, eEF2 activity is inhibited when AMPK is activated.

Summary and Practical Implications for Nutrition and Exercise

IGF can activate translation initiation and elongation via the PI3K-PKB-TSC2-mTOR pathway and the GSK-3β side track. Figure 6.5 should help you to understand this confusing cascade of signalling proteins. The stimulation of most of these proteins in muscle has been shown to increase protein synthesis and/or muscle growth. It is not entirely clear whether IGF-1 splice variants mediate the activation of the PKB-TSC2-mTOR pathway by resistance training or whether there is another link.

5. Satellite Cell Proliferation and Differentiation

An up-regulation of translation or protein synthesis is one major response to the signalling wave that is activated by resistance training. This will increase the size of a muscle fibre but leave the nuclei – and thus the DNA content of muscle fibres – unaffected. In this section we will discuss how resistance training leads to an increased number of nuclei and DNA.

Muscle fibres are, after α-motor neurons, the second largest cells of our body. Muscle fibres can reach lengths of more than 20 cm in some muscles (Heron & Richmond 1993). During myogenesis (i.e. the development of muscle), so-called myoblasts fuse and form a muscle fibre. If nuclei-per-length values for rat fibres are used then a 10 cm long skeletal muscle fibre contains between 4000 and 12 000 nuclei with a higher nuclear density found in type I than type II fibres. If we assume that our vastus lateralis muscle contained 500 000 muscle fibres per cross-section and if the muscle was 30 cm long then the total fibre length would be 15 km (almost 10 miles) and we shall have very roughly 1 billion nuclei in this muscle.

Skeletal muscle fibres can be seen as an exception to the rule that organ growth requires both cell growth and cell division. Normally, cells grow to a critical size and then divide, which ensures that DNA is not 'diluted' in a growing cell. Skeletal muscle fibres are different: The nuclei within a muscle fibre do not divide after development (i.e. they remain post-mitotic) even if muscle fibres grow. The production of DNA, however, is 'outsourced' to satellite cells which are developmental muscle cells that retain an ability to divide. Satellite cells and muscle fibres thus act as a functional unit: during muscle growth or regeneration satellite cells produce additional nuclei whereas the muscle fibres grow. This ensures a tight relationship between the number of nuclei and the volume of a fibre. This relationship has been conceptualized as the 'myonuclear domain' which refers to the amount of sarcoplasm controlled by a single myonucleus (Allen et al 1999).

Satellite cells were first discovered by Mauro using electron microscopy (Mauro 1961). He described that satellite cells are wedged between the plasma membrane of the muscle fibre and the sarcolemma. It was then shown that only satellite cells synthesized new DNA and divided and that some satellite cells were then incorporated into skeletal muscle fibres. Satellite cells are likely to increase the number of nuclei during hypertrophy induced by resistance training and during longitudinal growth, for example during adolescence. During longitudinal growth, satellite cells are active at the ends of muscle fibres, which is where fibres grow.

Various studies suggest that satellite cells proliferate during exercise and that some satellite cells then add their nuclei to growing muscle fibres. Satellite cell proliferation appears to be critical for the muscle growth response. In response to synergist ablation (a powerful muscle growth stimulus), first satellite cells and then myonuclei increase in the hypertrophying muscle, adding further support to the hypothesis that satellite cells proliferate first and that then some satellite cells fuse with muscle fibres (Snow 1990). If mild γ-irradiation is used to block satellite cell proliferation then rat muscle does not hypertrophy any more in response to synergist ablation (Rosenblatt et al 1994). In another study it was confirmed that mild γ-irradiation could prevent most hypertrophy induced by overload over the longer period of 3 months. However, γ-irradiation is a crude way of inhibiting satellite cells because it may have numerous other effects. A knockout of satellite cells in adult muscle – for example, by the specific knockout of a crucial satellite cell gene – would be the ideal model to investigate whether satellite cell proliferation is essential for muscle growth. However, this model has yet to be achieved.

Several studies suggest that satellite cell proliferation and nuclear uptake into muscle fibres occurs in response to resistance training in human muscles. People who resistance train have hypertrophied muscles and a larger number of nuclei per fibre, suggesting that resistance training can increase the number of nuclei in human muscle. After 10 weeks of resistance training in women, the fibre hypertrophy was accompanied by both a ~70% increase in the number of nuclei and a 46% increase in the number of satellite cells (Kadi & Thornell 2000), suggesting satellite cell proliferation and fusion with growing muscle fibres. Finally, satellite cells increase by 19% and 31% after 30 and 90 days of resistance training and decrease afterwards, confirming that satellite cells respond with proliferation to resistance training (Kadi et al 2004).

Regulation of the Satellite Cell Cycle by Myostatin and IGF-1

Satellite cells develop from muscle precursor cells. Paired box gene 7 (Pax7) was initially proposed to be a critical regulator of satellite cells (Seale et al 2000) but a subsequent paper showed that Pax7 knockout mice still possess some satellite cells (Oustanina et al 2004). Satellite cells in adult muscle are quiescent until stimulated by growth factors and mitogens. Stimulation activates two events which go hand in hand. First, satellite cells will progress through the cell cycle, which is necessary for the increase in satellite cell number. Second, satellite cells differentiate and fuse with existing muscle fibres.

The cell cycle is a tightly controlled process that is much studied by cancer researchers and cell biologists. It consists of four phases:

1. Gap_1 (G_1) phase
2. Synthesis (S) phase: DNA is replicated
3. Gap_2 (G_2)
4. Mitosis (M): nuclear and cytoplasm divide into two cells.

The cell cycle is regulated by signal transduction pathways that regulate so-called 'cyclin-dependent kinases' (Cdks) which form complexes with proteins that are called 'cyclins' (Roberts 1999). Cyclins regulate the kinase activity of Cdks, and active Cdks phosphorylate target proteins that regulate the mechanics of the cell cycle.

The second event is satellite cell differentiation. Satellite cell differentiation repeats many steps of muscle development, where the so-called primary myogenic regulatory factors myogenic factor 5 (Myf5) and myoblast determination protein 1 (MyoD) regulate development of muscle precursors into myoblasts whereas the secondary myogenic factors myogenin and muscle regulatory factor 4 (MRF4) regulate the terminal differentiation (Buckingham 2001). When placed in culture, quiescent satellite cells initially do not express myogenic regulatory factors. After 12 hours in culture MyoD mRNA appears, followed by MRF4 mRNA and myf-5 mRNA after 48 hours and finally myogenin mRNA after 72 hours.

Satellite cell proliferation (i.e. progression through the cell cycle) and differentiation responds to a plethora of growth factors and mitogens (factors that sitmulate mitosis), including IGF-1 and myostatin. IGF-1 has been shown to activate and myostatin to inhibit cyclin-dependent kinase-2 (cdk2). Cdk2 regulates whether cells will start to replicate DNA or remain quiescent in the G_1 phase of the cell cycle. IGF-1 stimulates satellite cell cdk2 and cell proliferation by down-regulating cyclin-dpendent kinase inhibitor 1 (p27[Kip1]; p27 indicates that the weight of this protein is 27 kDa). p27[Kip1] inhibits cdk2, which results in a G_1 arrest in the satellite cell cycle (Chakravarthy et al 2000). These data suggest that IGF-1 stimulates satellite cell proliferation via this mechanism. Myostatin increases the expression of the cyclin-dependent kinase inhibitor 1A (p21) and down-regulates cdk2 levels in cultured muscle cells and satellite cells. Furthermore, myostatin has been shown to inhibit differentiation of cultured muscle cells by down-regulating the expression of MyoD, Myf5 and myogenin (Langley et al 2002).

A second link between resistance training and satellite cell regulation is muscle injury, reviewed in detail by Vierck et al (2000). Accordingly, it has been hypothesized that resistance training induces injury, which changes the concentrations of cytokines, growth factors and mitogens and these stimulate the proliferation and differentiation of satellite cells.

Practical Recommendations

Signal transduction knowledge would hardly be relevant for coaches, gym instructors and clinical exercise physiologists if there were no resulting practical recommendations. We have thus produced a list with recommendations summarizing practical implications of the research presented in this chapter. Much of the underlying research is recent and most recommendations are thus based on limited evidence and should be viewed as recommendations that are likely to work:

1. The effects of resistance training and feeding protein on signalling (Karlsson et al 2004) and muscle growth (Esmarck et al 2001, Levenhagen et al 2001) are additive. We recommend to consume the equivalent of a pint of milk directly after resistance

training in order to further activate mTOR, regulators of translation initiation and elongation and thus protein synthesis.

2. If you have used resistance training to stimulate protein synthesis, avoid endurance training for the same muscle group afterwards if you want to maximize muscle growth. The activation of AMPK by endurance training is likely to inhibit translation initiation and elongation and thus protein synthesis (Browne et al 2004, Inoki et al 2003).

3. You should probably avoid glycogen depletion if you want to maximize protein synthesis: AMPK is more activated when glycogen is low (Wojtaszewski et al 2002) and is likely to reduce the increase of protein synthesis after resistance training.

4. Protein synthesis and the signalling in the lower half of the PKB-TSC2-mTOR pathway are activated for 48 hours or more after resistance training (Hernandez et al 2000, Rennie & Tipton 2000). Thus not each muscle group needs to be trained every day. So-called 'split routine' programmes (focusing on a different muscle group in each training session) should suffice for high muscle growth.

5. Resistance training stimulates protein synthesis for much longer (Rennie & Tipton 2000) than protein feeding (Bohe et al 2001). Thus, resistance training targeting all major muscle groups should be effective in increasing the basic metabolic rate for 48 hours or more by the increased thermogenesis resulting from elevated protein synthesis. Therefore, resistance training should be an effective fat loss (due to a higher energy turnover) treatment for overweight and obese subjects.

KEY POINTS

1. Resistance training is used to stimulate muscle growth for appearance, athletic performance, disease prevention, treatment and rehabilitation. 8–12 concentric/eccentric repetitions per set and ~3-minute breaks between sets are usually recommended for beginners. Such training will increase protein synthesis for 48 hours or more, which is much longer than nutrient-activated protein synthesis: this is increased for only ~2–3 hours even if the amino acid concentration is kept elevated.

2. Resistance training is likely to stimulate muscle growth via a five-step cascade of events: (1) sensing of a yet unknown anabolic signal associated with resistance exercise; (2) changed expression of skeletal muscle growth factors or another mechanism; (3) changed global transcriptional regulation; (4) activation of the PKB-TSC2-mTOR signalling cascade and of regulators of translation initiation and elongation resulting in increased protein synthesis; (5) increased satellite cell proliferation and differentiation.

3. Energy stress (sensed as increased [AMP]) or glycogen depletion lead to AMPK activation and the inhibition of protein synthesis. Therefore, energy stress should be limited during and after resistance training and glycogen depletion should be avoided. Protein should be ingested either directly after or possibly just before or during resistance training.

References

Allen D L, Roy R R, Edgerton V R 1999 Myonuclear domains in muscle adaptation and disease. Muscle Nerve 22(10): 1350–1360

Antonio J, Gonyea W J 1993 Skeletal muscle fiber hyperplasia. Medicine and Science in Sports and Exercise 25(12): 1333–1345

Atherton P J, Babraj J A, Smith K et al 2005 Selective activation of AMPK-PGC-1alpha or PKB-TSC2-mTOR signaling can explain specific adaptive responses to endurance or resistance training-like electrical muscle stimulation. FASEB Journal. 19(7):786–788.

Baar K, Esser K 1999 Phosphorylation of p70(S6k) correlates with increased skeletal muscle mass following resistance exercise. American Journal of Physiology 276(1 Pt 1): C120–C127

Baar K, Torgan C E, Kraus W E et al 2000 Autocrine phosphorylation of p70(S6k) in response to acute stretch in myotubes. Molecular Cell Biology Research Communications 4(2): 76–80

Bamman M M, Shipp J R, Jiang J et al 2001 Mechanical load increases muscle IGF-I and androgen receptor mRNA concentrations in humans. American Journal of Physiology 280(3): E383–E390

Berg H E, Dudley G A, Haggmark T et al 1991 Effects of lower limb unloading on skeletal muscle mass and function in humans. Journal of Applied Physiology 70(4): 1882–1885

Biolo G, Maggi S P, Williams B D et al 1995 Increased rates of muscle protein turnover and amino acid transport after resistance exercise in humans. American Journal of Physiology 268(3 Pt 1): E514–E520

Bodine S C, Stitt T N, Gonzalez M et al 2001 Akt/mTOR pathway is a crucial regulator of skeletal muscle hypertrophy and can prevent muscle atrophy in vivo. Nature Cell Biology 3(11): 1014–1019

Bogdanovich S, Krag T O, Barton E R et al 2002 Functional improvement of dystrophic muscle by myostatin blockade. Nature 420(6914): 418–421

Bohe J, Low J F, Wolfe R R et al 2001 Latency and duration of stimulation of human muscle protein synthesis during continuous infusion of amino acids. Journal of Physiology 532(Pt 2): 575–579

Bolster D R, Kubica N, Crozier S J et al 2003 Immediate response of mammalian target of rapamycin (mTOR)-mediated signalling following acute resistance exercise in rat skeletal muscle. Journal of Physiology 553(Pt 1): 213–220

Browne G J, Finn S G, Proud C G 2004 Stimulation of the AMP-activated protein kinase leads to activation of eukaryotic elongation factor 2 kinase and to its phosphorylation at a novel site, serine 398. Journal of Biological Chemistry 279(13): 12220–12231

Browne G J, Proud C G 2002 Regulation of peptide-chain elongation in mammalian cells. European Journal of Biochemistry 269(22): 5360–5368

Buckingham M 2001 Skeletal muscle formation in vertebrates. Current Opinion in Genetics and Development 11(4): 440–448

Butler A A, Le Roith D 2001 Control of growth by the somatropic axis: growth hormone and the insulin-like growth factors have related and independent roles. Annual Review of Physiology 63 141–164

Carlson C J, Booth F W, Gordon S E 1999 Skeletal muscle myostatin mRNA expression is fiber-type specific and increases during hindlimb unloading. American Journal of Physiology 277(2 Pt 2): R601–R606

Carson J A, Wei L 2000 Integrin signaling's potential for mediating gene expression in hypertrophying skeletal muscle. Journal of Applied Physiology 88(1): 337–343

Carter C S, Ramsey M M, Sonntag W E 2002 A critical analysis of the role of growth hormone and IGF-1 in aging and lifespan. Trends in Genetics 18(6): 295–301

Chakravarthy M V, Abraha T W, Schwartz R J et al 2000 Insulin-like growth factor-I extends in vitro replicative life span of skeletal muscle satellite cells by enhancing G1/S cell cycle progression via the activation of phosphatidylinositol 3'-kinase/Akt signaling pathway. Journal of Biological Chemistry 275(46): 35942–35952

Chen Y W, Nader G A, Baar K R et al 2002 Response of rat muscle to acute resistance exercise defined by transcriptional and translational profiling. Journal of Physiology 545(Pt 1): 27–41

Chesley A, MacDougall J D, Tarnopolsky M A et al 1992 Changes in human muscle protein synthesis after resistance exercise. Journal of Applied Physiology 73(4): 1383–1388

Clarkson P M, Hubal M J 2002 Exercise-induced muscle damage in humans. American Journal of Physical Medicine and Rehabilitation 81(11 Suppl): S52–S69

Cuthbertson D, Smith K, Babraj J et al 2004 Anabolic signaling deficits underlie amino acid resistance of wasting, aging muscle. FASEB Journal 19(3):422–424

Esmarck B, Andersen J L, Olsen S et al 2001 Timing of postexercise protein intake is important for muscle hypertrophy with resistance training in elderly humans. Journal of Physiology 535(Pt 1): 301–311

Fowles J R, MacDougall J D, Tarnopolsky M A et al 2000 The effects of acute passive stretch on muscle protein synthesis in humans. Canadian Journal of Applied Physiology 25(3): 165–180

Gibson J N, Halliday D, Morrison W L et al 1987 Decrease in human quadriceps muscle protein turnover consequent upon leg immobilization. Clinical Science (London) 72(4): 503–509

Goldberg A L, Etlinger J D, Goldspink D F et al 1975 Mechanism of work-induced hypertrophy of skeletal muscle. Medicine and Science in Sports 7(3): 185–198

Goldspink D F 1977 The influence of immobilization and stretch on protein turnover of rat skeletal muscle. Journal of Physiology 264(1): 267–282

Gonzalez-Cadavid N F, Taylor W E, Yarasheski K et al 1998 Organization of the human myostatin gene and expression in healthy men and HIV-infected men with muscle wasting. Proceedings of the National Academy of Sciences of the USA 95(25): 14938–14943

Grater F, Shen J, Jiang H et al 2005 Mechanically induced titin kinase activation studied by force-probe molecular dynamics simulations. Biophysical Journal 88(2): 790–804

Groppe J, Greenwald J, Wiater E et al 2002 Structural basis of BMP signalling inhibition by the cystine knot protein Noggin. Nature 420(6916): 636–642

Guo S, Rena G, Cichy S et al 1999 Phosphorylation of serine 256 by protein kinase B disrupts transactivation by FKHR and mediates effects of insulin on insulin-like growth factor-binding protein-1 promoter activity through a conserved insulin response sequence. Journal of Biological Chemistry 274(24): 17184–17192

Hameed M, Orrell R W, Cobbold M et al 2003 Expression of IGF-I splice variants in young and old human skeletal muscle after high resistance exercise. Journal of Physiology 547(Pt 1): 247–254

Hather B M, Tesch P A, Buchanan P et al 1991 Influence of eccentric actions on skeletal muscle adaptations to resistance training. Acta Physiologica Scandinavica 143(2): 177–185

Haussinger D, Roth E, Lang F et al 1993 Cellular hydration state: an important determinant of protein catabolism in health and disease. Lancet 341(8856): 1330–1332

Hernandez J M, Fedele M J, Farrell P A 2000 Time course evaluation of protein synthesis and glucose uptake after acute resistance exercise in rats. Journal of Applied Physiology 88(3): 1142–1149

Heron M I, Richmond F J 1993 In-series fiber architecture in long human muscles. Journal of Morphology 216(1): 35–45

Hickson R C 1980 Interference of strength development by simultaneously training for strength and endurance. Europeam Journal of Applied Physiology and Occupational Physiology 45(2-3): 255–263

Hikida R S, Staron R S, Hagerman F C et al 1983 Muscle fiber necrosis associated with human marathon runners. Journal of Neurological Sciences 59(2): 185–203

Hill J J, Qiu Y, Hewick R M et al 2003 Regulation of myostatin in vivo by GASP-1: a novel protein with protease inhibitor and follistatin domains. Molecular Endocrinology 17(6):1144–1154

Hornberger T A, Stuppard R, Conley K E et al 2004 Mechanical stimuli regulate rapamycin-sensitive signaling by a phosphoinositide 3-kinase, protein kinase B and growth factor independent mechanism. Biochemical Journal 380(Pt 3):795–804

Inoki K, Zhu T, Guan K L 2003 TSC2 mediates cellular energy response to control cell growth and survival. Cell 115(5): 577–590

Kadi F, Schjerling P, Andersen L L et al 2004 The effects of heavy resistance training and detraining on satellite cells in human skeletal muscles. Journal of Physiology 558(Pt 3): 1005–1012

Kadi F, Thornell L E 2000 Concomitant increases in myonuclear and satellite cell content in female trapezius muscle following strength training. Histochemistry and Cell Biology 113(2): 99–103

Karlsson H K, Nilsson P A, Nilsson J et al 2004 Branched-chain amino acids increase p70S6k phosphorylation in human skeletal muscle after resistance exercise. American Journal of Physiology Endocrinol Metab 287(1): E1–E7

Kelley G 1996 Mechanical overload and skeletal muscle fiber hyperplasia: a meta-analysis. Journal of Applied Physiology 81(4): 1584–1588

Kim D H, Sarbassov d D, Ali S M et al 2003 GbetaL, a positive regulator of the rapamycin-sensitive pathway required for the nutrient-sensitive interaction between raptor and mTOR. Molecular Cell 11(4): 895–904

Kraemer W J, Adams K, Cafarelli E et al 2002 American College of Sports Medicine position stand. Progression models in resistance training for healthy adults. Medicine and Science in Sports and Exercise 34(2): 364–380

Lai K M, Gonzalez M, Poueymirou W T et al 2004 Conditional activation of akt in adult skeletal muscle induces rapid hypertrophy. Molecular and Cellular Biology 24(21): 9295–9304

Lang C H, Frost R A, Svanberg E et al 2004 IGF-I/IGFBP-3 ameliorates alterations in protein synthesis, eIF4E availability, and myostatin in alcohol-fed rats. American Journal of Physiology Endocrinol Metab 286(6): E916–E926

Lange S, Xiang F, Yakovenko A et al 2005 The kinase domain of titin controls muscle gene expression and protein turnover. Science 308(5728): 1599–1603

Langley B, Thomas M, Bishop A et al 2002 Myostatin Inhibits Myoblast Differentiation by Down-regulating MyoD Expression. Journal of Biological Chemistry 277(51): 49831–49840

Lee S J, McPherron A C 2001 Regulation of myostatin activity and muscle growth. Proceedings of the National Academy of Sciences of the USA 98(16): 9306–9311

Levenhagen D K, Gresham J D, Carlson M G et al 2001 Postexercise nutrient intake timing in humans is critical to recovery of leg glucose and protein homeostasis. American Journal of Physiology 280(6): E982–E993

Lexell J, Taylor C C, Sjostrom M 1988 What is the cause of the ageing atrophy? Total number, size and proportion of different fiber types studied in whole vastus lateralis muscle from 15- to 83-year-old men. Journal of Neurological Sciences 84(2-3): 275–294

Liu W, Thomas S G, Asa S L et al 2003 Myostatin is a skeletal muscle target of growth hormone anabolic action. Journal of Clinical Endocrinology and Metabolism 88(11): 5490–5496

Low S Y, Rennie M J, Taylor P M 1997 Signaling elements involved in amino acid transport responses to altered muscle cell volume. FASEB Journal 11(13): 1111–1117

Low S Y, Taylor P M 1998 Integrin and cytoskeletal involvement in signalling cell volume changes to glutamine transport in rat skeletal muscle. Journal of Physiology 512 (Pt 2) 481–485

Ma K, Mallidis C, Artaza J et al 2001 Characterization of 5'-regulatory region of human myostatin gene: regulation by dexamethasone in vitro. American Journal of Physiology Endocrinol Metab 281(6): E1128–E1136

Ma K, Mallidis C, Bhasin S et al 2003 Glucocorticoid-Induced Skeletal Muscle Atrophy is Associated with Upregulation of Myostatin Gene Expression. American Journal of Physiology, 285(2):E363–371

Martineau L C, Gardiner P F 2001 Insight into skeletal muscle mechanotransduction: MAPK activation is quantitatively related to tension. Journal of Applied Physiology 91(2): 693–702

Matoba H, Gollnick P D 1984 Response of skeletal muscle to training. Sports Medicine 1(3): 240–251

Mauro A 1961 Satellite cell of skeletal muscle fibers. Journal of Biophysical and Biochemical Cytology, 9: 493–495

McPherron A C, Lawler A M, Lee S J 1997 Regulation of skeletal muscle mass in mice by a new TGF-beta superfamily member. Nature 387(6628): 83–90

Metges C C, Barth C A 2000 Metabolic consequences of a high dietary-protein intake in adulthood: assessment of the available evidence. Journal of Nutrition 130(4): 886–889

Millward D J 1995 A protein-stat mechanism for the regulation of growth and maintenance of the lean-body mass. Nutrition Research Reviews 8: 93–120

Nair K S, Halliday D, Garrow J S 1983 Thermic response to isoenergetic protein, carbohydrate or fat meals in lean and obese subjects. Clinical Science (London) 65(3): 307–312

Nygren A T, Kaijser L 2002 Water exchange induced by unilateral exercise in active and inactive skeletal muscles. Journal of Applied Physiology 93(5): 1716–1722

Ohanna M, Sobering A K, Lapointe T et al 2005 Atrophy of S6K1(-/-) skeletal muscle cells reveals distinct mTOR effectors for cell cycle and size control. Nature Cell Biology 7(3): 286–294

Oustanina S, Hause G, Braun T 2004 Pax7 directs postnatal renewal and propagation of myogenic satellite cells but not their specification. EMBO Journal 23(16): 3430–3439

Pallafacchina G, Calabria E, Serrano A L et al 2002 A protein kinase B-dependent and rapamycin-sensitive pathway controls skeletal muscle growth but not fiber type specification. Proceedings of the National Academy of Sciences of the USA 99(14): 9213–9218

Parsons S A, Millay D P, Wilkins B J et al 2004 Genetic loss of calcineurin blocks mechanical overload-induced skeletal muscle fiber-type switching but not hypertrophy. Journal of Biological Chemistry 279(25): 26192–26200

Phillips S M 2004 Protein requirements and supplementation in strength sports. Nutrition 20(7-8): 689–695

Phillips S M, Tipton K D, Aarsland A et al 1997 Mixed muscle protein synthesis and breakdown after resistance exercise in humans. American Journal of Physiology 273(1 Pt 1): E99–107

Phillips S M, Tipton K D, Ferrando A A et al 1999 Resistance training reduces the acute exercise-induced increase in muscle protein turnover. American Journal of Physiology 276(1 Pt 1): E118–E124

Price G M, Halliday D, Pacy P J et al 1994 Nitrogen homeostasis in man: influence of protein intake on the amplitude of diurnal cycling of body nitrogen. Clinical Science (London) 86(1): 91–102

Psilander N, Damsgaard R, Pilegaard H 2003 Resistance exercise alters MRF and IGF-I mRNA content in human skeletal muscle. Journal of Applied Physiology 95(3):1038–44

Putman C T, Xu X, Gillies E et al 2004 Effects of strength, endurance and combined training on myosin heavy chain content and fibre-type distribution in humans. European Journal of Applied Physiology 92(4-5): 376–384

Rand W M, Pellett P L, Young V R 2003 Meta-analysis of nitrogen balance studies for estimating protein requirements in healthy adults. American Journal of Clinical Nutrition 77(1): 109–127

Rena G, Guo S, Cichy S C et al 1999 Phosphorylation of the transcription factor forkhead family member FKHR by protein kinase B. Journal of Biological Chemistry 274(24): 17179–17183

Rena G, Woods Y L, Prescott A R et al 2002 Two novel phosphorylation sites on FKHR that are critical for its nuclear exclusion. EMBO Journal 21(9): 2263–2271

Rennie M J 2003 Claims for the anabolic effects of growth hormone: a case of the Emperor's new clothes? British Journal of Sports Medicine 37(2): 100–105

Rennie M J, Tipton K D 2000 Protein and amino acid metabolism during and after exercise and the effects of nutrition. Annual Review of Nutrition 20: 457–483

Rennie M J, Wackerhage H, Spangenburg E E et al 2004 Control of the size of the human muscle mass. Annual Review of Physiology 66: 799–828

Ritz P, Salle A, Simard G et al 2003 Effects of changes in water compartments on physiology and metabolism. European Journal of Clinical Nutrition 57 Supplement 2: S2–S5

Roberts J M 1999 Evolving ideas about cyclins. Cell 98(2): 129–132

Rome S, Clement K, Rabasa-Lhoret R et al 2003 Microarray profiling of human skeletal muscle reveals that insulin regulates approximately 800 genes during a hyperinsulinemic clamp. Journal of Biological Chemistry 278(20): 18063–18068

Rommel C, Bodine S C, Clarke B A et al 2001 Mediation of IGF-1-induced skeletal myotube hypertrophy by PI(3)K/Akt/mTOR and PI(3)K/Akt/GSK3 pathways. Nature Cell Biology 3(11): 1009–1013

Rosenblatt J D, Yong D, Parry D J 1994 Satellite cell activity is required for hypertrophy of overloaded adult rat muscle. Muscle Nerve 17(6): 608–613

Roth S M, Martel G F, Ferrell R E et al 2003 Myostatin gene expression is reduced in humans with heavy-resistance strength training: a brief communication. Experimental Biology and Medicine (Maywood) 228(6): 706–709

Sandri M, Sandri C, Gilbert A et al 2004 Foxo transcription factors induce the atrophy-related ubiquitin ligase atrogin-1 and cause skeletal muscle atrophy. Cell 117(3): 399–412

Schuelke M, Wagner K R, Stolz L E et al 2004 Myostatin mutation associated with gross muscle hypertrophy in a child. New England Journal of Medicine 350(26): 2682–2688

Seale P, Sabourin L A, Girgis-Gabardo A et al 2000 Pax7 is required for the specification of myogenic satellite cells. Cell 102(6): 777–786

Sjostrom M, Lexell J, Eriksson A et al 1991 Evidence of fibre hyperplasia in human skeletal muscles from healthy young men? A left-right comparison of the fibre number in whole anterior tibialis muscles. European Journal of Applied Physiology and Occupational Physiology 62(5): 301–304

Snow M H 1990 Satellite cell response in rat soleus muscle undergoing hypertrophy due to surgical ablation of synergists. Anatomical Record 227(4): 437–446

Souchelnytskyi S, Tamaki K, Engstrom U et al 1997 Phosphorylation of Ser465 and Ser467 in the C terminus of Smad2 mediates interaction with Smad4 and is required for transforming growth factor-beta signaling. Journal of Biological Chemistry 272(44): 28107–28115

Svanberg E, Ohlsson C, Kimball S R et al 2000 rhIGF-I/IGFBP-3 complex, but not free rhIGF-I, supports muscle protein biosynthesis in rats during semistarvation. European Journal of Clinical Investigation 30(5): 438–446

Taylor W E, Bhasin S, Artaza J et al 2001 Myostatin inhibits cell proliferation and protein synthesis in C2C12 muscle cells. American Journal of Physiology 280(2): E221–E228

Tipton K D, Ferrando A A, Phillips S M et al 1999 Postexercise net protein synthesis in human muscle from orally administered amino acids. American Journal of Physiology 276(4 Pt 1): E628–E634

Tschumperlin D J, Dai G, Maly I V et al 2004 Mechanotransduction through growth-factor shedding into the extracellular space. Nature 429(6987): 83–86

Vandenburgh H, Kaufman S 1979 In vitro model for stretch-induced hypertrophy of skeletal muscle. Science 203(4377): 265–268

Vanhaesebroeck B, Alessi D R 2000 The PI3K-PDK1 connection: more than just a road to PKB. Biochemical Journal 346 Pt 3: 561–576

Vierck J, O'Reilly B, Hossner K et al 2000 Satellite cell regulation following myotrauma caused by resistance exercise. Cell Biology International 24(5): 263–272

Walker K S, Kambadur R, Sharma M et al 2004 Resistance training alters plasma myostatin but not IGF-1 in healthy men. Medicine and Science in Sports and Exercise 36(5): 787–793

Willoughby D S 2004 Effects of heavy resistance training on myostatin mRNA and protein expression. Medicine and Science in Sports and Exercise 36(4): 574–582

Wojtaszewski J F, Jorgensen S B, Hellsten Y et al 2002 Glycogen-dependent effects of 5-aminoimidazole-4-carboxamide (AICA)-riboside on AMP-activated protein kinase and glycogen synthase activities in rat skeletal muscle. Diabetes 51(2): 284–292

Yang S, Alnaqeeb M, Simpson H et al 1996 Cloning and characterization of an IGF-1 isoform expressed in skeletal muscle subjected to stretch. Journal of Muscle Research and Cellular Motility 17(4): 487–495

Yarasheski K E, Campbell J A, Smith K et al 1992 Effect of growth hormone and resistance exercise on muscle growth in young men. American Journal of Physiology 262(3 Pt 1): E261–E267

Yu J G, Carlsson L, Thornell L E 2004 Evidence for myofibril remodeling as opposed to myofibril damage in human muscles with DOMS: an ultrastructural and immunoelectron microscopic study. Histochemistry and Cell Biology 121(3): 219–227

Zambon A C, McDearmon E L, Salomonis N et al 2003 Time- and exercise-dependent gene regulation in human skeletal muscle. Genome Biology 4(10): R61

Appendix, Section 1

Histochemical methods

GENERAL

The following outline procedures are applicable to transverse sections of human/mammalian skeletal muscle, cut in a cryostat at ~10 μm thickness, picked up on coverslips, air dried and then reacted promptly and without fixation, unless otherwise indicated.

Abbreviation DCM = 'Dehydrate, Clear and Mount'. The section, on its coverslip, is taken through a series of two or three increasing concentrations of ethanol, finishing at 100% (= Dehydration), then taken to an anhydrous Mounting medium via xylol (which is not only miscible with both ethanol and mounting media but leaves unstained tissue components translucent; for this last reason it is termed Clearing).

DEHYDROGENASES

Based on the particularly simple formulae in:

Martin TP, Bodine-Fowler S, Roy R et al 1988 American Journal of Physiology 255:C43–C50.

For lucid discussion of principles, with slightly more complex formulae, see:

Kiernan JA 1999 Histological and Histochemical Methods; Theory and Practice, 3rd.edn. Butterworth Heinemann, Oxford, p 312–324.

Storable component solutions

Store in refrigerator or, better, as pre-measured aliquots in freezer.

100 mM Phosphate buffers
(A) 0.2 M $NaH_2PO_4.H_2O$ = 27.6 g/L
(B) 0.2 M $Na_2HPO_4.2H_2O$ = 35.6 g/L

pH 7.4 = 9.5 mL **A** + 40.5 mL **B** + 50 mL distilled water
pH 7.6 = 6.5 mL **A** + 43.5 mL **B** + 50 mL distilled water

1 mM Sodium azide
Sodium azide = 0.065 g
Distilled water = dissolve, then make up to 1 L

1 mM Phenazine methosulphate (PMS)
PMS (*Care – toxic!*) = 0.03 g
Distilled water = dissolve, then make up to 100 mL
Prepare quickly and store in dark

Incubation media
Prepare quickly and store in dark
Succinate dehydrogenase (SDH) medium
Phosphate buffer, pH 7.6 = 80 mL

1 mM Sodium azide	=	1 mL
Nitro B.T. (*Toxic!*)	=	0.12 g
EDTA	=	0.19 g
Disodium succinate	=	1.3 g
Check pH and adjust to 7.6 if necessary		
1 mM PMS*	=	2 mL
Phosphate buffer, pH 7.6	=	to 100 mL

For **NADH–tetrazolium reductase** ('NADH diaphorase') substitute 200 mg NADH for 1.3 g succinate in the above, or proportionately in smaller volumes for better economy.

α-Glycerol-phosphate dehydrogenase (αGPDH) medium

Phosphate buffer, pH 7.4	=	80 mL
Nitro B.T. (*Toxic!*)	=	0.1 g
Sodium glycerophosphate	=	0.3 g
Check pH and adjust to 7.4 if necessary.		
1 mM PMS*	=	2 mL
Phosphate buffer, pH 7.4	=	to 100 mL

*Note in both the above that PMS harms pH electrodes, so is added after adjustment.

Method
For each of the above:
  (1) Incubate sections at 37°C (or room temperature), preferably in the dark, for 15–60 min (until at least some fibres are strongly blue in colour)
  (2) For best preservation, fix sections 10–15 min in 'formol saline' (4% formalin in normal saline)
  (3) In any case now wash in water (tap or distilled)
  (4) DCM

Result
Blue-purple formazan deposits indicate enzyme activity.

PHOSPHORYLASE
(Variously also known as 'glycogen-', 'amylo-' or 'myo-phosphorylase'.)
  Procedure modified by I Montgomery (personal communication 2005) from:
  Lojda Z, Gossrau R, Schiebler TH 1979 Enzyme histochemistry: a laboratory manual. Springer-Verlag, Berlin, p 218–222.

Storable component solutions

0.2 M Sodium acetate

| Sodium acetate (anhydrous) | = | 1.64 g |
| Distilled water | = | dissolve and make to 100 mL |

0.2 M Acetic acid

| Glacial acetic acid | = | 1.16 mL |
| Distilled water | = | make to 100 mL while stirring |

0.2 M Acetate buffer pH 5.9

| 0.2 M Sodium acetate | = | 87.5 mL |
| 0.2 M Acetic acid | = | 12.5 mL |

1% Periodic acid (*pronounced 'per-iodic'– per as in 'person'*)

Schiff reagent
Purchase commercially or make as follows:
Basic fuchsin   =   0.5 g
N–HCl   =   15 mL
Shake until completely dissolved (do not warm)
0.6% potassium metabisulphite   =   85 mL
Stand in dark at room temperature at least 24 hours until solution becomes yellow. Add animal charcoal and shake vigorously; filter. Repeat charcoal stage if necessary, till solution colourless.

Incubation medium
Add in the following order (dextran *must* be last):
0.2 M Acetate buffer pH 5·9   =   80 mL
Glucose-1-phosphate   =   0.2 g
Adenosine monophosphate   =   0.66 g
EDTA   =   0.1 g
Sodium fluoride (*Toxic!*)   =   0.08 g
Ethanol 100%   =   20 mL
Dextran   =   4 g (MW 200–275 000)
Check pH and adjust to 5.9 before use

Method
(1) Incubate sections for 1 hour at 37°C
(2) Shake off excess medium
(3) Wash briefly in 40% alcohol
(4) Absolute alcohol   =   15–30 min
(5) 1% Periodic acid   =   10 min
(6) Wash in running tap water   =   5 min
(7) Schiff reagent   =   10 min minimum
(8) Wash in running tap water   =   10 min minimum
(9) Mount directly in aqueous mountant or DCM (more permanent)

Result
Red stained reaction product; typically, in laboratory mammals and untrained humans:
Type 1 fibres +   Type 2A ++   Type 2B/X +++

MYOFIBRILLAR ATPASES

Myosin ATPase
Guth L, Samaha FJ 1970 Experimental Neurology 28:365–367.
This is the 'gold standard' method, from the start of the modern era of mammalian fibre typing.

Storable solutions
Fixative (*stable if stored at 4°C*)
Paraformaldehyde   =   5 g
Distilled water   =   80 mL
N–NaOH   =   a few drops
Dissolve at 60°C, cool to room temperature
Sodium cacodylate   =   3.1 g
1 M Calcium chloride   =   4.56 mL
Sucrose   =   11.5 g

Adjust to pH 7.6
Distilled water   =   to 100 mL

Rinsing solution (*stable if stored at 4°C*)
Trizma base   =   6.05 g
1 M Calcium chloride   =   9 mL
Distilled water   =   450 mL
Adjust to pH 7.8
Distilled water   =   to 500 mL

1.5 M 2-Amino-2-methyl-1-propanol (2A-2M-1P)
2-Amino-2-methyl-1-propanol   =   13.37 g
Distilled water   =   to 100 mL
(*Or use Sigma 221 buffer solution*)

N Potassium hydroxide (KOH)
Potassium hydroxide   =   5.6 g
Distilled water   =   to 100 mL

Working solutions
Alkaline pre-treatment ('alkali pre-incubation')
Prepare just before use
1.5 M 2A-2M-1P   =   6.7 mL
1 M Calcium chloride   =   1.8 mL
Distilled water   =   to 80 mL
Adjust with N HCl to pH 10.2–10.8 (*originally 10.4, but optimum varies with species*)
Distilled water   =   to 100 mL

Alkaline wash
Prepare just before use
1.5 M 2A-2M-1P   =   33.3 mL
Distilled water   =   to 450 mL
Adjust to pH 9.4
Distilled water   =   to 500 mL

Acid pre-treatment ('acid pre-incubation')
Prepare shortly before use
M Calcium chloride   =   1.8 mL
Glacial acetic acid   =   0.3 mL
Distilled water   =   80 mL
Adjust with N KOH to pH 4.3–4.75 (originally 4.35 but may be varied according to species and required fibre-type discrimination)
Distilled water   =   to 100 mL

Incubation medium
Prepare just before use
1.5 M 2A-2M-1P   =   6.7 mL
M Calcium chloride   =   1.8 mL
Potassium chloride   =   0.37 g
ATP (Disodium)   =   0.15 g
Distilled water   =   80 mL
Adjust to pH 9.4 with N HCl
Distilled water   =   to 100 mL

Post-incubation wash

1 M Calcium chloride	=	4.56 g
Distilled water	=	to 100 mL

1% Cobalt chloride

1% Ammonium sulphide (*prepare just before use*)

Method

Alkali-stable ATPase

(1) Fixative	=	5 min
(2) Rinsing solution	=	rinse for 1 min
(3) Alkaline pre-treatment	=	15 min
(4) Rinsing solution	=	2 × 1 min
(5) Incubation medium at 37°C	=	15–60 min
(6) Post-incubation wash	=	3 × 30 s
(7) 1% Cobalt chloride	=	3 min
(8) Alkaline wash	=	4 × 30 s
(9) 1% Ammonium sulphide	=	3 min
(10) Running tap water	=	3–5 min
(11) DCM		

Acid-stable ATPase

(1) Acid pre-treatment	=	5–30 min
(2) Rinsing solution	=	2 × 1 min
(3) Incubation medium* at 37°C	=	15–60 min
(4)–(9) as steps (6)–(11) above		

Use separate jars of incubation medium for acid- and alkali-pre-treated sections.

Results

After alkaline pre-treatment, type 2B/2X fibres dark brown, 2A medium, 1 pale
After most extreme acid (typically pH 4.3–4.4) type 1 dark brown, type 2 unstained
After less extreme acid (typically pH 4.6–4.75) 1 dark, 2B/2X light-medium brown

MYOSIN ATPase

Slightly simpler variant, working well for human muscle, which relies for distinctions among type 2 fibres on the comparison of two acid pre-treatments:
Round JM, Matthews Y, Jones DA 1980 Histochemical Journal 12:707–710

Solutions

Glycine buffer

Distilled water	=	150 mL
Glycine	=	1.5 g
Sodium chloride	=	1.16 g
Distilled water	=	to 200 mL

Buffered calcium chloride (BCC)

Glycine buffer	=	100 mL
1 M Calcium chloride	=	20 mL
Distilled water	=	60 mL
Adjust to pH 9.4 with N NaOH		
Distilled water	=	to 200 mL

Dilute BCC
BCC   =   100 mL
Distilled water   =   to 500 mL

0.2 M sodium acetate and 0.2 M acetic acid
Make as for Phosphorylase (above)

pH 4.3 Pre-treatment
0.2 M Sodium acetate   =   13.2 mL
0.2 M Acetic acid   =   36.8 mL
Distilled water   =   50 mL
Check pH and adjust to 4.3

pH 4.6 Pre-treatment
0.2 M Sodium acetate   =   24.5 mL
0.2 M Acetic acid   =   25.5 mL
Distilled water   =   50 mL
Check pH and adjust to 4.6

1 mM Dithiothreitol (DTT)
Dithiothreitol   =   0.03 g
Distilled water   =   to 100 mL

1% Calcium chloride
1 M Calcium chloride. =   10 mL
Distilled water   =   to 220 mL

2% Cobalt chloride
1% Ammonium sulphide (*prepare just before use*)

Routine incubation medium
ATP (disodium)   =   10 mg
Dissolve in a few drops of distilled water
BCC   =   20 mL
DTT   =   2 drops
Do not check pH – DTT ruins electrodes!

Reverse method incubation medium
ATP (disodium)   =   10 mg
Dissolve in a few drops of distilled water
Dilute BCC   =   20 mL
DTT   =   2 drops
Do not check pH – DTT ruins electrodes!

Methods
Alkali (routine method – pH 9.4)
(1) Incubate at 37°C for 30 min
(2) Wash well in 1% calcium chloride for 3 × 2 min
(3) 2% cobalt chloride for 2 min
(4) Wash very thoroughly in running tap water
(5) 1% ammonium sulphide
(6) Wash very thoroughly in running tap water
(7) Mount in glycerogel or DCM

Acid (reverse method – with pH 4.6 or 4.3 pre-treatments)
(1) Pre-treat in acetate buffer, pH 4.6 or 4.3, at 37°C for 10 min

(2) Wash quickly in dilute BCC
(3) Incubate in reverse method medium at 37°C for 30 min
(4)–(9) as steps **(2)–(7)** above

Results

After routine method, type 2 fibres dark brown
After reverse method, type 1 fibres dark brown; pH 4.6 leaves 2B/2X medium brown also

ACTOMYOSIN ATPASE

Mabuchi K, Sreter F 1980 Muscle and Nerve 3:233–239.
Also known as 'Ca, Mg-ATPase'

Solutions

Standard incubation medium ('Ca, Mg–ATPase')

Distilled water	=	80 mL
Sodium barbital*	=	0.41 g
1 M Calcium chloride*	=	1 mL
1 M Magnesium chloride*	=	1 mL
ATP	=	0.083 g
Sodium azide.	=	0.032 g
Ouabain (*optional*	=	0.018 g
Adjust to pH 9.4		
Distilled water	=	to 100 mL

*For amphibian muscle use double these amounts of barbital, Ca and Mg chlorides
(Rowlerson AM, Spurway NC 1988 Histochemical Journal 20:657–673).
This may pay also with other poikilotherm specimens.

Medium for ethanol-modified actomyosin ATPase

Distilled water	=	75 mL
Sodium barbital	=	0.41 g
1 M Calcium chloride	=	1 mL
1 M Magnesium chloride	=	0.5 mL
ATP	=	0.055 g
Sodium azide	=	0.032 g
Ethanol (analytical grade)	=	add to 16–20%

(*Original recommendations: cat muscle 16%, human 17–18%, rat 19–20%*) *Note that mixture becomes turbid when ethanol concentration reaches 18%*
Adjust to pH 9.4

Distilled water	=	to 100 mL

2% Cobalt chloride

1% Ammonium sulphide (*prepare just before use*)

Method

Actomyosin ATPase, step 1

Basic procedure:
Leave fresh-cut sections at room temperature 5–15 min, then incubate (human muscle 30 min, animal muscle 20 min), agitating every few min. (Alternatively use a rotary shaker or mixer.)
If sections wrinkle, and/or detach from coverslips, either:
(a) use sections stored 3–4 days at 0°C before incubating, *or*

(b) add ethanol to standard medium, to the extent of 10%, and experiment with reduced incubation time (13 min for human and 9 min for animal specimens). This can be sufficient to inhibit cross-bridge activity and consequent movement within sections, but is not regarded as giving an 'ethanol-modified ATPase' reaction.

Ethanol–modified actomyosin ATPase, step 1

Incubate at room temperature: 40–60 min for human and 30–50 min for animal specimens. After any of the above:

- **(2)** Rinse in distilled water
- **(3)** 2% cobalt chloride   =   4 min
- **(4)** Rinse gently in running tap water
- **(5)** 1% ammonium sulphide   =   2 min
- **(6)** Rinse well in running tap water
- **(7)** Mount in Glycerogel or DCM

Result

Dark grey-brown deposits indicate Actomyosin ATPase activity.

Order of staining intensity in mammalian fibres: types 2B/X > 2A > 1

Appendix, Section 2

RNA extraction and quantitative RT–PCR

1 RNA Extraction

1.1 RNA Extraction Protocol

Protocol for extracting RNA from skeletal muscle samples:

1. *Preparation.* Wipe pipettes, spatulas with RNAse inhibiting solution (can be purchased from Ambion, Qiagen, Sigma, Aldrich) and use RNAse-free pipette tips and Eppendorf tubes.
2. (a) For frozen muscle: add 50–100 mg of frozen muscle (store samples on dry ice; never let thaw, use liquid N_2-cooled spatulas, wear gloves) to mortar and pulverize in liquid N_2. Quickly add 1 mL of Trizol and immediately homogenize on ice for 90 s using a Polytron homogenizer or for 3 min with RNAse-free scissors. (b) For fresh muscle: add muscle 50–100 mg to 1 mL of Trizol, chop with RNAse-free scissors for 1 min and then homogenize on ice for 90 s using a Polytron homogenizer. (c) For cultured muscle: wash three times quickly with PBS, add 1 mL of Trizol to 10 cm diameter dish, scrape cells off, pipette three times up and down.
3. Leave at room temperature for 5 minutes.
4. Add 100 μL chloroform (or bromochloropropane), vortex briefly and leave for 5 minutes.
5. Centrifuge at 12 000 r.p.m. for 15 min at 4°C.
6. Transfer supernatant (~500 μL) to fresh, RNAse-free tube. Be sure to suck up only the clear supernatant – do not suck up the interface.
7. Add the same volume of isopropanol to the supernatant (i.e. add 500 μL of isopropanol if you have recovered 500 μL of supernatant). Invert tubes and then leave at room temperature for 10 min.
8. Centrifuge at 12 000 r.p.m. for 8 min at 4°C.
9. Remove supernatant and wash pellet in 1 mL of 80% ethanol made up in diethylpyrocarbonate (DEPC)-treated water.
10. Centrifuge at 7500 r.p.m. for 5 min at 4°C.
11. Remove supernatant; do not touch white pellet at bottom.
12. Flash spin (quick spin) and remove more of the ethanol with a smaller pipette tip.
13. Optional: Repeat steps 8 and 9 three times for a better wash of RNA.
14. Air dry until ethanol has evaporated and RNA becomes translucent.
15. Dissolve pellet in 50 μL DEPC-treated water (more if the pellet is large).

1.2 RNA Concentration Measurement

The RNA now needs to be quantified and quality-tested. RNA is measured using spectrophotometry and its quality is tested by running a non-denaturing agarose gel or using an RNA analyser. Two buffers, a TE and a 10× TBE buffer need to be prepared:

TE (TRIS-EDTA) buffer (pH 8):

- 1.576 g TRIS HCl
- 0.372 g EDTA
- Add double distilled H_2O to make up 1 L.

10× TBE TRIS-boric acid-EDTA buffer (pH 8.3):

- 108 g TRIS base
- 55 g boric acid
- 9.3 g EDTA
- Add double distilled H_2O to make up 1 L.

RNA concentration measurement protocol:

1. Take 1 μL of RNA in DEPC-treated water and add 99 μL of TRIS/EDTA (TE-) buffer at pH 8. Transfer to a 100 μL quartz cuvette, and measure optical density (OD) at 260 nm (OD_{260}) and 280 nm (OD_{280}) in a spectrophotometer.
2. Wash cuvette with distilled water between measurements. (a) Calculate RNA concentration as follows: RNA concentration (in μg/μL) = optical density (OD_{260}) × 40 × dilution factor[1]. (b) A ratio of OD260:OD280 ≥ 2 is one indicator for good quality RNA.
   [1]*Explanation*. The result has to be multiplied by '40' because 40 μg/mL RNA gives a OD260 of 1. The 'dilution factor' refers to the dilution of the RNA sample in the TE-buffer; for example if you added 1 μL of RNA solution to 99 μL of TE-buffer then it is 100 times diluted compared to the original sample. In this case the 'dilution factor' is 100.
3. Aliquot and store RNA in DEPC-treated water at −80°C.

1.3 RNA Quality Check

RNA can degrade quickly and its integrity needs to be determined. A horizontal gel electrophoresis apparatus and a power pack are required:

1. Add 1 g agarose to 90 mL of distilled water and 10 mL of 10× TBE buffer.
2. Microwave on full power for 2 min and swirl gently. Microwave further until solution is clear. Remove, cool for 1 minute and swirl while adding ethidium bromide (dangerous mutagen) to a final concentration of 0.5 μg/mL. Pour in to gel tray and place in comb to form wells. Remove any bubbles with a pipette. Place a box over the gel to reduce loss of fluorescence. Slowly remove comb after >45 min.
3. Prepare RNA samples by mixing the equivalent of 1 μg of RNA in DEPC-treated water with an equal volume of non-denaturing RNA sample buffer (purchase ready made gel loading solution).
4. A DNA ladder (DNA fragments of known size used as a size standard) is used to confirm size of bands. Mix 5 μL of DNA ladder with an equal volume of RNA loading buffer.
5. Run gel at 80 V at least 4 cm along the gel.
6. Visualize under UV light. Ribosomal 28 S rRNA (5.9 kilobases) should be twice as dense as 18 S (1.9 kilobases) rRNA. DNA contamination is indicated by 'streaking' in the lane, especially above the 28 s band. Streaking between the 18 S and 28 S rRNA bands indicates RNA degradation.

1.4 DNA Digestion

A potential problem of RT-PCR is the contamination of the RNA sample with genomic DNA. The treatment of the RNA sample with DNAse (an enzyme that degrades DNA) before reverse transcription is strongly recommended. The protocol using the Sigma DNAse I (AMP-D1) kit is:

1. Prepare two tubes by diluting 1 μg RNA in 8 μL of DEPC-treated water.
2. To each tube containing diluted RNA add 1 μL of 10 × reaction buffer (part of the kit) and 1 μL of amplification grade DNAse I. One tube should contain reverse transcriptase and one should not (negative control; nothing should be amplified).
3. Incubate for 15 min at room temperature for the digestion of DNA by DNAse I.

4. Add 1 μL of stop solution (part of the kit) and heat at 70°C for 10 min to destroy the DNAse I (the DNAse would otherwise destroy newly built cDNA during the reverse transcription step).
5. Chill on ice before proceeding with the reverse transcription of RNA into cDNA.
   Outcome. You should now have 1 μg of RNA in 10 μL of DNA-free solution per tube.

1.5 Reverse Transcription
The remaining RNA is reverse transcribed using the following protocol (using iScript Reverse Transcriptase):

6. The iScript cDNA synthesis kit contains RNase H+ iScript reverse transcriptase, a premixed RNAse inhibitor to prevent indiscriminate degradation of RNA template, and a blend of oligo (dT) and random primers. To each tube add:
   - 4 μL 5× iScript Reaction mix:
   - 1 μL of iScript Reverse Transcriptase
   - 10 μL DNAse-treated RNA
   - 5 μL nuclease free water.
7. Incubate samples using a thermal cycler (or heating block):
   - 5 min at 25°C
   - 30 min at 42°C for reverse transcription
   - 5 min at 85°C to denature iScript reverse transcriptase.
8. All RNA should have been converted to cDNA in the first tube and only RNA should be present in the second, negative control tube. Store both tubes at –80°C.

Outcome. You should now have ~1 μg of cDNA (concentration depends on the efficiency of reverse transcription) in 20 μL of DNA-free solution per tube.

2 Quantitative RT–PCR
2.1 RT–PCR Primer Design
The following steps should be followed in order to get primers using freely available primer design software programmes:

1. Visit the website: www.ensembl.org/homo_sapiens and type the gene name into the search box and press enter. Search the results for the correct search result (different names may be used, isoforms may exist).
2. Open the gene page, scroll down and select 'transcript information'. On the new website, scroll down to 'transcript cDNA sequence' (leave this page open as you will need it later). Select 'no markup' and 'no numbers'. All exons will now be shown alternating in black and blue (first exon black, second exon blue and so on; no introns). Copy the entire blue/black exon sequence.
3. Paste the exon sequence into a primer design website such as http:// frodo.wi.mit.edu/cgi-bin/ primer3/primer3_www.cgi. Select the variables shown in Table 1 in order to avoid amplifying artefacts and to allow quality checks (similar variables can be selected in other programmes; leave other boxes untouched).

Table 1

Variable	Minimum	Maximum
Primer size (in base pairs)	18	22
Primer T_m (in °C)	50	65
Primer GC content (in %)	45	55
Product size (in base pairs)	100	300
Product T_m (in °C)	70	95

4. Several sets of primers will be displayed; in each set one primer is named 'right', 5' or 'forward' and the second 'left', 3' or reverse primer. Now undertake a quality control and exclude primers.

5. *Quality control.* Step 1: copy the forward primer, go back on the blue/black exon site and paste the primer sequence into 'find on page' in the 'edit' folder. The primers should ideally cross the blue/black boundary between two exons. Such primers will amplify only intron-less cDNA but not genomic DNA as the latter contains introns.

6. *Quality control.* Step 2: enter both primers into the *in silico* PCR simulator www.genome.ucsc.edu/cgi-bin/hgPcr and press 'submit'. On the results page you can click the genomic location link 'chr . . .' and this should show the region of the gene you wish to amplify.

7. *Quality control.* Step 3: go to http://www.ncbi.nlm.nih.gov/BLAST/ and select 'nucleotide search'. Paste your primer sequence, select the species from which you have obtained your sample, take off the low complexity filter and press 'BLAST'. You will receive a list of homologous (i.e. similar) sequences. You should find the exact primer sequence on the locus of your target (there may be several nucleotides that have been published). Any other results with E-values <0.05 are a concern and the primer should be excluded.

8. Order primers from an oligonucleotide producer.

Some genes may have limited numbers of exons and thus it is not possible to find appropriate sequences. Rather than going through the laborious task of attempting to find your own and fit the criteria, try a set of primers listed and run melt curve analysis (see later) and an agarose gel following PCR in order to check for individual products.

2.2 Primer Validation

The selected primers now need to be validated experimentally. The aim is to test (a) whether the primers actually amplify cDNA (successful cDNA amplification), (b) whether the sample was contaminated by DNA (shown if negative control RNA sample is amplified) or (c) whether the primers amplify themselves (shown if a negative control water sample is amplified). The protocol is described for the Biorad iCycler:

1. Keep forward and reverse primers both as a stock solution of 100 pmol μL^{-1}.

2. On the day of the PCR experiment dilute primers to 10 pmol μL^{-1} (i.e. add 1 μL of primer to 9 μL of DNAse-free water). You will need 0.75 μL of each primer for each reaction.

3. To validate two primer sets: Take six PCR tubes and add 8 μL DNase free water into each and label 1–6.

4. Take a 2 μL aliquot of cDNA (which resulted from reverse-transcribing the RNA) template and place into tube 1.

5. Remove 2 μL from tube 1 and add into tube 2 (mix with tip).

6. Remove 2 μL from tube 2 and add into tube 3 (mix with tip) and so on until tube 6. You now have a serial, 5-fold dilution of cDNA in tubes 1–6.

7. Make 23 μL of a complete Supermix (Biorad) per reaction. Test two primers with five dilutions (original, 1 in 5, 1 in 25, 1 in 125, 1 in 625) in duplicates (i.e. each dilution twice) plus a negative control (RNA not cDNA) and blank (water not cDNA) per primer. Thus, you will need to prepare the supermix for 12 wells for forward and reverse primer set 1 and another 12 wells for primer set 2 (i.e. 24 wells altogether).

8. If you have six tubes with cDNA dilutions then you will have to make 12 times the following (see amounts in brackets) for 12 wells for the first forward and reverse primer set and because you will have two additional wells for negative controls. Once you have calculated the required quantity of each constituent then add 10 % to allow for error in pipetting:

- 12.5 µL (165 µL for 12 wells) of basic Supermix (contains nucleotides, fluorescent, DNA-binding dye, DNA polymerase and $MgCl_2$)
- 0.75 µL (9.9 µL for 12 wells) of forward primer (10 pmol $µL^{-1}$)
- 0.75 µL (9.9 µL for 12 wells) of reverse primer (10 pmol $µL^{-1}$)
- 9 µL (118.8 µL for 12 wells) of DNAse-free water.

9. Place 23 µL of the Supermix solution in each of the 24 wells of the plate. Add 2 µL of the 1-in-5 serial dilution of cDNA into wells 1–5, 7–11, 13–17 and 19–23. Add two negative controls: 1 µg RNA to wells 6 and 18 and 2 µL of DNAse-free water to wells 12 and 24 (Table 2)

10. Programme the Biorad iCycler for two step with melt curve (annealing/extension and melting curve analysis with increment in temperature of 0.5°C each 10 s (there are protocols on the cycler already). In **'view results'** label the genes against which the primers were designed. State the 5-fold, serial dilution. Indicate the fluorescence dye used (for example SYBR green; part of Supermix).

    Following PCR and subsequent melt curve analysis, the programme will produce a standard curve of temperature versus fluorescence. There will also be a 'PCR efficiency' value. Good efficiency is indicated by a high value (>85%), and good linearity across the dilution range. The negative control and blank should have no amplification. If there is amplification in the blank then this indicates primer dimers. Furthermore, if there is any amplification in the negative control then this probably indicates genomic DNA contamination. When looking at the melt curve there should be one specific peak, generally at >80°C because non-specific products will usually have lower melting temperatures. Here is a list of the criteria to apply in the lab before accepting the data for efficiency from a dilution curve:

    - Use PCR baseline subtraction (not curve fitting default option)
    - Set the threshold manually to 'lab standard'
    - Check that all melting curves are OK
    - Check that slopes are parallel in log view
    - Delete samples if multiple dilutions cross line together (usually at dilute end of curve)
    - Delete samples if you can detect amplification at cycle 10 or earlier
    - Ensure that there are at least five points
    - Check that the correlation coefficient is more than 0.990 ·

11. If primers satisfy these criteria then they are suitable for gene expression analyses. If they are not then they should be redesigned.

Table 2 Well loading for testing two primer sets (reverse and forward primer) in duplicates.

	Primer set 1		Primer set 2	
Basic cDNA	1	7	13	19
5-fold diluted	2	8	14	20
25-fold diluted	3	9	15	21
125-fold diluted	4	10	16	22
625-fold diluted	5	11	17	23
Negative controls	6 RNA	12 water (blank)	18 RNA	24 water (blank)

2.3 Quantitative RT-PCR

The cDNA samples can now be measured and compared against a standard. Thus, each sample needs to be amplified using primers against the target and primers against a standard. Typical standards are actin and glyceraldehyde 3-phosphate dehydrogenase (GAPDH) and should not be affected by the treatment investigated. Thus, scrutinize the literature for standards used when similar treatments were applied.

For each reaction, add:

1. 2 μL of each cDNA sample
2. 23 μL of a complete Supermix (Biorad):
   - 12.5 μL of basic Supermix (contains nucleotides, fluorescent, DNA-binding dye, DNA polymerase and $MgCl_2$)
   - 0.75 μL (9.9 μL for 12 wells) of forward primer (10 pmol $μL^{-1}$)
   - 0.75 μL (9.9 μL for 12 wells) of reverse primer (10 pmol $μL^{-1}$)
   - 9 μL (118.8 μL for 12 wells) of DNAse-free water.

Run PCR for a sufficient number of cycles so that all samples are beyond their linear phase of amplification. Melting curve analysis should be performed starting at 60°C for 10 s and increasing 0.5°C each 10 s up to 99°C. Check melting curve for specificity. Quantify expression of your target relative to the expression of the standard.

Appendix, Section 3

Muscle extraction and western blotting protocol

1 Muscle Extraction Protocol

This protocol is used to prepare protein extracts from animal or human muscle samples for Western blotting.

1.1 Solutions

Basic homogenisation buffer (pH 7.5). Add to 100 ml:

- 0.788 g Tris-HCl
- 0.0372 g EDTA
- 0.0380 g EGTA
- 1 ml Triton X-100
- 0.1 ml 2-mercaptoethanol

Protease and phosphatase inhibitors are expensive and should only be added to the basic homogenisation buffer on the day of the extraction. Produce the complete homogenisation buffer by adding the following to 10 ml of basic homogenization buffer (only produce enough for the numbers of samples you whish to extract):

- 1 protease inhibitor cocktail tablet (Roche)
- 0.108 g β-glycerophosphate (Ser/Thr phosphatase inhibitor)
- 10 μl of 2 mM okadaic acid stock (Ser/Thr phosphatase inhibitor)
- 250 μl of 200mM sodium orthovanadate stock (Tyr phosphatase inhibitor)[1]

Phosphatase (pp) inhibitors only need to be added for phospho-blots.

[1]Sodium orthovanadate stock solution needs to be prepared by adjusting the pH to 10. Boil solution until it turns colourless from yellowish and cool to room temperature. Adjust pH again to 10 and repeat the boil-cool cycle until the solution remains colourless.

Table 3 Homogenization buffer.

Chemical	FW	Concentration	Per 100 mL
TRIS-HCl	157.6	50 mM	0.788 g
EDTA	372.2	1 mM	0.0372 g
EGTA	380.4	1 mM	0.0380 g
Triton X-100	–	1 %	1 mL
2-mercaptoethanol (cleaves disulphide bonds)	–	0.1 %	0.1 mL

Table 4

Chemical	FW	Concentration	Per 10 mL
Protease inhibitor cocktail (Aprotinin, leupeptin)	–	–	1 tablet
β-glycerophosphate (Ser/Thr pp inhibitor)	216.0	10 mM	0.108 g
Okadaic acid (Ser/Thr pp inhibitor)	822.04	2 μM	10 μL of 2 mM stock
Sodium orthovanadate (Tyr pp inhibitor)	183.91	0.5 mM	250 μL of 200 mM stock[1]

Phosphatase (pp) inhibitors need to be added only for phospho-blots.
[1]Sodium orthovanadate stock solution needs to be prepared by adjusting the pH to 10. Boil solution until it turns colourless from yellowish and cool to room temperature. Adjust pH again to 10 and repeat the boil–cool cycle until the solution remains colourless.

0.5% bromophenol blue:
- 0.1 g bromophenol blue
- 10 ml water
- Vortex and filter at 0.45 μm
- Combine 6.3 g glycerol with 5 ml of filtered bromophenol blue (steps 1-3 above).

0.625 M Tris buffer, pH 6.8:
- Add 37.84 g Tris (0.625 M) to 500 ml of water; pH to 6.8 (store at room termperature).

2X Laemmli SDS Sample Buffer (you will need to use the above solutions):
- 2.52 g (20 %) of glycerol (weigh out)
- 1.6 ml 0.625 M Tris, pH 6.8 (see above)
- 4 ml 10% (w/v) SDS (Sodium dodecyl sulphate, stock, store at room temp)
- 0.5 ml 0.5 % (w/v) bromophenol blue (stock, store at room temperature)
- 1.4 ml water
- Prior to use add 100 μl of β-mercaptoethanol to 900 μl of sample buffer.

1.2 Muscle Extraction Protocol
Use the solutions to extract protein from muscle samples. Human muscle biopsy samples should be washed before freezing to remove blood. Blood contamination will affect the protein readings and cause problems! Be quick and reproducible: Washing may increase AMPK activity.

1. Take a small piece of muscle (>20 mg) and homogenize on ice in 0.2 mL of homogenization buffer per 10 mg of muscle (i.e 0.6 mL for 30 mg of muscle; does not need to be very precise because actual protein content will be measured later).
2. Additional step for blood contaminated samples: before adding homogenization buffer, add ice-cold buffer (for example TRIS-HCl of the extraction buffer) and shake or vortex muscle until surface blood is washed off. Quickly spin (~10 s) to get muscle to the bottom of the Eppendorf. Remove buffer quickly and proceed as described under step 1.
3. Homogenize in Eppendorf tube with small scissors for 2 min (very effective) and then with a Polytron homogeniser (use scissors for 5 min if you don't have a homogenizer). Alternatively, use a Fastprep extraction instrument.

4. Shake samples for 60 minutes at 4°C. (If you worry about dephosphorylation, consider shaking for shorter periods or not at all especially if the sample is well homogenized).
5. Centrifuge at 13 000 r.p.m. and 4°C for 10 min.
6. Take supernatant (protein extract with unknown protein concentration).
7. Measure concentration using Bradford assay as follows:
   (a) Add 200 µL of Bradford assay to each cuvette
   (b) Then add 2 µL of the supernatant obtained in step 4. Fill 2 µL into two cuvettes (measure duplicates)
   (c) Fill up to 1 mL with 798 µL of water
   (d) Fill one control cuvette (blank) with 200 µL of Bradford assay and 800 µL of water (no protein)
   (e) Produce a standard curve using 1 µg, 2 µg, 5 µg, 10 µg, 15 µg 20 µg, 25 µg of albumin unless you have produced one within the last months
   (f) Switch on spectrophotometer, calibrate and change wavelength to 595 nm
   (g) Add blank and zero spectrophotometer
   (h) Read all your samples. If the OD595 is above 1 then add less sample, read again and recalculate
   (i) Use 'best-fit' formula to calculate protein content for each extract.
8. Prepare 1–2 µg/µL protein (normally 2 µg/µL for human and 1 µg/µL for rat) in 2× Laemmli SDS sample as follows:
   (a) Add 300 µg of protein (600 µg for human muscle) for 300 µL. Example: If your have 2 µg/µl protein then add 150 µL.
   (b) Add 100 µL of Laemmli SDS sample buffer.
   (c) Top up to 300 µL with basic homogenization buffer. *Example*: You have added 150 µL extract, 100 µL Laemmli SDS sample buffer and you will now need to add 50 µL homogenization buffer.
9. Use a small bore syringe to push a hole into each Eppendorf cuvette. Heat at 95°C for 4 minutes.

2 Western Blot Protocol
2.1 Solutions
Several solutions (SDS-PAGE running buffer, Towbin Western blot transfer buffer and TRIS-buffered Saline) are usually prepared as 10-fold (10×) concentrated stock solutions. These solutions are then diluted on the day. We suggest filtering some of these solutions but they work without filtering; shelflife, however, may be shorter. Use MilliQ purified water.

SDS-PAGE running buffer, pH 8.3 (usually prepare as 10× stock).
For 1 litre (check but do not adjust pH; make up 1 L for two gels):
- 3.03 g TRIS base (60.6 g for 2 L of 10× stock)
- 14.4 g Glycine (288 g for 2 L of 10× stock)
- 1.0 g SDS (20 g for 2 L of 10× stock).
Usually produce a 10-fold concentrated solution and dilute on the day. Store at room temperature.

Towbin Western blot transfer buffer, pH 8.3 (usually prepare as 10× stock).
For 1 litre (check but do not adjust pH; make up 2 L for 2–4 gels (1 tank)):
- 3.03 g TRIS base (60.6 g for 2 L of 10× stock)
- 14.4 g glycine (288 g for 2 L of 10× stock)
- 200 mL of methanol (20% w/v; stabilizes membrane).
Usually produce a 10-fold concentrated solution without the methanol and dilute on the day. Store at room temperature. Do not forget to add the methanol.

TRIS-buffered saline, pH 7.6 (usually prepare as 10× stock).
For 1 litre (check and adjust pH; make up 10 fold concentrated stock and dilute 1 in 10 on day of use):
- 2.42 g TRIS base (48.4 g for 2 L of 10× stock)
- 8 g NaCl (160 g for 2 L of 10× stock).

Store at room temperature.

Wash buffer.
Make on day of use (1 L for two gels):
- TRIS-buffered saline
- 0.1 % Tween-20.

Store at room temperature.

Blocking buffer.
Make on day of use (20 mL for two gels):
- TRIS-buffered saline
- 0.1 % Tween-20
- 5 % w/v non-fat dry milk powder (Marvel) or 5% bovine serum albumin (BSA).

Cell Signaling recommend the use of 5% BSA instead of milk powder for polyclonal antibodies (Marvel). Make up fresh every day.

2.2 Gel Casting

Casting SDS acrylamide gels is much cheaper than purchasing ready-made gels. The procedure is safe if pre-cast acrylamide solution is purchased.

Basic stock solutions

1.875 M TRIS buffer, pH 8.8, prepare beforehand:
- Add 113.5 g TRIS (1.875 M) to 500 mL of water; pH to 8.8 (store at room temperature).

0.625 M TRIS buffer, pH 6.8, prepare beforehand (also use for Laemmli SDS sample buffer):
- Add 37.84 g TRIS (0.625 M) to 500 mL of water; pH to 6.8 (store at room temperature).

10% SDS, prepare beforehand:
- Add 10 g of SDS to 100 mL of water.

10% AMPS (ammonium persulphate), prepare beforehand:
- Add 1 g of AMPS to 10 mL of water. Important: make up daily or at least weekly.

Combine stock solutions to make up the following:
Prepare two 50 mL falcon tubes with 4× TRIS/SDS buffer; prepare the first one using the 1.875 M TRIS buffer, pH 8.8 and the second one using the 0.625 M TRIS buffer, pH 6.8 (store both at 4°C for up to 3 months):
- 40 mL of 1.875 M (pH 8.8) or 0.625 M (pH 6.8) TRIS buffer (see above)
- 2 mL 10% SDS
- 8 mL H_2O
- filter at 0.45 μm.

30% acrylamide (37.5:1 acrylamide:bisacrylamide; store at 4°C for 3 months; ideally purchase pre-made solution because it is toxic, carcinogenic; treat with utmost care):
- 30 g acrylamide
- 0.8 g bis-acrylamide
- fill to 100 mL with H_2O
- filter at 0.45 μm.

Table 5   7.5 % gel (use for most proteins; generally >~30 kDa) stacking and running gel solutions.

	1 gel		2 gels		4 gels	
	Stack	Run	Stack	Run	Stack	Run
4XTRIS/SDS, pH 6.8	1 mL		2 mL		4 mL	
4XTRIS/SDS, pH 8.8		1.25 mL		2.5 mL		5 mL
30% acrylamide	0.665 mL	1.25 mL	1.33 mL	2.5 mL	2.66 mL	5 mL
dd H$_2$0	2.35 mL	2.45 mL	4.7 mL	4.9 mL	9.4 mL	9.8 mL
10% AMPS	33 µL	50 µL	66 µL	100 µL	130 µL	200 µL
Cast running buffer, add butanol to smoothen surface and wash off with water. Then wash again with 2 mL of stacking buffer without the TEMED. Finally, add TEMED to start polymerization.						
TEMED[1]	5 µL	4 µL	10 µL	8 µL	20 µL	16 µL

Table 6   12.5 % gels (use for small proteins like 4E-BP1 <~30 kDa) stacking and running gel solutions.

	1 gel		2 gels		4 gels	
	Stack	Run	Stack	Run	Stack	Run
4XTRIS/SDS, pH 6.8	1mL		2 mL		4 mL	
4XTRIS/SDS, pH 8.8		1.25 mL		2.5 mL		5 mL
30% acrylamide	0.665 mL	2.08 mL	1.33 mL	4.2 mL	2.66 mL	8.3 mL
dd H$_2$0	2.35 mL	1.62 mL	4.7 mL	3.2 mL	9.4 mL	6.5 mL
10% AMPS	33 µL	50 µL	66 µL	100 µL	130 µL	200 µL
Cast running buffer, add butanol to smoothen surface and wash off with water. Then wash again with 2 mL of stacking buffer without the TEMED. Finally, add TEMED to start polymerization.						
TEMED[1]	5 µL	4 µL	10 µL	8 µL	20 µL	16 µL

AMPS ammonium persulphate. Make up fresh every week.
[1]The TEMED concentration in the running gel has been doubled since the previous protocol because the polymerization was too slow.

1. Clean gel casting plates with tissue soaked in 70% ethanol. Place in stands ensuring that plates are flush and even.
2. Add TEMED, vortex running gel solution thoroughly and add ~4.5 mL between the casting plates.
3. Add a layer of H$_2$0 saturated butanol 50/50 (v/v) immediately on top of the separating layer. Once the separating layer has polymerized the H$_2$0 saturated butanol is poured off. Wash (a) with water and (b) with 2 mL of stacking buffer without TEMED.
4. Add TEMED to stacking layer, briefly vortex and fill between casting plates to the top. Add 1 mm combs immediately and leave stacking layer to polymerize.

2.3 Western Blotting Protocol
The procedure takes $1^1/_2$ days and the gels need to be prepared on the evening before day 1 or in the morning of day 1. We describe the procedure for the Biorad mini protean gel and power

pack system for running the SDS acrylamide gels and a Scie-plas transfer tank, which is a budget option for a transfer tank.

Day 1. Assemble Western setup and fill middle (in-between gels) with SDS-PAGE running buffer. The buffer will overflow; fill until the whole tank is filled. You will need ~1 L or SDS-PAGE running buffer per tank.

1. Load samples from left to right. Load 10 µl of coloured reference proteins in lane 1 and the required amount of protein per lane (you usually need to load 20 µg of rat protein and 40 µg of human protein). Briefly vortex all samples prior to use. Precise and reproducible pipetting is crucial for good results.
2. Run for ~20 min at 100 V through the stacking layer of the gel. This will focus the proteins as a narrow band on top of the running layer.
3. Run for ~40 min at 200 V through the running layer of the gel to separate the proteins according to weight. Stop when the bromophenol blue is about to run off the gel.
4. While the gel is running, prepare the following:
   (a) Cut 85 mm × 60 mm large PVDF membrane (0.2 µm pores; some protein will slip through if the pores are larger). Wet in 100% methanol for 5 min; wash in MilliQ water for another 5 min. Mark right bottom corner of membrane with pencil. Touch only with tweezers and never allow to dry.
   (b) Prepare ~2 L of Towbin western blot transfer buffer per tank.
   (c) Cut six 90 mm × 70 mm large blotting paper pieces (thick blotting paper; Whatman 3MM) per gel.
5. At the end of electrophoresis, take out the gel cassette, take off glass plate and immerse gel into small tray with transfer buffer.
6. Fill a plastic box with Towbin transfer buffer (described for a Scie-plas tank) and wet fibre pads, and blotting paper prior to preparing the gel 'sandwich' as follows:
   (a) black casing plate
   (b) fibre pad
   (c) three pieces of blotting paper
   (d) gel (try to place gel as straight as possible on the blotting paper using a glass plate moistened in Towbin transfer buffer)
   (e) PVDF membrane. The pencil-marked side should face gel. Use tweezer to drive out air bubbles between PVDF membrane and gel
   (f) three pieces of blotting paper
   (g) fibre pad. Use pencil or round pipette to carefully roll out air bubbles
   (h) white casing plate.
7. Place cartridges into transfer tank filled with transfer buffer (do not forget to add the methanol to the transfer buffer). The black casing plate must face the cathode (−) so that the negatively charged proteins will migrate towards the anode (+), the direction where the PVDF membrane is.
8. Run the transfer for 2 hours at 100 V and between 200 and 300 mA (after ~90 min prepare blocking buffer).
9. If you are using frozen, previously used antibodies then thaw them now on ice.
10. This step confirms a successful transfer by temporarily staining the proteins on the membrane but can be omitted: Add ~ 3 mL (enough to cover membrane) Ponceau S stain to PVDF membrane. If the transfer was successful then the proteins should be stained. Check for equal loading.
11. Rinse three times with double-distilled H_2O.
12. Incubate PVDF membrane in 30 mL of blocking buffer with gentle agitation for 1 hour.
13. Incubate membrane with primary antibody overnight at 4°C with gentle agitation. Initially use all primary antibodies at a 1 in 1000 dilution. Make up in appropriate amount of

blocking buffer (use 5% BSA for polyclonal and 5% milk for monoclonal antibodies in TBS). The choice of a good antibody is crucial for Western blotting experiments. Ensure that the antibody has been successfully used for probes of your species (i.e. scan of Western result available).

Day 2. Time required (assuming stock solutions are available): ~2.5 hours: preparation 15 min; secondary antibody 1 hour; washes 15 min; ECL incubation plus Saran wrap 15 min; exposure and development 30 min.

14. Wash PVDF membrane three times for 5 min in 30 mL of wash buffer with gentle agitation at room temperature.
15. Incubate PVDF membrane for 1 hour at room temperature with gentle agitation in ~10 mL of blocking buffer containing HRP-conjugated secondary antibody.
16. Wash PVDF membrane three times for 5 min in 30 mL of wash buffer with gentle agitation at room temperature.
17. Incubate PVDF membrane with a total of ~3 mL (50:50 v/v) ECL reagents per membrane for 1 min.
18. Drain PVDF membrane of excess fluid but do not allow it to completely dry.
19. Wrap membrane in Saran wrap ensuring no air pockets are formed and place in and tape to X-ray cassette. Alternatively, add membranes between two OHP acetates which can be reused.
20. Expose membrane to X-ray film (18 × 24 cm is ideal) in dark room for as long as necessary e.g. 1 min, 5 min etc. You may even expose overnight. Begin with a 1 min exposure.
21. Place film in developer or develop by hand like photo film in dark room.

Glossary

Definitions of terms which may be unfamiliar to the expected readers of this book. In accordance with the assumptions of prior knowledge stated in the Preface, basic terms from muscle anatomy, physiology and biochemistry are not included. Nor is the terminology of the main skeletal muscle fibre types, for which see Table 3.2 (p 000)

ACE
In heritability studies, adjective indicating a model in which Additive genetic, Common environmental and non-common Environmental contributions to phenotypic variance are considered. In enzymology, angiotensin-converting enzyme (noun).

Allele
Chromosomal locus where people or other organisms vary in their DNA sequence.

Allometry
Quantitative study of scale effects in biology, expressing them as power functions of body mass.

amATPase
Actomyosin ATPase: enzymic function of myosin interacting with actin; requires presence of Mg^{2+} ions.

Angiogenesis
Development of new blood vessels. New microvasculature develops in muscles in response to endurance training.

Archaebacteria
Group of bacteria different from eubacteria, many of which live in extreme conditions such as high temperatures or strongly sulphurous environments.

Assortative mating
Mate-selection which is non-random in respect of the trait investigated.

Athlete's heart
Enlarged heart resulting from protracted training, particularly of endurance type.

Autosome
Any chromosome which is not a sex (X or Y) chromosome.

BETA analysis
In heredity studies, form of path analysis in which biological and cultural inheritances are not distinguished.

Bioinformatics
Informatics applied to biological research. Important examples are genome browsers and programs that allow the user to analyse DNA, RNA and protein data.

Calmodulins
Highly conserved group of intracellular calcium-binding proteins, mediating many signalling functions.

Candidate gene
Gene hypothesized as having influence on a quantitative trait.

Carboloading (also carbohydrate or glycogen loading)
Dietary and exercise intervention aimed at increasing the body's amount of glycogen. Used before endurance competitions.

Cardiac hypertrophy
Physiological or pathological enlargement of the heart. Can be due to protracted training, usually but not always of endurance type (physiological, healthy and reversible: athlete's heart) or disease (pathological, can lead to heart failure). Hypertrophy resulting from endurance training consists of both internal and external ventricular enlargement, without wall thickening; that resulting from resistance training consists only of external enlargement, the hypertrophied wall being thicker.

cDNA
Complimentary DNA. Refers usually to DNA obtained by reverse transcribing RNA. cDNA obtained from RNA is commonly used to clone genes because it is free of introns.

Cell cycle
Period from one cell division to the next.

Chloroplast
Membrane-bound, chlorophyll-containing organelle which is the site of photosynthesis in all plants, but not in bacteria or algae.

Cluster analysis
Computerized search for statistically significant groupings in multiple ('multi-dimensional') data-sets.

Codon
Three nucleotides in mRNA that code for one amino acid.

Competitive/competition period
A period in which major competitions take place. Usually low-volume but high-intensity training.

Conservation (biochemical)
Similarity of molecular structure in different organisms, attributable to shared evolutionary history.

Constant proportion group
Group of enzymes on single or closely related metabolic pathway(s), whose activities in different cells vary in close proportion one to another.

Cryostat
Refrigerated chamber containing microtome.

Cytosol
Fluid/jelly-like substance within cells; the non-organelle component of cytoplasm.

DAB
Di-amino benzidine: reagent for producing visible deposit in immunoperoxidase technique.

Discriminative ratio
Ratio of activities of representative enzymes from two different constant proportion groups indicating contrasting functions, such as aspects of aerobic and anaerobic metabolism respectively.

Dizygous (DZ) twins
Formed from different zygotes, so not 'identical'.

DNA microarray
Method used to compare the concentrations of thousands of mRNAs.

Downstream, 3′ direction
The sugar molecules in DNA have a 5′ carbon on one side and a 3′ carbon on the other. Downstream refers to the direction from 5′ to 3′ and is the direction in which transcription takes place.

EMSA
Electromobility shift assay; method for quantifying the binding of a protein (usually a transcription factor) to a small stretch of DNA.

Endosymbiosis
Form of symbiosis in which one organism is taken up into the other.

Epitope
Small synthetic section of a protein, carrying (one of) its antigenic site(s).

Eubacteria
The major group of bacteria; they are prokaryotes with rigid cell walls.

Eukaryote/eucaryote
Single- or multicellular organism, whose cells have their genetic material contained within nuclear envelopes.

Exon
Protein-coding sequence of a gene.

Fartlek
Swedish term that can be literally translated as 'speed play'. Endurance-runners' training method in which the intensity is varied during the run.

Fluorescent antibody technique
Immunocytochemical procedure for visualizing the primary or secondary antibody by coupling it to a fluorescent dye which can then be viewed, usually under UV illumination; sensitive but impermanent.

Fraternal (of twins)
Dizygous.

Gene–environment interaction
Situation in which both genes and environmental influences (e.g. training) affect the phenotype, but in ways which cannot simply be added together.

Genome browser
Website or other computer software enabling user to access information resulting from various genome mapping projects.

Genotype
Genetic make-up of an organism.

Heritability (H_{est}, h^2)
Proportion of total variance in a phenotype attributable to genetic differences; estimated quantitatively as percentage (H_{est}) or decimal (h^2). Usually based on studies of twins.

Heterozygous
Possessing two different variants of an allele.

Histochemical profile
Characterization of tissue or cells in terms of a battery of separate histochemical reactions; in muscle studies these will minimally include at least one reaction indicating each of aerobic, anaerobic and myofibrillar ATPase capacities respectively.

Histochemistry
Study by chemical methods of molecular (usually enzymic) contents of tissues and their component cells, normally performed on sections prepared by quench-freezing followed by cutting in a cryostat.

Homology
Phenotypic: fundamental similarity and shared evolutionary origin between two organs in different species, even if dissimilarly used. *Genetic*: similarity of chromosomal location of genes with equivalent function in different species. *Molecular*: degree of identity between DNA, RNA or amino acid sequences of different species.

Homozygous
Possessing identical alleles.

Hybrid (of muscle fibres)
Containing more than one type of MHC.

Hyperplasia
Increase in the number of cells.

Hypertrophy
Increase in the size of cells.

Immunocytochemistry/immunohistochemistry
Study of molecular contents of tissues and their component cells by immunological methods, commonly but not always performed on sections prepared as described for histochemistry.

Immunoperoxidase technique
Immunocytochemical procedure for visualizing a primary or secondary antibody by coupling it to horse-radish peroxidase, then reacting this with DAB to produce a permanent dark brown deposit.

in vitro
Latin 'in glass'; experiment involving organs or cells removed from the body.

in vivo
Experiment carried out in a living organism.

Intron
DNA sequence of a gene that is cut out during splicing.

Isoenzyme (isozyme)
One of two or more differences in structure but having the same catalytic action.

Isoform
Version of a protein.

Isometric
Contraction of a muscle at constant length.

Isotonic
Contraction of a muscle where tension is constant during the movement.

Kinase
Enzyme that transfers a phosphate group onto another molecule, usually a protein.

Knockout
Inactivation of a gene by transgenic methods.

Linkage analysis
Method used to determine the chromosomal region responsible for a trait.

Lymphoblast
Precursor cell of lymphocyte.

mATPase
Myosin ATPase: enzymic function of myosin alone; requires presence of Ca^{2+} ions in highly non-physiological concentration, but not Mg^{2+}.

Mechanotransduction
Conversion of mechanical signals into signal transduction reactions.

MHC
Myosin heavy chain: one of the two large component proteins of a myosin molecule, which principally determine both its ATPase (and hence contractile) characteristics and its antigenicity.

Microphotometer/microdensitometer
Instrument for measuring the intensity of light emitted or transmitted (in the case of densitometer, only transmitted) by a microscopical region of a specimen.

Mitosis
Nuclear division resulting in two daughter nuclei.

Monoclonal antibody
Antibody recognizing one antigen (usually a part of a protein). Produced by cells created by fusing antibody-producing B lymphocytes with cancer cells.

Monozygous (MZ) twins
Formed by division of a single zygote; 'identical'.

mRNA
messenger RNA; synthesized from DNA template by RNA polymerase.

Myofibrillar ATPase
mATPase or amATPase.

Myogenesis
Development and differentiation of skeletal muscle.

Myr
Million years.

Needle biopsy
Technique for rapid sampling of a few mm^3 of tissue from sites close to the surface of a living animal or human subject: also specimen so obtained.

Northern blot
Technique to quantity mRNAs; now largely superseded by RT-PCR. Involves separation of RNAs by electrophoresis, transfer of RNAs from gel to nitrocellulose and detection with a suitable probe.

Nuclear localization signal
Short amino acid sequence in a protein that determines the nuclear localization of the protein.

PAP
Peroxidase–antiperoxidase: sophisticated and highly sensitive immunocytochemical technique in which the second antibody is peroxidase-labelled and a third is an antibody to it.

Path analysis
Technique for investigating relative contributions of inheritance and environment to a phenotype, in which a series of different assumptions about the interactions between pre-identified variables is explored, till the simplest effective model emerges. Not limited to twin data.

PCR
Polymerase chain reaction. Sequence of temperature-controlled reactions used to amplify DNA.

Peptide
Small chain of amino acids linked via peptide bounds.

Periodization
Structuring a training year into training periods with different intensity, volume and contents.

Plyometric (of exercise)
Invoking a large element of elastic rebound.

Phenotype
Observable traits of an organism.

Phosphatase
Enzyme that removes a phosphate group from a molecule, usually a protein.

Phosphatidylinositols
Phospholipids that are modified by phosphorylation and dephosphorylation; part of signal transduction.

Plasma membrane
Cell membrane proper, as distinct from any extracellular coat such as the muscle fibre's sarcolemma.

Pleiotropy
Situation in which one gene has many effects.

Polyclonal antibody
Mixture of antibodies which recognize several parts of a protein; generated by injecting antigen into an antibody-producing host.

Polygenic
Influenced by several or many genes.

Polymorphism
Common variation of DNA resulting from mutations.

Preparatory period
A training period usually with high volume, low intensity and few or no competitions.

Primer
Nucleic acid strand that serves as starting point for DNA replication. Essential for PCR.

Prokaryote/procaryote
Unicellular organism whose genetic material is free in the cytoplasm, not enclosed within a nucleus.

Promoter
DNA sequence important for the transcription of the gene. Contains the binding site for RNA polymerase II.

Protein domain
Structurally and functionally defined protein region.

PWC$_{150}$
Physical work capacity at heart rate of 150 beats·min^{-1}.

Quantitative trait
In genetics, a trait (characteristic) which is continuously variable, like $\dot{V}O_2$max or % slow fibres, in contrast to a qualitative one such as sex or blood group. All quantitative traits are polygenic.

Quantitative trait locus (QTL)
Region of the genome (usually, of an identified chromosome) containing a gene or genes influencing the trait being measured.

Quench–freezing
Very rapid freezing of tissue sample, usually to the temperature of liquid nitrogen but requiring use of intermediate liquid or other technique to maximize heat conduction from tissue to nitrogen.

Ribosome
Cellular organelle where protein synthesis happens; consists of ribosomal RNA and about 80 proteins.

RNA polymerase
Enzyme that transcribes DNA into RNA.

RT–PCR
Reverse transcriptase polymerase chain reaction; RNA is first reverse transcribed into cDNA. cDNA is then amplified using the polymerase chain reaction. Used to quantify concentrations of RNA.

Sarcolemma
Extracellular coat surrounding muscle fibre. Sometimes mis-named 'basement membrane', which is a term correctly applied only to the extracellular layer between an epithelium and underlying tissue.

Sarcopterygians
Lobe-finned subgroup of early bony fish, from which the earliest land animals descended.

Satellite cell
Mono-nucleated muscle cell located between the plasma membrane and sarcolemma of a muscle fibre. Retains capacity to divide, making it important for muscle growth and repair.

Sibling
Sister or brother.

Signal transduction
Sensing of intracellular and extracellular signals, computation of this information inside the cell and regulation of cellular output.

Single nucleotide polymorphism (SNP)
DNA sequence variation between individuals involving only one nucleotide.

Southern blot
Technique to detect and quantify DNA. Involves separation of DNA by electrophoresis, transfer of DNA from gel to a membrane and detection with probes. Named after its inventor, Edwin Southern. ('Northern' and 'Western' blots are subsequent wordplays).

Splice variants
Variations of a protein generated by alternative splicing (splicing of different parts of the gene).

Splicing
Removal of introns and joining of exons in DNA.

Split routine
Method of structuring strength/resistance training; muscle groups are trained on different days.

Stable isotope
Isotope that does not undergo radioactive decay.

Stereology
Quantitive study of tissue components in microscopical sections; involving deduction of surface-area and volume information, not merely counting.

Stromatolite
Multilayered colony of photosynthetic bacteria.

Symbiosis
Close, mutually beneficial relationship between two organisms.

Taper, tapering period
Reduction of training volume before a competition.

Thermogenesis
Metabolic generation of heat.

Transcription
Process of copying DNA into complimentary RNA by RNA polymerase.

Transcription factor
Protein that binds to regulatory regions of the DNA and controls gene expression.

Transgenic
Containing foreign genes.

Transition period
Period following that of competition, focusing on recovery.

Translation
Synthesis of an amino acid chain (peptide or protein) using mRNA as a template.

Trilobites
Ancestors of crustaceans: family of bilaterally symmetrical marine animals, flourishing for about 100 Myr from Cambrian times onward, which have left numerous strikingly preserved fossils.

Ultrastructure
Structure of cells, or other tissue components, beyond the resolution of the light microscope.

Upstream, 5′ direction
The sugar molecules in DNA have a 5′ carbon at the head and a 3′ carbon at the end. Upstream refers to the direction from 3′ to 5′ and is opposite to the direction of transcription.

Western blot
Technique to detect and quantify proteins. Involves separation of proteins by electrophoresis, their transfer from gel to a membrane and detection with antibodies.

Zygosity
Number of zygotes contributing to a multiple birth.

Zygote
Fertilized ovum.

Index